STUDY GUIDE
CLINICAL
PSYCHOPHARMACOLOGY

A Companion to
The American Psychiatric Publishing
Textbook of Psychopharmacology,
Third Edition

STUDY GUIDE TO
CLINICAL
PSYCHOPHARMACOLOGY

A Companion to
The American Psychiatric Publishing
Textbook of Psychopharmacology,
Third Edition

Kelly L. Cozza, M.D.

Civilian Consulting Psychiatrist, Department of Psychiatry, Walter Reed Army Medical Center, Washington, D.C.; Associate Professor, Department of Psychiatry, Uniformed Services University of the Health Sciences, Bethesda, Maryland; Fellow, Academy of Psychosomatic Medicine

Scott C. Armstrong, M.D.

Medical Director, Tuality Center for Geriatric Psychiatry, Forest Grove, Oregon; Associate Clinical Professor of Psychiatry, Oregon Health and Science University, Portland, Oregon

Jessica R. Oesterheld, M.D.

Medical Director, Spurwink, Portland, Maine; Department of Psychiatry, Maine Medical Center, Portland, Maine; Clinical Associate Professor, Department of Psychiatry, University of Vermont College of Medicine, Burlington, Vermont; Instructor in Family Medicine, University of New England School of Osteopathy, Biddeford, Maine

Neil B. Sandson, M.D.

Director, Division of Education and Residency Training, Sheppard Pratt Health System, Towson, Maryland; Associate Director, University of Maryland/Sheppard Pratt Psychiatry Residency Program; Clinical Assistant Professor, Department of Psychiatry, University of Maryland Medical System, Baltimore, Maryland

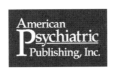

American Psychiatric Publishing, Inc.

Washington, DC
London, England

Note: The authors have worked to ensure that all information in this publication is accurate at the time of publication and consistent with general psychiatric and medical standards, and that information concerning drug dosages, schedules, and routes of administration is accurate at the time of publication and consistent with standards set by the U.S. Food and Drug Administration and the general medical community. As medical research and practice continue to advance, however, therapeutic standards may change. Moreover, specific situations may require a specific therapeutic response not included in this publication. For these reasons and because human and mechanical errors sometimes occur, we recommend that readers follow the advice of physicians directly involved in their care or the care of a member of their family.

Publications of American Psychiatric Publishing, Inc. (APPI), represent the views and opinions of the individual authors and do not necessarily represent the policies and opinions of APPI or the American Psychiatric Association.

If you would like to buy between 25 and 99 copies of this or any other APPI title, you are eligible for a 20% discount; please contact APPI Customer Service at appi@psych.org or 800-368-5777. If you wish to buy 100 or more copies of the same title, please email us at bulksales@psych.org for a price quote.

Manufactured in the United States of America on acid-free paper
11   10   09   08   07   5   4   3   2   1

First Edition

Typeset in Revival BT and Adobe's The Mix

American Psychiatric Publishing, Inc.
1000 Wilson Boulevard
Arlington, VA 22209-3901
www.appi.org

Contents

Answer Guide

Page numbers in the Answer Guide refer to *The American Psychiatric Publishing Textbook of Psychopharmacology,* Third Edition.

Visit **www.appi.org** for more information about this textbook.

| | | |

Purchase the online version of this Study Guide at

www.cme.psychiatryonline.org

and receive instant scoring and CME credits.

C H A P T E R   1

Neurotransmitters, Receptors, Signal Transduction, and Second Messengers in Psychiatric Disorders

Select the single best response for each question.

1.1   Which of the following compounds is able to rapidly penetrate lipid bilayer membranes and directly interact with cytoplasmic receptors inside cells to regulate gene transcription?

   A. Salts such as lithium.
   B. Hormones such as glucocorticosteroids.
   C. Amino acids such as L-tryptophan.
   D. All of the above.
   E. None of the above.

1.2   Where are the majority (>50%) of the serotonin (5-hydroxytryptamine [5-HT])–producing cell bodies located in the brain?

   A. Dorsal raphe nucleus.
   B. Tuberoinfundibular system.
   C. Nucleus basalis of Meynert.
   D. Throughout the cerebral cortex.
   E. Medial raphe nucleus.

1.3   Which of the following is the only low-molecular-weight neurotransmitter substance that is not derived from an amino acid?

   A. Dopamine.
   B. Serotonin.
   C. Norepinephrine.
   D. Glutamate.
   E. Acetylcholine.

1.4   How do benzodiazepines function?

   A. By binding to a potentiator site on the γ-aminobutyric acid A (GABA$_A$) receptor, increasing the amplitude and duration of inhibiting postsynaptic currents in response to GABA binding.
   B. By limiting production of GABA α-oxoglutarate transaminase.
   C. By antagonistic binding of the GABA$_B$ receptor, decreasing the amplitude and duration of excitatory postsynaptic currents in response to GABA binding.
   D. By inhibiting potentiation of γ subunits of GABA receptors.
   E. None of the above.

1.5   Which of the following peptides are regulated by lithium?

   A. Vasoactive intestinal peptide and corticotropin-releasing factor.
   B. Leptin and cholecystokinin.
   C. Neuromedin N and calcitonin gene–related peptide.
   D. Vasopressin and gastrin.
   E. Dynorphin and melanocyte-stimulating hormone.

CHAPTER 2

Basic Principles of Molecular Biology and Genomics

Select the single best response for each question.

2.1 What is the function of chromatin?

   A. Provides structure to chromosomes.
   B. Represses gene expression by inhibiting the ability of transcription factors to access DNA.
   C. Ensures that enzyme genes are inactive until their expression is commanded.
   D. All of the above.
   E. None of the above.

2.2 *Transcription* is best described as

   A. The process of making proteins from mRNA codons.
   B. The process of synthesizing, in a 5′ to 3′ direction, an RNA molecule that is complementary to one strand of a gene's DNA and that becomes a template for translation.
   C. The process of synthesizing, in a 3′ to 5′ direction, an RNA molecule that is complementary to one strand of a gene's DNA.
   D. The process of making cloverleaf tRNA in ribosomes.
   E. None of the above.

2.3 Which of the following statements about polymerase chain reaction (PCR) is *true?*

   A. PCR is a rapid procedure for replicating segments of DNA, utilizing bacteriophages.
   B. PCR is a procedure for cloning DNA, utilizing *Escherichia coli.*
   C. PCR is a linkage analysis procedure for localizing genes via examining cosegregation of phenotypes, using genetic markers.
   D. PCR is an in vitro procedure, generally requiring heat, that allows for enzymatic amplification of specific segments of DNA without using living organisms.
   E. None of the above.

2.4 Which of the following statements about antisense oligonucleotides (AOs) is *false?*

   A. AOs are useful in studying gene and protein function because of their irreversibility.
   B. AOs are short sequences of DNA that are complementary to regions of mRNA and block specific protein production when taken up by cells.
   C. AOs are useful in studying gene and protein function because they are specific, effective, and reversible.
   D. AOs have been injected into mice to limit overexpression of amyloid β to reverse deficits in learning and memory that are similar to those seen in Alzheimer's disease.
   E. Unmodified AOs are rapidly degraded.

2.5 The term *knockout* in transgenic studies in mice refers to

A. Mice euthanized for use in antisense oligonucleotide studies.
B. The use of viral vectors with low toxicity and high infection rates to deliver gene sequences to mice.
C. The study of allelic variations (polymorphisms) by comparing wild type to "diseased" genotype in mice.
D. The use of bacteriophage techniques to study "blank" stretches of DNA in mice.
E. Mice in which an existing gene is inactivated or "knocked out" by replacing it or disrupting it with a "construct sequence" or artificial piece of DNA.

CHAPTER 3

Chemical Neuroanatomy of the Primate Brain

Select the single best response for each question.

3.1 Which of the following statements about the dopaminergic system is *false*?

A. Dopamine neurotransmission is terminated through the actions of the dopamine transporter (DAT).

B. The mediodorsal nucleus of the thalamus and the posterior vermis of the cerebellum (areas reported to be dysfunctional in schizophrenia) contain low densities of dopamine axons.

C. The majority of dopamine cells, which synthesize approximately three-fourths of all the dopamine in the brain, are located in the anterior midbrain (mesencephalon).

D. Primary sensory cortices (e.g., the visual cortex) generally have low densities of dopamine axons, and these are present only in layers 1 and 6.

E. The major projection target of dopamine neurons in the substantia nigra is the striatum.

3.2 Which of the following statements about the noradrenergic system is *false*?

A. Primary somatosensory and visual cortices have a very low density of norepinephrine neurons.

B. Norepinephrine-containing neurons in the central nervous system are located predominantly in the medulla and pons.

C. In the hypothalamus, the paraventricular nucleus contains the highest density of norepinephrine axons.

D. In the amygdala, the basolateral nuclei contain the highest density of norepinephrine axons.

E. Norepinephrine elicits responses in the postsynaptic cell via G-protein–mediated second-messenger systems.

3.3 What percentage of serotonin (5-hydroxytryptamine [5-HT]) in the body is found in the brain?

A. 95%.

B. 70%.

C. 25%–40%.

D. 10%.

E. 2%.

3.4 Of the serotonin (5-hydroxytryptamine [5-HT]) receptors, 5-HT$_3$ is the only 5-HT subtype that does not belong to the G-protein receptor superfamily. To which receptor family does this subtype belong?

A. G-protein subfamily.

B. Ligand-gated ion channels.

C. Nuclear receptors.

D. Ionotropic receptors.

E. Hormone-responsive elements.

3.5   Which of the following statements about neuropeptide Y is *true*?

    A. Neuropeptide Y has a role in regulating eating behaviors.
    B. Cerebrospinal fluid (CSF) levels of neuropeptide Y are higher in patients with depression.
    C. Plasma levels of neuropeptide Y are higher in patients with depression.
    D. CSF and plasma levels of neuropeptide Y decrease after electroconvulsive therapy.
    E. All of the above.

CHAPTER 4

Electrophysiology

Select the single best response for each question.

4.1   Regarding the opening of chloride ion channels in a neuron, which of the following statements is *false*?

   A. Neuronal activity decreases.
   B. Chloride ions leave the neuron.
   C. The neuron becomes hyperpolarized.
   D. Chloride ions enter the neuron.
   E. γ-Aminobutyric acid (GABA) is often the neurotransmitter involved in opening neuronal chloride channels.

4.2   Which of the following statements regarding extracellular/neuronal ion concentrations is *true*?

   A. Calcium exists in equal concentrations both intra- and extracellularly.
   B. Calcium's concentration gradient is less extreme than sodium's gradient.
   C. Calcium ion concentrations are very low within the cell in order to use the ion for specialized purposes.
   D. Calcium ion concentrations are very high within the cell in order to use the ion for specialized purposes.
   E. The extracellular fluid contains much more calcium than sodium.

4.3   An ion channel that opens in response to a neurotransmitter is referred to as a

   A. Ligand-gated channel.
   B. Voltage-gated channel.
   C. Ion-gated channel.
   D. Voltage-dependent channel.
   E. Neurotransmitter-gated channel.

4.4   In research examining actual neuronal response to stimuli, such as from a drug, the least invasive method is

   A. Field potential recordings.
   B. Electroencephalograms.
   C. Single-unit extracellular recordings.
   D. Patch clamp recordings.
   E. Whole-cell recordings.

4.5   The most complete model of a neuronal system's functioning or of its response to drug application can be derived by

   A. Using in vitro findings.
   B. Using only in vivo findings.
   C. Using the best in vitro findings that correlate with in vivo findings.
   D. Comparing the results obtained in vitro with those obtained from the intact organism.
   E. Examining the intact organism and ignoring the in vitro findings.

4.6   Electrophysiological measurements of drug response are best used for detecting

   A. Neurotransmitter release over long periods of time.
   B. Transient electrophysiological events.
   C. Neurotransmitter release over both short and long periods of time.
   D. Both transient and sustained electrophysiological events.
   E. None of the above.

CHAPTER 5

Animal Models

Select the single best response for each question.

5.1 Learned helplessness was one of the earliest studied animal models for depression. Animal models exposed to uncontrollable stress have been shown to exhibit all of the following *except*

A. Changes in noradrenergic and serotonergic brain systems.
B. Altered sleep patterns.
C. Ability to learn avoidance–escape behavior.
D. Diminished consumption of food and water.
E. Social impairments.

5.2 Avoidance–escape deficits in rats are reversed by subchronic administration of which of the following drug classes?

A. Neuroleptics.
B. Anxiolytics.
C. Stimulants.
D. Antidepressants.
E. Sedatives.

5.3 Which of the following statements regarding chronic stress models in rats is *true*?

A. Behavioral measures of anhedonia are restored to normal by administration of antidepressants.
B. Chronic stress levels of glucocorticoids in rodents are easy to maintain.
C. There is evidence that antidepressants work by decreasing dopamine potentiation in the nucleus accumbens.
D. Glucocorticoid levels always decrease.
E. None of the above.

5.4 Regarding animal and human studies on hypercortisolism, cognition, and depression, which of the following statements is *true*?

A. Chronic administration of hydrocortisone in humans improves prefrontal cognitive performance.
B. Drugs that block glucocorticoids at the receptor level are being tested as possible antidepressants.
C. Hypercortisolism enhances cognition.
D. Hypercortisolism improves stress-induced depression in squirrel monkeys.
E. None of the above.

5.5   Mice genetically engineered to lack serotonin$_{1A}$ (5-hydroxytryptamine [5-HT$_{1A}$]) receptors throughout the brain demonstrate

A. Decreased food and water consumption.
B. Increased anxiety-like behaviors on a variety of tests.
C. Improved inhibitory control of the line-of-sight response.
D. Decreased anxiety-like behaviors on a variety of tests.
E. Reduced inhibitory control of the line-of-sight response.

5.6   An advantage of using animal models to study psychiatric disorders is that

A. Animals are very similar genetically and behaviorally to humans.
B. Humans are often too difficult to study.
C. Animal life spans are generally shorter than human life spans, thereby facilitating longitudinal research.
D. Animals are simpler to study.
E. There are no advantages to using animals to better understand human psychiatric disorders.

CHAPTER 6

Psychoneuroendocrinology

Select the single best response for each question.

6.1 The anterior pituitary gland secretes all of the following hormones *except*

A. Adrenocorticotropic hormone (ACTH).
B. Follicle-stimulating hormone (FSH).
C. Thyrotropin-releasing hormone (TRH).
D. Prolactin.
E. Growth hormone.

6.2 In depression, increased hypothalamic-pituitary-adrenal (HPA) axis activity has been shown to be

A. Initially mediated by increased secretion of adrenal cortisol.
B. Found in only a handful of studies and difficult to replicate.
C. Associated with increased hypothalamic-pituitary drive that is primarily mediated by hypersecretion of corticotropin-releasing hormone (CRH).
D. Continuous throughout a depressed person's life span and unchanged by treatment.
E. None of the above.

6.3 Evidence that increased endogenous hypothalamic-pituitary-adrenal (HPA) axis activity is associated with alterations in emotions includes all of the following *except*

A. Exogenous corticosteroids cause alterations in emotions.
B. Patients with severe depression show elevated serum cortisol concentrations over a 24-hour period.
C. Depressed patients have a blunted response on the dexamethasone suppression test (DST).
D. Depressed patients show a blunted adrenocorticotropic hormone (ACTH) response to corticotropin-releasing hormone (CRH).
E. Depressed patients have high evening cortisol levels.

6.4 Antidepressants may exert their action in part by

A. Upregulating the hypothalamic-pituitary-adrenal (HPA) axis.
B. Downregulating the HPA axis.
C. Increasing mRNA synthesis of hypothalamic corticotropin-releasing hormone (CRH).
D. Increasing adrenocorticotropic hormone (ACTH).
E. Increasing cortisol.

6.5 Regarding the finding that most patients with depression show some alterations in thyroid function, which of the following is *true*?

   A. Changes include decreased levels of thyroxine (T$_4$).
   B. Changes include increased levels of triiodothyronine (T$_3$).
   C. Changes include a more pronounced nocturnal rise in thyroid-stimulating hormone (TSH).
   D. An enhanced response of TSH secretion to thyrotropin-releasing hormone (TRH) stimulation is seen in 25% of patients with depression.
   E. A blunted response of TSH secretion to TRH stimulation is seen in 25% of patients with depression.

6.6 Regarding the thyrotropin-releasing hormone (TRH) stimulation test in depression, which of the following statements is *true*?

   A. The thyroid-stimulating hormone (TSH) response to TRH stimulation in depressed patients does not change after a course of treatment.
   B. Successful treatment of depression is always predicated on normalization of the TSH response to TRH stimulation.
   C. Relapse rates following successful treatment of depression are independent of the posttreatment results of the TRH stimulation test.
   D. A higher rate of relapse is seen after a successful course of depression treatment in those patients whose TRH stimulation of TSH does not normalize.
   E. None of the above.

6.7 Blunting of growth hormone (GH) in response to challenge agents has been found in all of the following psychiatric disorders *except*

   A. Schizophrenia.
   B. Obsessive-compulsive disorder.
   C. Bipolar disorder/mania.
   D. Panic disorder.
   E. Depression.

6.8 In depression, altered levels or blunted responses to various challenge agents have been found for all of the following *except*

   A. Prolactin.
   B. Thyroid-stimulating hormone (TSH).
   C. Luteinizing hormone (LH).
   D. Growth hormone.
   E. Adrenocorticotropic hormone (ACTH).

CHAPTER 7

Principles of Pharmacokinetics and Pharmacodynamics

Select the single best response for each question.

7.1 Which of the following statements about presystemic elimination is *true*?

   A. A first-pass or presystemic elimination effect is indicated by an increased amount of parent drug reaching the systemic circulation after oral administration.
   B. A first-pass effect is indicated by a reduced quantity of metabolites after oral administration.
   C. Presystemic metabolism of drugs is minimally accomplished by cytochrome P450 enzymes in the luminal epithelium of the small intestine.
   D. Cytochrome P450 3A4 has a profound effect on presystemic drug metabolism.
   E. First-pass metabolism is not associated with P-glycoproteins.

7.2 Which of the following statements about protein binding is *false*?

   A. Drug binding in the tissues cannot be directly measured in vivo.
   B. Displacement of drug from plasma protein binding sites may result from drug–drug interactions.
   C. Plasma protein binding displacement interactions are a major source of variability in psychopharmacology.
   D. Compensatory change occurs in the body to buffer the impact of drug-binding interactions.
   E. None of the above.

7.3 The time required from the first administered dose to the point at which approximate steady state occurs is equivalent to

   A. 9–10 half-lives.
   B. 1–2 half-lives.
   C. 2 weeks.
   D. 2 days.
   E. 4–5 half-lives.

7.4 The time course of tolerance to psychoactive drug effects varies from minutes to weeks. The operative elements in the development of tolerance include which of the following?

   A. Homeostatic changes in receptor sensitivity from blockade of various transporters.
   B. Acute depletion of a neurotransmitter or cofactor.
   C. Receptor agonist or antagonist effects.
   D. All of the above.
   E. None of the above.

7.5 Which of the following statements concerning the metabolic consequences of genetic polymorphisms is *false*?

A. Genetic polymorphism in a drug-metabolizing enzyme results in a subpopulation of individuals who are poor or rapid metabolizers of substrates of the affected enzyme.

B. When an active drug is administered to a person who is a poor metabolizer of the enzyme responsible for the drug's metabolism, higher drug concentrations can be expected, leading to an exaggerated response or potential toxicity.

C. When a drug whose therapeutic effect depends on formation of an active metabolite is administered to a person who is a poor metabolizer of the enzyme responsible for the drug's metabolism, high concentrations of the metabolite can be expected, leading to an exaggerated response or potential toxicity.

D. The most serious consequences of genetic polymorphisms occur in poor metabolizers who are administered active drugs with narrow therapeutic windows.

E. For cytochrome P450 2D6, poor metabolizer status is inherited as an autosomal recessive trait.

CHAPTER 8

Brain–Immune System Interactions: Relevance to the Pathophysiology and Treatment of Neuropsychiatric Disorders

Select the single best response for each question.

8.1   Examples of the innate immunity response include all of the following *except*

   A. Phagocytes.
   B. Complement C3.
   C. Tumor necrosis factor–α (TNF-α).
   D. T lymphocytes.
   E. Acute-phase reactants.

8.2   Which of the following immune system changes are seen in major depression?

   A. Decreased white blood cells.
   B. Decreased interleukin-6.
   C. Increased natural killer (NK) cell activity.
   D. Decreased haptoglobin.
   E. Decreased lymphocyte percentage.

8.3   Which of the following statements about how glucocorticoids modulate immune functioning is *true*?

   A. They increase cytokine production and function.
   B. They inhibit cytokine production and function.
   C. They facilitate arachidonic acid pathways.
   D. They increase production of T cells.
   E. They inhibit production of haptoglobin.

8.4   Which of the following statements best describes the effect of antidepressants on immune responsiveness?

   A. Antidepressants increase immune responsiveness.
   B. Antidepressants have no effect on immune responsiveness.
   C. Antidepressants decrease immune responsiveness.
   D. Antidepressants of different types either increase or decrease immune responsiveness.
   E. Only antidepressants of the selective serotonin class increase immune responsiveness.

8.5   Which of the following statements is *true*?

   A. The increased prevalence of major depression in the United States may be caused in part by the increased consumption of omega-3 fatty acids.
   B. The increased prevalence of bipolar disorder in the United States may be caused in part by the increased consumption of omega-3 fatty acids, which have anti-inflammatory effects.
   C. The decreased prevalence of bipolar disorder in the United States may be caused in part by the increased consumption of omega-3 fatty acids, which increase prostaglandins and proinflammatory cytokines.
   D. The increased prevalence of major depression in the United States may be caused in part by the decreased consumption of omega-3 fatty acids, which increase prostaglandins and proinflammatory cytokines.
   E. The increased prevalence of major depression in the United States may be caused in part by the decreased consumption of omega-3 fatty acids, which inhibit prostaglandins and proinflammatory cytokines.

CHAPTER 9

Brain Imaging in Psychopharmacology

Select the single best response for each question.

9.1   Regarding brain imaging technologies now in common use, which of the following statements is *true*?

   A. Positron emission tomography (PET) has gained rapid acceptance because of the widespread availability of tomography units.
   B. PET has gained rapid acceptance because it does not involve radioactive exposure.
   C. Functional magnetic resonance imaging (fMRI) has gained rapid acceptance because of the lack of radioactive exposure and the availability of MRI units.
   D. PET has gained rapid acceptance because it can be repeated within a short time on the same subject.
   E. PET has gained acceptance because it does not employ injectable substances.

9.2   Which of the following statements best describes an advantage of positron emission tomography (PET) over functional magnetic resonance imaging (fMRI)?

   A. PET is less expensive than MRI.
   B. PET allows for event-related design experiments.
   C. PET allows for longitudinal studies of the same subject.
   D. PET allows for metabolic and receptor mapping.
   E. PET is easier to perform and can be conducted by one person.

9.3   Which of the following statements best characterizes a major difference between electroencephalography (EEG) and magnetoencephalography (MEG)?

   A. MEG uses relatively simple equipment.
   B. MEG requires cutting-edge technology.
   C. EEG requires cutting-edge technology.
   D. EEG requires a higher density of scale electrodes.
   E. Only MEG is a surface technology.

9.4   Which of the following statements best describes the limitations of functional brain imaging techniques for diagnosis?

   A. Functional brain imaging has a high rate of false negatives.
   B. Functional brain imaging is relatively insensitive, because there are few ways a brain scan may appear to be abnormal.
   C. Functional brain imaging has a high rate of false positives.
   D. Functional brain imaging studies in clinical populations have been characterized by excessively large sample sizes.
   E. None of the above.

9.5   The isotopes most commonly used in positron emission tomography (PET) are

    A. Carbon-11, chlorine-18, and nitrogen-14.
    B. Carbon-11, oxygen-15, fluorine-18, and nitrogen-13.
    C. Carbon-12, oxygen-14, fluorine-18, and nitrogen-13.
    D. Carbon-11 and oxygen-14.
    E. Carbon-12, oxygen-15, and lithium-18.

C H A P T E R 1 0

Statistics and Clinical Trial Design in Psychopharmacology

Select the single best response for each question.

10.1 "Statistical significance" is an indicator of

  A. The validity of a study.
  B. The clinical relevance of a study.
  C. The quality of a study.
  D. A double-blind, placebo-controlled study design.
  E. An odds ratio greater than one.

10.2 A "negative study" is a study in which

  A. The study drug produces a negative outcome.
  B. It is demonstrated that the study drug produces no significant effect compared with the control (i.e., placebo).
  C. The study findings generate P values greater than 0.05.
  D. Bias has been introduced into the study design.
  E. The study produces a negative NNT (number needed to treat) value.

10.3 A "failed study" is a study in which

  A. The study fails to get published in a peer-reviewed journal.
  B. A high dropout rate requires modification of the study design.
  C. Investigators fail to maintain the blind.
  D. The results are eventually discovered to have been fabricated.
  E. The effects of a study drug are not "statistically significant."

10.4 *Number needed to treat* (NNT) is defined as

  A. The number of subjects that need to be exposed to a treatment in order to average one more response than would be achieved with the control drug.
  B. The number of subjects that need to be treated in order to ensure an odds ratio greater than one.
  C. The number of subjects that need to be exposed to a treatment in order to achieve a P value of less than 0.05.
  D. Equal to 1 minus the risk difference.
  E. The ratio of sensitivity to specificity.

10.5 Which of the following is a necessary feature of a "clinically significant effect"?

A. An effect size greater than 20% of baseline measures.
B. An odds ratio greater than 1.
C. The demonstration of statistical significance.
D. The ability of this statistic to alter the practice patterns of clinicians who are made aware of these study results.
E. A number needed to treat (NNT) of less than 100.

CHAPTER 11

Pharmacoeconomics

Select the single best response for each question.

11.1 Cost comparison of two or more treatment strategies of equal efficacy is termed

A. Cost-effectiveness analysis.
B. Cost minimization analysis.
C. Cost utility analysis.
D. Cost–benefit analysis.
E. Cost correlation analysis.

11.2 According to a British study by Guest and Cookson (1999), which of the following accounted for the largest portion of costs attributable to schizophrenia in the 5 years following initial diagnosis?

A. Inpatient hospitalization costs.
B. Medication costs.
C. Property damage caused during acute exacerbations of illness.
D. Lost productivity.
E. Treatment of iatrogenic complications.

11.3 Factors that contribute to the superior cost-effectiveness of atypical versus typical antipsychotic agents include all of the following *except*

A. More benign side-effect profiles.
B. Reduced levels of acute extrapyramidal side effects (EPS) and tardive dyskinesia.
C. Improved medication compliance.
D. Reduction in inpatient hospitalization days.
E. Less weight gain.

11.4 According to pharmacoeconomic studies, which of the following antidepressants is the *least* cost-effective?

A. Imipramine.
B. Fluoxetine.
C. Mirtazapine.
D. Venlafaxine.
E. Bupropion.

11.5 According to a pharmacoeconomic analysis by Greenberg et al. (1999), which of the following accounted for the largest portion of costs attributable to anxiety disorders?

A. Lost productivity.
B. Psychiatric treatment costs.
C. Nonpsychiatric medical treatment costs.
D. Prescription medication costs.
E. Mortality costs.

11.6 According to various pharmacoeconomic studies, the class of illnesses with the highest associated total costs in the United States is

A. Schizophrenia spectrum disorders.
B. Dissociative disorders.
C. Anxiety disorders.
D. Depressive disorders.
E. Bipolar spectrum disorders.

CHAPTER 12

Tricyclic and Tetracyclic Drugs

Select the single best response for each question.

12.1   Which of the following is a secondary-amine tricyclic antidepressant (TCA)?

   A. Amitriptyline.
   B. Maprotiline.
   C. Protriptyline.
   D. Clomipramine.
   E. Doxepin.

12.2   Tertiary-amine tricyclic antidepressants (TCAs), as distinguished from their secondary-amine TCA metabolites, are more potent in blocking the reuptake of which of the following neurotransmitters?

   A. Serotonin.
   B. Norepinephrine.
   C. Dopamine.
   D. Acetylcholine.
   E. Glutamate.

12.3   The least anticholinergic of the tricyclic antidepressants (TCAs) is

   A. Protriptyline.
   B. Nortriptyline.
   C. Doxepin.
   D. Desipramine.
   E. Imipramine.

12.4   The tricyclic antidepressant (TCA) least likely to cause orthostatic hypotension is

   A. Desipramine.
   B. Nortriptyline.
   C. Trimipramine.
   D. Clomipramine.
   E. Amitriptyline.

12.5 The cytochrome P450 enzyme chiefly responsible for hydroxylation of nortriptyline and desipramine is

A. 1A2.
B. 2C9.
C. 2C19.
D. 2D6.
E. 3A4.

12.6 Which of the following cytochrome P450 enzymes is involved in the demethylation of tertiary-amine tricyclic antidepressants (TCAs) to secondary-amine TCAs?

A. 2B6.
B. 2C9.
C. 2C19.
D. 2D6.
E. 2E1.

12.7 Which of the tricyclic antidepressants (TCAs) is most effective in the treatment of obsessive-compulsive disorder (OCD)?

A. Imipramine.
B. Amitriptyline.
C. Doxepin.
D. Desipramine.
E. Clomipramine.

12.8 The most potent histamine$_1$ (H$_1$) receptor blocker among the tricyclic antidepressants (TCAs) is

A. Amitriptyline.
B. Clomipramine.
C. Doxepin.
D. Imipramine.
E. Trimipramine.

12.9 The principal cause of death following tricyclic antidepressant (TCA) overdose is

A. Cardiac arrhythmia.
B. Status epilepticus.
C. Aspiration leading to adult respiratory distress syndrome.
D. Hemorrhagic cerebrovascular accident.
E. Hepatorenal syndrome.

CHAPTER 13

Fluoxetine

Select the single best response for each question.

13.1   The selective serotonin reuptake inhibitor with active metabolites and the longest half-life is

  A. Paroxetine.
  B. Sertraline.
  C. Citalopram.
  D. Escitalopram.
  E. Fluoxetine.

13.2   What is the washout period for fluoxetine before a monoamine oxidase inhibitor (MAOI) may be safely administered?

  A. 1 day.
  B. 5 days.
  C. 30 days.
  D. 5 weeks.
  E. 3 months.

13.3   Which cytochrome P450 enzyme(s) does fluoxetine inhibit to any degree?

  A. 2C9 and 2C19.
  B. 2D6.
  C. 3A3/4.
  D. All of the above.
  E. None of the above.

13.4   Acute treatment of fluoxetine overdose includes which of the following?

  A. Hemodialysis.
  B. Supportive care only.
  C. Ipecac and charcoal.
  D. Alkalinization of the urine.
  E. Naltrexone.

13.5   Fluoxetine does not generally require a taper to avoid a withdrawal syndrome, because

  A. It has active metabolites with long half-lives.
  B. It has no active metabolites.
  C. It is rapidly and fully metabolized, leading to fewer adverse events.
  D. All of the above.
  E. None of the above.

CHAPTER 14

Sertraline

Select the single best response for each question.

14.1 Sertraline has been approved by the U.S. Food and Drug Administration (FDA) for which of the following indications?

A. Major depressive disorder.
B. Obsessive-compulsive disorder (OCD).
C. Posttraumatic stress disorder.
D. Premenstrual dysphoric disorder.
E. All of the above.

14.2 The most common adverse effect of sertraline is

A. Tinnitus.
B. Gastrointestinal disturbances.
C. Sexual dysfunction.
D. Weight gain.
E. Acne.

14.3 The elimination half-life of sertraline is

A. 2 weeks.
B. 5 weeks.
C. 125 hours.
D. 26–32 hours.
E. 5–10 hours.

14.4 Which of the following cytochrome P450 enzymes is responsible for the metabolism of sertraline?

A. 1A2.
B. 2C9, 2C19, 2D6, and 3A4.
C. 1A2 and 2E1.
D. 2E1.
E. 2D6.

14.5 Sertraline's metabolite, desmethylsertraline, has which of the following characteristics?

A. It is an inactive compound.
B. It has greater activity and potency than sertraline in blocking reuptake of serotonin (5-hydroxytryptamine [5-HT]).
C. It is one-tenth as active as sertraline in blocking reuptake of 5-HT.
D. It is a prodrug.
E. None of the above.

CHAPTER 15

Paroxetine

Select the single best response for each question.

15.1   Which selective serotonin reuptake inhibitor (SSRI) is the most potent inhibitor of the norepinephrine transporter (NET)?

    A. Fluoxetine.
    B. Sertraline.
    C. Citalopram.
    D. Escitalopram.
    E. Paroxetine.

15.2   Which SSRI is the most anticholinergic (with anticholinergic effects similar to those of desipramine)?

    A. Fluoxetine.
    B. Sertraline.
    C. Citalopram.
    D. Escitalopram.
    E. Paroxetine.

15.3   In prescribing paroxetine for elderly patients, which of the following pharmacokinetic properties of this drug should be taken into consideration?

    A. Paroxetine is the least anticholinergic of the selective serotonin reuptake inhibitors (SSRIs).
    B. Paroxetine is the least potent inhibitor of cytochrome P450 2D6 among the SSRIs.
    C. There is a threefold increase in maximum plasma concentration in elderly subjects.
    D. The drug's half-life is reduced by 50% in elderly patients.
    E. Paroxetine is associated with type 2 diabetes.

15.4   Which selective serotonin reuptake inhibitor (SSRI) is the most potent inhibitor of cytochrome P450 2D6?

    A. Paroxetine.
    B. Sertraline.
    C. Citalopram.
    D. Escitalopram.
    E. Fluoxetine.

15.5 For patients with obsessive-compulsive disorder (OCD), optimal treatment with paroxetine typically requires

A. 10 mg/day, 3–12 weeks until response.
B. ≥60 mg/day, 3–12 weeks until response.
C. 20 mg/day, 2–4 weeks until response.
D. 40 mg/day, less than 2 weeks until response.
E. None of the above.

CHAPTER 16

Fluvoxamine

Select the single best response for each question.

16.1 Fluvoxamine is approved by the U.S. Food and Drug Administration (FDA) for use in treating which of the following?

A. Major depression.
B. Panic disorder.
C. Obsessive-compulsive disorder (OCD).
D. Posttraumatic stress disorder.
E. OCD in adults only.

16.2 Which of the following statements accurately describes fluvoxamine's pharmacokinetic profile?

A. Well absorbed orally, long half-life, high protein binding, metabolized to active metabolites.
B. Well absorbed, moderate half-life, low protein binding, excreted unchanged by the renal system.
C. Well absorbed, moderate half-life, low protein binding, metabolized to inactive metabolites.
D. Poorly absorbed, short half-life, high protein binding, metabolized to inactive metabolites.
E. Poorly absorbed, long half-life, low protein binding, metabolized to active metabolites.

16.3 Steady-state fluvoxamine levels are reported to be

A. Two- to fourfold higher in children than in adolescents.
B. Two- to fourfold lower in children than in adolescents.
C. The same in children as in adolescents.
D. Lower in female children compared with male children.
E. None of the above.

16.4 Fluvoxamine has been demonstrated in placebo-controlled studies to be efficacious in which of the following?

A. Trichotillomania.
B. Relapse of alcohol dependence.
C. Anxiety disorders in the elderly.
D. Social phobia.
E. Pathological gambling.

16.5 Which of the following statements about sexual side effects of fluvoxamine is *true*?

A. Sexual side effects with fluvoxamine are similar in frequency to those with other selective serotonin reuptake inhibitors (SSRIs).
B. Sexual side effects with fluvoxamine are fewer in frequency than with other SSRIs.
C. Fluvoxamine provokes more delayed orgasm than does paroxetine.
D. Investigators find an increased incidence of sexual dysfunction when spontaneous reporting rather than direct questioning is used.
E. Sexual dysfunction may persist for a long period after discontinuation of fluvoxamine.

16.6 Fluvoxamine shows potent inhibition of which cytochrome P450 enzyme?

A. 2C19.
B. 3A4.
C. 2D6.
D. 2E1.
E. 1A2.

CHAPTER 17

Citalopram and *S*-Citalopram

Select the single best response for each question.

17.1 Comparisons of *S*-citalopram and *R*-citalopram have revealed all of the following *except*

 A. *S*-Citalopram is 30-fold more potent than *R*-citalopram in inhibiting the serotonin transporter (5-HTT).
 B. *S*-Citalopram's half-life is the same as that of *R*-citalopram.
 C. *S*-Citalopram's half-life is shorter than that of *R*-citalopram.
 D. *S*-Citalopram may have less propensity to inhibit cytochrome P450 enzymes than does *R*-citalopram.
 E. *S*- and *R*-citalopram undergo similar metabolism by cytochrome P450 enzymes.

17.2 Citalopram has been shown in double-blind, placebo-controlled trials to have efficacy in the treatment of which of the following?

 A. Major depression, obsessive-compulsive disorder (OCD), and bulimia.
 B. Major depression, OCD, and trichotillomania.
 C. OCD, panic disorder, and poststroke depression.
 D. Panic disorder, poststroke depression, and pathological gambling.
 E. Major depression and panic disorder only.

17.3 The most common side effects of citalopram are

 A. Nausea, increased sweating, and dry mouth.
 B. Sexual side effects, tremor, and somnolence.
 C. Nausea, headache, and diarrhea.
 D. Sexual side effects.
 E. Cardiac conduction effects, nausea, and dry mouth.

17.4 Citalopram has a low likelihood of drug–drug interactions because

 A. It is highly protein-bound.
 B. It is metabolized mainly by cytochrome P450 2C19.
 C. It is eliminated primarily via renal clearance.
 D. It is a potent inhibitor of several cytochrome P450 enzymes; therefore, it increases the levels of coadministered drugs.
 E. It is metabolized by three different cytochrome P450 enzymes; therefore, inhibition of any one of these enzymes by another drug is unlikely to significantly affect citalopram's metabolism.

17.5   The side effects of *S*-citalopram differ from those of citalopram in which of the following ways?

   A. *S*-Citalopram is associated with greater cardiovascular effects.
   B. *S*-Citalopram is associated with fewer sexual side effects.
   C. *S*-Citalopram is associated with greater gastrointestinal effects.
   D. *S*-Citalopram and citalopram have similar side-effect profiles.
   E. *S*-Citalopram is associated with greater weight gain.

CHAPTER 18

Monoamine Oxidase Inhibitors

Select the single best response for each question.

18.1   Endogenous substrates for monoamine oxidase (MAO) isoenzymes include

    A. Acetylcholine, dopamine, and epinephrine.
    B. Tyramine, serotonin, and histamine.
    C. Epinephrine, dopamine, and serotonin.
    D. Histamine, acetylcholine, and serotonin.
    E. Tyramine, acetylcholine, and dopamine.

18.2   The therapeutic effect of monoamine oxidase inhibitors (MAOIs) is believed to be due to

    A. Amine accumulation in stored vesicles.
    B. Increases in amine levels at the synapse.
    C. Indirect norepinephrine and dopamine effects similar to those of stimulants.
    D. Amine accumulation in the cytoplasm, which leads to secondary adaptive mechanisms.
    E. Decreases in amine levels at the synapse.

18.3   Classic and irreversible monoamine oxidase inhibitors (MAOIs) have been shown in double-blind, placebo-controlled studies to be efficacious in all of the following *except*

    A. Major depressive disorder.
    B. Obsessive-compulsive disorder (OCD).
    C. Panic disorder.
    D. Dysthymia.
    E. "Atypical" depression.

18.4   Dietary restrictions with irreversible monoamine oxidase inhibitors (MAOIs) can be a challenge for patients. Which of the following groupings of foods/drinks can be ingested in moderation when taking an MAOI?

    A. Cream cheese, coffee, chocolate, and beer.
    B. Red wine, cheese, tea, and soy sauce.
    C. Chicken liver, colas, cream cheese, and soy sauce.
    D. Sherry, monosodium glutamate, and chocolate.
    E. None of the above.

18.5 The most common and problematic side effect with phenelzine and isocarboxazid—both hydrazine-type, irreversible monoamine oxidase inhibitors (MAOIs)—is

A. Hypertensive crisis if tyramine is consumed.
B. Hepatitis.
C. Postural hypotension.
D. Headache.
E. Urinary hesitancy.

18.6 All of the following statements regarding headaches with the use of monoamine oxidase inhibitors (MAOIs) are correct *except*

A. Headaches may occur with tyramine ingestion.
B. Headaches may be a result of a hypertensive crisis, in which case treatment with nifedipine is indicated.
C. Headaches may be due to low blood pressure (i.e., histamine headache).
D. Headaches are a common side effect of taking MAOIs and are not serious.
E. A severe headache after consuming food in someone taking an MAOI should receive prompt medical attention, given the potential risk of serious consequences such as cerebral hemorrhage.

18.7 Drug–drug interactions are a potential drawback to use of irreversible monoamine oxidase inhibitors (MAOIs). Concomitant use with an MAOI must be avoided for all of the following drugs *except*

A. Carbamazepine.
B. Stimulants.
C. Selective serotonin reuptake inhibitors.
D. Meperidine.
E. L-Tryptophan.

18.8 Regarding moclobemide, a reversible monoamine oxidase A (MAO-A) inhibitor, which of the following statements is *true*?

A. Moclobemide is effective as an adjunct treatment for Parkinson's disease.
B. Moclobemide has been shown to be effective for both endogenous and nonendogenous depression.
C. Dietary restrictions for moclobemide are similar to those for classic monoamine oxidase inhibitors (MAOIs).
D. Side effects of moclobemide are similar to those of classic MAOIs.
E. None of the above.

CHAPTER 19

Trazodone and Nefazodone

Select the single best response for each question.

19.1 Which of the following statements best describes the receptor profile of trazodone?

    A. It is a mixed serotonin antagonist/agonist.
    B. It is a serotonin agonist.
    C. It is a serotonin antagonist.
    D. It is a serotonin, norepinephrine, and dopamine agonist.
    E. It is a serotonin, norepinephrine, and dopamine antagonist.

19.2 A 25-year-old man has been treated with trazodone 50 mg/day for sleep. If fluoxetine is added for the treatment of major depression, which of the following is likely to occur?

    A. Blood levels of trazodone's active metabolite will decrease.
    B. Blood levels of trazodone's active metabolite will increase.
    C. Blood levels of trazodone will decrease.
    D. Blood levels of both trazodone and its active metabolite will decrease.
    E. None of the above.

19.3 In which of the following circumstances is the serotonin syndrome likely to develop?

    A. When a monoamine oxidase inhibitor (MAOI) is added to trazodone.
    B. When paroxetine is added to trazodone.
    C. When venlafaxine is added to trazodone.
    D. When duloxetine is added to trazodone.
    E. All of the above.

19.4 A patient with major depression is prescribed nefazodone at a starting dosage of 200 mg twice a day. If the total daily dose is doubled, which of the following is likely to occur?

    A. Blood levels of nefazodone will be doubled.
    B. Plasma half-life will remain steady.
    C. Blood levels of nefazodone's four active metabolites will be decreased.
    D. Blood levels of nefazodone will be more than doubled.
    E. Blood levels of nefazodone will increase by 125%.

CHAPTER 20

Bupropion

Select the single best response for each question.

20.1 Bupropion has been approved by the U.S. Food and Drug Administration (FDA) for which of the following indications?

A. Major depression and panic disorder.
B. Generalized anxiety disorder and smoking cessation.
C. Major depression and smoking cessation.
D. Panic disorder and smoking cessation.
E. Obsessive-compulsive disorder and major depression.

20.2 A patient who is taking bupropion SR (sustained release) 300 mg daily for major depression develops rash, joint pain, fever, and lymphadenopathy. What is the likely diagnosis?

A. An allergic reaction to the red dye in bupropion SR.
B. A toxic drug interaction with caffeine.
C. A toxic drug interaction with nicotine.
D. Serum sickness.
E. An unrelated medical illness.

20.3 Bupropion differs from the selective serotonin reuptake inhibitors (SSRIs) in which of the following ways?

A. It has a higher incidence of sexual side effects and a lower incidence of sedation and weight gain.
B. It has a lower incidence of sexual side effects and a lower incidence of sedation and weight gain.
C. It has a lower incidence of sexual side effects and a higher incidence of sedation and weight gain.
D. It has a lower incidence of sexual side effects and weight gain and a higher incidence of sedation.
E. It has a higher incidence of sexual side effects and sedation and a lower incidence of weight gain.

20.4 Which of the following statements about bupropion and attention-deficit/hyperactivity disorder (ADHD) is *true*?

A. Bupropion is U.S. Food and Drug Administration approved for the treatment of ADHD in persons younger than 18 years.
B. In clinical studies, bupropion has been found to be more effective than methylphenidate products for the treatment of ADHD.
C. Bupropion is a second-line agent in the treatment of ADHD.
D. Bupropion is less effective in the treatment of the inattentive form than of the combined form of ADHD.
E. Bupropion is less effective in the treatment of girls than it is in boys with ADHD.

20.5   Which of the following adverse effects of bupropion are clinically most common?

    A. Weight gain.

    B. Agitation, tremor, and insomnia.

    C. Dry mouth.

    D. Sexual dysfunction.

    E. All of the above.

CHAPTER 21

Mirtazapine

Select the single best response for each question.

21.1   Mirtazapine is classified as...

   A. A selective serotonin reuptake inhibitor (SSRI).
   B. A noradrenergic and specific serotonergic antidepressant (NaSSA).
   C. A serotonergic and noradrenergic reuptake inhibitor (SNRI).
   D. A phenylpiperazine antidepressant.
   E. A monoamine oxidase inhibitor (MAOI).

21.2   A 27-year-old man who is taking mirtazapine for generalized anxiety disorder and major depression experiences significant sedation at a dosage of 7.5 mg/day. Which neurotransmitter receptor is most likely being affected?

   A. Histamine$_1$ (H$_1$).
   B. Serotonin$_2$ (5-hydroxytryptamine [5-HT]$_2$).
   C. Dopamine$_2$ (D$_2$).
   D. Serotonin$_3$ (5-HT$_3$).
   E. None of the above.

21.3   Mirtazapine is primarily metabolized by which cytochrome P450 enzymes?

   A. 2E1.
   B. 3A5.
   C. 1A2, 2D6, and 3A4.
   D. 1A2 and 2E1.
   E. 2C9 and 2C19.

21.4   A 49-year-old woman has major depression with a significant anxiety component. She is currently taking valproate for a seizure disorder. She has lost 8 kg in the past 2 months, and she reports great difficulty in falling asleep. Which of the following antidepressants would be the best choice for this patient?

   A. Bupropion.
   B. Fluoxetine.
   C. Desipramine.
   D. Selegiline.
   E. Mirtazapine.

21.5   A 19-year-old woman takes 150 mg of mirtazapine in a suicide attempt. Which of the following consequences is likely?

A. Stevens-Johnson syndrome.
B. Prolonged QTc.
C. Seizure.
D. Renal failure.
E. Disorientation and drowsiness, with tachycardia.

CHAPTER 22

Venlafaxine

Select the single best response for each question.

22.1 Which of the following drugs is minimally protein-bound?

A. Olanzapine.
B. Fluoxetine.
C. Warfarin.
D. Venlafaxine.
E. All of the above.

22.2 What is venlafaxine's primary route of excretion?

A. Pulmonary.
B. Hepatic.
C. Renal.
D. None of the above.
E. Unknown.

22.3 Which of the following drugs may produce a greater antidepressant response than selective serotonin reuptake inhibitors (SSRIs)?

A. Venlafaxine.
B. Lithium.
C. St. John's wort.
D. Mirtazapine.
E. Trazodone.

22.4 Which of the following statements regarding treatment-emergent adverse effects of venlafaxine is *true*?

A. Nausea is the most frequent treatment-emergent side effect, but it diminishes markedly after the first few weeks of therapy.
B. Nausea is rarely a side effect.
C. Nausea is the most frequent treatment-emergent side effect and rarely diminishes over time.
D. The incidence and intensity of nausea are greater with extended-release (XR) venlafaxine than with immediate-release (IR) venlafaxine.
E. None of the above.

22.5 Which of the following statements regarding potential hypertensive adverse effects of venlafaxine is *true*?

A. All patients develop transient hypertension.
B. Sustained hypertension is dose related with the immediate-release (IR) formulation.
C. All treatment-emergent hypertension requires the addition of antihypertensive agents.
D. Treatment-emergent hypertension requires discontinuation of venlafaxine.
E. None of the above.

CHAPTER 23

Duloxetine and Milnacipran

Select the single best response for each question.

23.1   Duloxetine and milnacipran are classified as

    A. Selective serotonin reuptake inhibitors (SSRIs).
    B. Tricyclic antidepressants (TCAs).
    C. Monoamine oxidase inhibitors (MAOIs).
    D. α_2-Adrenergic antagonists.
    E. Serotonergic and noradrenergic reuptake inhibitors (SNRIs).

23.2   Regarding potential drug interactions, blood levels of duloxetine are most likely to be increased when it is coadministered with drugs that potently inhibit which cytochrome P450 enzyme?

    A. 1A2.
    B. 2D6.
    C. 3A4.
    D. 2C9.
    E. 2C19.

23.3   Serious drug interactions can result if duloxetine or milnacipran is coadministered with which of the following?

    A. Selective serotonin reuptake inhibitors (SSRIs).
    B. Monoamine oxidase inhibitors (MAOIs).
    C. St. John's wort.
    D. All of the above.
    E. None of the above.

23.4   Conditions for which duloxetine may be beneficial include which of the following?

    A. Chronic pain.
    B. Stress urinary incontinence.
    C. Depression.
    D. All of the above.
    E. None of the above.

CHAPTER 24

Benzodiazepines

Select the single best response for each question.

24.1 When administered orally, the benzodiazepine that produces the most rapid onset of action is

A. Lorazepam.
B. Chlordiazepoxide.
C. Prazepam.
D. Diazepam.
E. None of the above.

24.2 When administered orally, the benzodiazepine with the longest elimination half-life is

A. Flurazepam.
B. Clonazepam.
C. Diazepam.
D. Prazepam.
E. Lorazepam.

24.3 When administered orally, the benzodiazepine with the shortest elimination half-life is

A. Lorazepam.
B. Oxazepam.
C. Triazolam.
D. Temazepam.
E. Alprazolam.

24.4 The triazolobenzodiazepines (i.e., alprazolam and triazolam) undergo phase I metabolism almost exclusively through which of the following cytochrome P450 enzymes?

A. 1A2.
B. 2B6.
C. 2C19.
D. 2D6.
E. 3A4.

24.5 All of the following pharmacological properties have been described for the benzodiazepine receptor *except*

A. Anticonvulsant effects.
B. Negative ionotropic effects.
C. Muscle relaxation effects.
D. Anxiolytic effects.
E. Sedative-hypnotic effects.

24.6 Phenytoin and barbiturates can precipitate benzodiazepine withdrawal through which of the following mechanisms?

    A. Delayed gastric emptying.
    B. Inhibition of hepatic conjugation.
    C. Hepatic enzyme induction.
    D. Inhibition of hepatic glucuronidation.
    E. None of the above.

CHAPTER 25

Buspirone and Gepirone

Select the single best response for each question.

25.1 Buspirone is thought to exert its anxiolytic actions through agonism of which of the following neurotransmitter receptors?

    A. Serotonin (5-hydroxytryptamine)$_{1A}$ (5-HT$_{1A}$).
    B. 5-HT$_{2A}$.
    C. 5-HT$_{2C}$.
    D. α_1-Adrenergic.
    E. α_2-Adrenergic.

25.2 Buspirone is metabolized principally by which of the following cytochrome P450 enzymes?

    A. 1A2.
    B. 2C19.
    C. 2D6.
    D. 2E1.
    E. 3A4.

25.3 The existing evidence base most strongly supports the effectiveness of buspirone in the treatment of

    A. Obsessive-compulsive disorder (OCD).
    B. Posttraumatic stress disorder (PTSD).
    C. Panic disorder.
    D. Generalized anxiety disorder (GAD).
    E. Social phobia.

25.4 All of the serotonin (5-hydroxytryptamine [5-HT]) receptors are members of the G protein–coupled superfamily *except*

    A. 5-HT$_{1A}$.
    B. 5-HT$_{2A}$.
    C. 5-HT$_{2C}$.
    D. 5-HT$_3$.
    E. 5-HT$_4$.

25.5 Buspirone's major metabolite, which lacks the parent drug's serotonergic effects, is

    A. *m*-Chlorophenylpiperazine (mCPP).
    B. 1-Pyrimidinyl-piperazine (1-PP).
    C. 5-Hydroxyindoleacetic acid (5-HIAA).
    D. 3-Hydroxy-4-methoxyphenylglycol (MHPG).
    E. Homovanillic acid (HVA).

25.6 The side effect most frequently encountered with buspirone is

    A. Nausea.
    B. Headache.
    C. Dizziness.
    D. Night sweats.
    E. Agitation.

CHAPTER 26

Investigational Treatments for Mood and Anxiety Disorders: CRH Receptor Antagonists, NK-1 Receptor Antagonists, and Glucocorticoid Receptor Antagonists

Select the single best response for each question.

26.1 Substance P receptor (neurokinin-1 [NK-1] receptor) antagonists are currently being investigated in the treatment of

A. Psychosis.
B. Obsessive-compulsive symptoms.
C. Depression.
D. Intractable pain.
E. Mania.

26.2 In animal models of depression, antidepressant response correlates with

A. Decreased transcription and translation of brain glucocorticoid receptors (GRs).
B. Increased activity of corticotropin-releasing hormone (CRH).
C. Enhancement of the activity of hypothalamic vasopressin.
D. Diminished mineralocorticoid receptor (MR) functioning.
E. Improved GR functioning.

26.3 The mechanism by which metyrapone and ketoconazole are thought to exert possible antidepressant activity is

A. Inhibition of corticosteroid synthesis.
B. Inhibition of cytochrome P450 3A4.
C. Corticotropin-releasing hormone (CRH) receptor antagonism.
D. Catecholamine reuptake blockade.
E. Antagonism of neurokinin-1 (NK-1) receptors.

26.4 In two open-label studies, mifepristone, also known as RU-486 or C-1073, demonstrated efficacy in treating which of the following?

A. Manic symptoms.
B. Posttraumatic stress disorder symptoms.
C. Obsessive-compulsive symptoms.
D. Binge eating.
E. Psychotic symptoms.

26.5 Corticotropin-releasing hormone receptor 1 (CRHR1) is found in all of the following brain structures *except*

A. Olfactory bulb.
B. Amygdala.
C. Cortex.
D. Locus coeruleus.
E. Anterior lobe of the pituitary gland.

CHAPTER 27

Classic Antipsychotic Medications

Select the single best response for each question.

27.1 A 42-year-old woman with a diagnosis of schizophrenia is unwilling to take any of the atypical antipsychotics because she has heard that they cause weight gain. She has a seizure disorder that is being treated with gabapentin. Which of the following classic antipsychotics would be a logical choice for this patient?

A. Thioridazine.
B. Chlorpromazine.
C. Molindone.
D. Pimozide.
E. Perphenazine.

27.2 A 28-year-old man with a diagnosis of Tourette's syndrome has failed to respond to trials with two different atypical antipsychotics. Which of the following classic antipsychotics would be a logical choice for this patient?

A. Thioridazine.
B. Chlorpromazine.
C. Molindone.
D. Pimozide.
E. Perphenazine.

27.3 According to positron emission tomography (PET) data, a dopamine$_2$ (D$_2$) receptor occupancy of what percentage correlates with the appearance of extrapyramidal side effects (EPS)?

A. 20%.
B. 40%.
C. 60%.
D. 80%.
E. None of the above.

27.4 Which traditional antipsychotic is effective for the treatment of nausea and intractable hiccups?

A. Haloperidol.
B. Chlorpromazine.
C. Molindone.
D. Pimozide.
E. Perphenazine.

27.5 An 18-year-old cocaine user is given intramuscular haloperidol in the emergency room to manage serious aggression. Medical personnel should actively monitor this patient for which of the following potential adverse effects?

A. Antipsychotic-induced parkinsonism.
B. Tardive dyskinesia.
C. Tardive dystonia.
D. Tardive dysmentia.
E. Dystonia.

27.6 A patient has received haloperidol for the acute treatment of aggression for 3 days in an inpatient unit in addition to his usual dose of olanzapine. He develops a fever, tachycardia, and extreme agitation. Which of the following laboratory studies should be ordered?

A. Creatinine.
B. Electrocardiogram.
C. Creatine phosphokinase.
D. Electroencephalogram.
E. None of the above.

CHAPTER 28

Clozapine

Select the single best response for each question.

28.1   What is the primary reason that clozapine is a second-line rather than a first-line treatment for schizophrenia in the United States?

   A.   Side effects such as sedation, constipation, and sialorrhea are very common and difficult to manage.
   B.   Other chemically related medications, such as olanzapine and quetiapine, are equally efficacious with fewer side effects.
   C.   Clozapine is not a second-line treatment for schizophrenia in the United States; it is a first-line treatment.
   D.   Use of clozapine carries a risk of agranulocytosis.
   E.   Clozapine is associated with a higher risk of extrapyramidal side effects (EPS).

28.2   What serum level of clozapine is associated with greater toxicity with no apparent clinical benefit?

   A.   >600 ng/mL.
   B.   Serum levels have not been associated with efficacy or toxicity with clozapine.
   C.   >350 ng/mL.
   D.   >250 ng/mL.
   E.   >1,000 ng/mL.

28.3   Which of the following statements best describes clozapine's unique receptor profile?

   A.   High affinity for dopamine$_2$ (D$_2$) receptors and low affinity for serotonin$_{2A}$ (5-hydroxytryptamine [5-HT]$_{2A}$) receptors.
   B.   Low affinity for both D$_2$ and 5-HT$_{2A}$ receptors.
   C.   Moderate affinity for D$_2$ receptors and a high affinity for 5-HT$_{2A}$ receptors.
   D.   Moderate affinity for both D$_2$ and D$_4$ receptors.
   E.   Low affinity for D$_2$ receptors and a moderate affinity for 5-HT$_{2A}$ receptors.

28.4   Clozapine has been shown to be effective in all of the following conditions *except*

   A.   Treatment-refractory schizophrenia.
   B.   Depression with psychotic features.
   C.   Mania.
   D.   Psychosis in Parkinson's disease.
   E.   Maintenance therapy in schizophrenia.

28.5   Regarding the monitoring of hematological parameters during clozapine treatment, which of the following statements is *false*?

A. Agranulocytosis occurs in less than 1% of patients taking clozapine in the United States.
B. If leukopenia occurs with clozapine use, a patient can be rechallenged several months later without an increased risk of redevelopment of leukopenia or agranulocytosis.
C. Agranulocytosis is defined as an absolute neutrophil count of <500/mm^3.
D. If leukopenia is identified early, most patients recover within 2–3 weeks following cessation of clozapine.
E. With early identification and proper management, most patients with clozapine-associated agranulocytosis fully recover.

28.6   Which of the following factors appears to be associated with a greater risk of clozapine-associated myocarditis and cardiomyopathy?

A. Male gender.
B. Female gender.
C. Older than 50 years of age.
D. Younger than 50 years of age.
E. No obvious risk factors have been associated with these rare side effects.

28.7   Regarding the metabolic side effects of clozapine, all of the following statements are true *except*

A. Serum triglyceride and cholesterol levels increase with clozapine treatment.
B. The average 6-month weight gain with clozapine treatment is 6.9 kg.
C. If diabetes occurs, it usually appears within the first 6 months of treatment.
D. Prescribing guidelines recommend regular monitoring of weight and glucose levels.
E. Weight gain can persist for several years after starting clozapine.

28.8   Clozapine is metabolized primarily by cytochrome P450 1A2. Which of the following drugs can substantially increase clozapine serum levels by inhibiting cytochrome P450 1A2?

A. Fluoxetine.
B. Sertraline.
C. Paroxetine.
D. Carbamazepine.
E. Fluvoxamine.

CHAPTER 29

Olanzapine

Select the single best response for each question.

29.1 Olanzapine's chemical structure is closest to that of which of the following drugs?

A. Diazepam.
B. Clozapine.
C. Quetiapine.
D. Risperidone.
E. None of the above; olanzapine's chemical structure is unique and not related to other approved drugs.

29.2 Many of olanzapine's receptor-binding properties are similar to those of clozapine. Which of the following statements is *false*?

A. Olanzapine nonselectively binds to many different dopamine receptors, whereas clozapine is only partially selective for dopamine$_2$ (D$_2$) receptors.
B. Olanzapine and clozapine both inhibit the firing of A10 neurons without significant inhibition of A9 tracts of the nigrostriatal projections.
C. Olanzapine and clozapine both have a high affinity for serotonin$_{2A}$ (5-hydroxytryptamine [5-HT]$_{2A}$) receptors.
D. Olanzapine and clozapine both have a low affinity for 5-HT$_1$ receptors.
E. Olanzapine and clozapine have moderate binding affinities for 5-HT$_3$ receptors.

29.3 All of the following statements about olanzapine's pharmacokinetics and disposition are true *except*

A. Olanzapine's clearance is decreased in the elderly.
B. Olanzapine's pharmacokinetics in children and adolescents is similar to that in nonsmoking adults.
C. Smoking decreases the clearance of olanzapine.
D. Cytochrome P450 1A2 is the main enzyme responsible for the formation of 4'-*N*-desmethyl-olanzapine.
E. Food has little effect on olanzapine's bioavailability after oral intake.

29.4 Olanzapine has been approved by the U.S. Food and Drug Administration for treatment of which of the following indications?

A. Schizophrenia, bipolar disorder, and depression associated with psychosis.
B. Schizophrenia, mania, and depression associated with psychosis.
C. Psychosis, bipolar disorder, and agitation and psychosis in the elderly.
D. Psychosis, schizophrenia, and bipolar mania.
E. Schizophrenia and schizoaffective disorder only.

29.5   Olanzapine has been demonstrated in placebo-controlled studies to be efficacious in which of the following?

    A. Posttraumatic stress disorder (PTSD).
    B. Borderline personality disorder.
    C. Schizoaffective disorder.
    D. Anorexia nervosa.
    E. Panic disorder.

29.6   The risk of tardive dyskinesia associated with olanzapine treatment has been reported as

    A. Negligible.
    B. An annual rate of 2%–3%.
    C. Similar to that associated with haloperidol.
    D. An annual rate of 5%.
    E. An annual rate of 0.5%.

CHAPTER 30

Quetiapine

Select the single best response for each question.

30.1 Given that quetiapine is metabolized primarily by cytochrome P450 3A4, which of the following statements is *false*?

  A. Coadministration of lithium with quetiapine has little or no effect on quetiapine levels.
  B. Quetiapine is not vulnerable to drug–drug interactions.
  C. Quetiapine's levels can be lowered by 3A4-inducing agents such as carbamazepine.
  D. Quetiapine has little effect on other drug levels.
  E. Erythromycin can raise quetiapine levels.

30.2 Which of the following statements regarding quetiapine and negative symptoms of schizophrenia is *true*?

  A. Overall, studies indicate that quetiapine is much more effective than haloperidol in treating negative symptoms, as measured by the Scale for the Assessment of Negative Symptoms (SANS).
  B. Negative symptoms do not improve with quetiapine.
  C. Quetiapine's high affinity for serotonin$_{1A}$ (5-hydroxytryptamine [5-HT]$_{1A}$) receptors may increase dopamine levels in the hypoactive mesocortical dopaminergic pathway, thereby improving negative symptoms.
  D. Both A and C are correct.
  E. None of the above.

30.3 In studies comparing quetiapine and haloperidol, for which cluster of symptoms did quetiapine show superior efficacy?

  A. Aggression and cognitive symptoms.
  B. Negative and cognitive symptoms.
  C. Positive and negative symptoms.
  D. Cognitive symptoms only.
  E. Negative symptoms only.

30.4 Quetiapine's risk for extrapyramidal side effects (EPS)

  A. Is similar to that of placebo.
  B. Is slightly higher than that of placebo.
  C. Is similar to that of risperidone.
  D. Is similar to that of haloperidol.
  E. Has not been established.

30.5   Regarding changes in prolactin levels with quetiapine use, which of the following statements is *true*?

   A. Prolactin levels begin to increase as the daily dose of quetiapine exceeds 300 mg.
   B. Prolactin levels begin to increase as the daily dose of quetiapine exceeds 500 mg.
   C. Prolactin levels show no difference compared to placebo over a wide range of daily doses of quetiapine (75–750 mg/day).
   D. Elevations in prolactin are common with quetiapine and are not necessarily dose related.
   E. None of the above.

30.6   Quetiapine, in common with other second-generation atypical antipsychotics, has been associated with weight gain. Which of the following orderings accurately represents these agents' relative propensity (from highest to lowest) to cause weight gain?

   A. Clozapine ~ olanzapine > quetiapine > ziprasidone > risperidone.
   B. Quetiapine > clozapine ~ olanzapine > risperidone > ziprasidone.
   C. Clozapine ~ olanzapine > quetiapine > risperidone > ziprasidone.
   D. Quetiapine > olanzapine > clozapine > risperidone > ziprasidone.
   E. Clozapine ~ olanzapine > risperidone > quetiapine > ziprasidone.

CHAPTER 31

Aripiprazole

Select the single best response for each question.

31.1 Which of the following statements best describes the receptor profile of aripiprazole?

    A. Dopamine$_2$ (D$_2$) partial antagonist, serotonin$_{1A}$ (5-hydroxytryptamine [5-HT]$_{1A}$) partial agonist, 5-HT$_{2A}$ agonist.

    B. D$_2$ and 5-HT$_{1A}$ partial agonist, 5-HT$_{2A}$ agonist.

    C. D$_2$ and 5-HT$_{1A}$ partial agonist, 5-HT$_{2A}$ antagonist.

    D. D$_2$ partial antagonist, 5-HT$_{1A}$ partial agonist, 5-HT$_{2A}$ antagonist.

    E. D$_2$ partial antagonist, 5-HT$_{1A}$ partial antagonist, 5-HT$_{2A}$ agonist.

31.2 Which of the following describes the likely outcome if carbamazepine is coadministered with aripiprazole?

    A. Carbamazepine will increase the blood levels of aripiprazole, and adverse effects from aripiprazole will ensue.

    B. Aripiprazole will increase the blood levels of carbamazepine, and adverse effects from carbamazepine will ensue.

    C. Aripiprazole will decrease the blood levels of carbamazepine.

    D. Carbamazepine will decrease the blood levels of aripiprazole.

    E. No drug–drug interaction will arise between aripiprazole and carbamazepine.

31.3 Aripiprazole is associated with which of the following potential adverse effects?

    A. Extreme weight gain.

    B. Increases in triglycerides.

    C. Increases in fasting blood glucose.

    D. Increases in prolactin levels.

    E. None of the above.

31.4 A 62-year-old woman with schizophrenia is about to begin a trial of aripiprazole. Which of the following dosing adjustments may be necessary?

    A. The initial dose must be lowered to 5 mg because of gender-related decreases in kidney function.

    B. The initial dose must be increased to 20 mg because of gender-related increases in cytochrome P450 1A2 activity.

    C. The initial dose must be increased to 20 mg if the patient smokes cigarettes.

    D. No specific changes in dosing requirements are necessary.

    E. Because she is older than 60 years, the initial dose must be increased because of the increased glomerular filtration rate.

CHAPTER 32

Risperidone

Select the single best response for each question.

32.1   Which of the following statements best describes the receptor profile of risperidone?

A. Serotonin$_{2A}$ (5-hydroxytryptamine [5-HT]$_{2A}$) and dopamine$_2$ (D$_2$) agonism.
B. 5-HT$_{2A}$ antagonism and D$_2$ agonism, modest histamine$_1$ (H$_1$) activity, and no affinity for α_1-adrenergic receptors.
C. 5-HT$_{2A}$ and D$_2$ agonism and no affinity for histamine or α_1-adrenergic receptors.
D. 5-HT$_{2A}$ and D$_2$ antagonism.
E. None of the above.

32.2   A patient with bipolar mania is about to begin a trial with risperidone. Which of the following describes the likely time course of risperidone's absorption following oral administration?

A. Peak plasma level of risperidone will be reached only after 8 hours.
B. Because of its active metabolite, peak plasma levels will be reached in 12 hours.
C. Peak plasma levels of risperidone will be reached only after 16 hours.
D. Peak plasma levels of risperidone will be reached within 1 hour.
E. Peak plasma levels of risperidone will be reached in 6 hours.

32.3   A 27-year-old man with schizophrenia is receiving risperidone 16 mg/day. Which of the following statements regarding likely side effects or interactions is *true*?

A. Because of his low dose of risperidone, he is likely to experience few adverse events.
B. If paroxetine is added, he is likely to have a decrease in his blood levels of risperidone.
C. He is unlikely to experience sexual adverse effects.
D. He is unlikely to experience parkinsonian symptoms.
E. He is at risk for parkinsonian symptoms.

32.4   In clinical studies, risperidone's efficacy has been demonstrated for which of the following conditions?

A. Schizophrenia, bipolar mania, and attention-deficit/hyperactivity disorder.
B. Generalized anxiety disorder, and attention-deficit/hyperactivity disorder.
C. Schizophrenia, bipolar mania, and autistic disorder.
D. Oppositional defiant disorder, trichotillomania, and schizophrenia.
E. None of the above.

32.5   Risperidone is metabolized by which cytochrome P540 enzyme?

A. 2C19.
B. 2D6.
C. 2E1.
D. 3A4.
E. None of the above.

CHAPTER 33

Ziprasidone

Select the single best response for each question.

33.1 Which of the following uniquely characterizes ziprasidone's receptor profile in comparison with other atypical antipsychotics?

A. Blockade of serotonin reuptake.
B. Blockade of norepinephrine reuptake.
C. Blockade of dopamine reuptake.
D. Blockade of serotonin and norepinephrine reuptake.
E. Blockade of serotonin, norepinephrine, and dopamine reuptake.

33.2 A 22-year-old man with schizophrenia is about to begin a trial of ziprasidone. Which of the following dosing considerations are important?

A. Monitoring of aldehyde oxidase levels will be needed.
B. Expect that doubling the ziprasidone dosage will produce a doubling of the drug's blood levels.
C. If the patient is taking warfarin, expect increases in the international normalized ratio (INR).
D. If the patient is a cigarette smoker, expect to decrease the dosage of ziprasidone.
E. If the patient is also taking a cytochrome P450 2D6 inhibitor, expect ziprasidone blood levels to be extremely elevated.

33.3 In which of the following patients would ziprasidone be a reasonable first-choice medication for treatment of schizophrenia?

A. A patient currently taking quinidine who is extremely thin.
B. A patient currently taking amiodarone who is extremely obese.
C. A patient currently taking warfarin who is extremely obese.
D. A patient who is a smoker and is extremely thin.
E. A patient currently taking carbamazepine who is extremely obese.

33.4 A 28-year-old man with schizophrenia has failed to respond to olanzapine, and a switch to ziprasidone is planned. Assuming that no contraindications exist, which of the following statements describes the best protocol?

A. Stop olanzapine and start ziprasidone the same day to avoid the sedating effects of ziprasidone.
B. Stop olanzapine and start ziprasidone the same day to avoid the hypotensive effects of ziprasidone.
C. Gradually cross-taper the two drugs to avoid the hypotensive effects of ziprasidone.
D. Gradually cross-taper the two drugs to avoid the activating effects of ziprasidone.
E. Gradually cross-taper the two drugs to avoid the parkinsonian effects of ziprasidone.

33.5 After successful use of parenteral ziprasidone (20 mg im) for acute agitation with psychosis in the emergency department, how is the transition to oral ziprasidone accomplished?

A. Cross-taper intramuscular preparation and oral preparation for 3–7 days as tolerated.
B. Initiate oral therapy the day after intramuscular therapy ceases, at 40 mg po twice a day.
C. Allow 36–48 hours after intramuscular therapy ceases before administering 40 mg po twice a day.
D. Initiate oral therapy the day after intramuscular therapy ceases, at 200 mg po twice a day.
E. None of the above.

CHAPTER 34

Drugs to Treat Extrapyramidal Side Effects

Select the single best response for each question.

34.1 The form of extrapyramidal side effects (EPS) most likely to appear within days of initiating an antipsychotic agent is

A. Akathisia.
B. Rabbit syndrome.
C. Acute dystonic reaction.
D. Tardive dyskinesia.
E. Pseudoparkinsonism.

34.2 Benztropine and trihexyphenidyl are able to prevent and treat antipsychotic-induced parkinsonism and acute dystonic reactions through blockade of which receptor?

A. Dopamine$_2$ (D$_2$).
B. Serotonin$_{2C}$ (5-hydroxytryptamine [5-HT]$_{2C}$).
C. Histamine$_1$ (H$_1$).
D. Muscarinic.
E. Nicotinic.

34.3 Benztropine, trihexyphenidyl, and other anticholinergic drugs can produce all of the following side effects *except*

A. Miosis.
B. Tachycardia.
C. Urinary retention.
D. Constipation.
E. Dry mouth.

34.4 Amantadine has demonstrated effectiveness in the treatment of which of the following?

A. Acute dystonic reactions.
B. Influenza A.
C. Akathisia.
D. Tardive dyskinesia.
E. Tardive dystonia.

34.5 Of the following drugs, the agent most effective in the treatment of akathisia is

    A. Benztropine.
    B. Lorazepam.
    C. Vitamin E.
    D. Atenolol.
    E. Propranolol.

34.6 Which of the following antipsychotic agents is *least* likely to produce extrapyramidal side effects?

    A. Risperidone.
    B. Chlorpromazine.
    C. Perphenazine.
    D. Clozapine.
    E. Olanzapine.

CHAPTER 35

Lithium

Select the single best response for each question.

35.1   Which of the following is a predictor of poor antimanic response to lithium?

   A. Late age at first manic episode.
   B. Grandiosity.
   C. Euphoria.
   D. Rapid cycling.
   E. Pregnancy.

35.2   Lithium has demonstrated efficacy for which of the following?

   A. Treatment of obsessive-compulsive disorder.
   B. Treatment of hyperthyroidism.
   C. Antidepressant augmentation in unipolar depression.
   D. Treatment of anorexia nervosa.
   E. Correction of syndrome of inappropriate antidiuretic hormone secretion (SIADH).

35.3   Lithium levels may be increased by all of the following *except*

   A. Osmotic diuretics.
   B. Thiazide diuretics.
   C. Nonsteroidal anti-inflammatory drugs (NSAIDs).
   D. Angiotensin-converting enzyme inhibitors.
   E. Sodium restriction.

35.4   The cardiac malformation most associated with the use of lithium during pregnancy is

   A. Patent ductus arteriosus.
   B. Dextrocardia.
   C. Ventricular septal defect.
   D. Atrial septal defect.
   E. Dysplastic tricuspid valve.

35.5   Lithium is associated with all of the following side effects *except*

   A. Cognitive dulling.
   B. Weight loss.
   C. Tremor.
   D. Hypothyroidism.
   E. Diabetes insipidus.

35.6 Which of the following is relatively contraindicated in combination with lithium?

    A. Olanzapine.
    B. Valproate.
    C. Electroconvulsive therapy (ECT).
    D. Nortriptyline.
    E. Gabapentin.

CHAPTER 36

Valproate

Select the single best response for each question.

36.1 U.S. Food and Drug Administration (FDA)–approved indications for the use of valproate include all of the following *except*

    A. Bipolar mania.
    B. Bipolar maintenance.
    C. Migraine prophylaxis.
    D. Monotherapy for absence seizures.
    E. Adjunctive therapy for other seizure types.

36.2 Valproate-induced hair loss may be minimized by taking a multivitamin containing which of the following?

    A. Magnesium.
    B. Calcium.
    C. Inositol.
    D. Danshen (*Salvia miltiorrhiza*).
    E. Zinc and selenium.

36.3 The greatest teratogenic risk posed by valproate is for which of the following?

    A. Tricuspid atresia.
    B. Cleft palate.
    C. Neural tube defects.
    D. Bone marrow suppression.
    E. Floppy baby syndrome.

36.4 The free concentration of valproate is most likely to be increased by which of the following?

    A. Aspirin.
    B. Fluvoxamine.
    C. Phenytoin.
    D. Risperidone.
    E. Lithium.

36.5 The ability of valproate to inhibit phase II glucuronidation can lead to increased levels of coadministered drugs. Which of the following drugs, if taken concomitantly with valproate, is susceptible to this effect?

A. Glyburide.
B. Warfarin.
C. Alprazolam.
D. Lamotrigine.
E. Zonisamide.

36.6 A 25-year-old medically healthy man who has been receiving valproate monotherapy for migraine prophylaxis for about 1 month experiences sudden, sharp midepigastric pain. Which of the following laboratory studies is most likely to reveal the cause of this pain?

A. Alkaline phosphatase.
B. Mean corpuscular volume.
C. Serum amylase.
D. Valproate blood level.
E. Creatine phosphokinase.

CHAPTER 37

Carbamazepine and Oxcarbazepine

Select the single best response for each question.

37.1   In the treatment of mood disorders, the oxcarbazepine dosage is gradually raised

    A. To a usual dose of 3,600 mg/day.
    B. To clinically desired effect.
    C. To a serum level of 50–150 µg/mL.
    D. Until the patient develops diplopia, at which point the dosage is gradually tapered until diplopia resolves.
    E. None of the above.

37.2   Which of the following is *not* considered a clinical action of carbamazepine?

    A. Decreasing sodium influx and glutamate release.
    B. Acting on peripheral benzodiazepine receptors.
    C. Acting on α_2-adrenergic receptors.
    D. Inhibiting monoamine reuptake.
    E. All of the above.

37.3   Which of the following statements concerning carbamazepine is *true*?

    A. Carbamazepine is ineffective in treating acute mania.
    B. Carbamazepine does not autoinduce its own metabolism.
    C. Carbamazepine has equal acute antimanic and antidepressant effects.
    D. Carbamazepine has equal prophylactic antimanic and antidepressant effects.
    E. None of the above.

37.4   Which of the following adverse events is *not* associated with the rapid titration of carbamazepine?

    A. Extrapyramidal side effects (EPS).
    B. Diplopia and nystagmus.
    C. Ataxia.
    D. Sedation.
    E. All of the above are associated with rapid carbamazepine titration.

37.5 During gradual titration of carbamazepine dosage, the emergence of dizziness, ataxia, and diplopia 1–2 hours after an individual dose may indicate that

A. The patient has misunderstood the dosing schedule.
B. The adverse-effect threshold has been exceeded, requiring dosage redistribution.
C. A drug–drug interaction has occurred.
D. The patient needs reassurance that the symptoms will subside.
E. None of the above.

37.6 Patients taking carbamazepine should be alerted to seek immediate medical attention if they experience which of the following symptoms?

A. Oral ulcers.
B. Petechiae.
C. Easy bruising and bleeding.
D. Rash.
E. All of the above.

37.7 Laboratory monitoring during carbamazepine therapy is performed after 2, 4, 6, and 8 weeks postinitiation and every 3 months thereafter. This laboratory testing includes which of the following?

A. Thyroid panel.
B. Clean-catch urinalysis.
C. Complete blood count (CBC) and liver-associated enzymes.
D. Electrocardiogram.
E. Urine metabolites.

37.8 Inhibition of which metabolic cytochrome P450 enzyme causes carbamazepine toxicity?

A. 1A2.
B. 2D6.
C. 3A3/4.
D. 2C19.
E. 2E1.

37.9 Which cytochrome P450 metabolic enzyme is induced by both carbamazepine and oxcarbazepine?

A. 1A2.
B. 2D6.
C. 3A3/4.
D. 2C19.
E. 2E1.

CHAPTER 38

Gabapentin

Select the single best response for each question.

38.1 Gabapentin is thought to exert its effects through which of the following mechanisms?

   A. Directly regulating the benzodiazepine receptor.
   B. Acting as a monoamine reuptake inhibitor.
   C. Blocking dopamine release primarily in limbic structures.
   D. Increasing brain intracellular γ-aminobutyric acid (GABA) via blood-brain barrier amino acid transporter and other enzymatic regulatory mechanisms.
   E. None of the above.

38.2 Gabapentin has a benign drug-interaction profile because

   A. It has no active metabolites.
   B. It has no protein binding.
   C. It has no cytochrome P450 interactions.
   D. All of the above.
   E. None of the above.

38.3 Controlled studies have shown that gabapentin is clearly beneficial in the treatment of which of the following?

   A. Migraine headaches.
   B. Diabetic neuropathy.
   C. Postherpetic neuralgia.
   D. All of the above.
   E. None of the above.

38.4 Gabapentin shows promise in the treatment of

   A. Bipolar disorder.
   B. Social phobia.
   C. Major depression.
   D. Schizophrenia.
   E. None of the above.

38.5 Although gabapentin has a benign side-effect profile, which serious adverse effect has been associated with use of gabapentin in pediatric epilepsy and adult mania?

   A. Torsades de pointes.
   B. Serotonin syndrome.
   C. Aggression.
   D. Tics.
   E. Sleepwalking.

CHAPTER 39

Lamotrigine

Select the single best response for each question.

39.1 Lamotrigine's mechanism of action is not fully understood but is presumed to be associated with

    A. Its effects on dopamine$_1$ (D$_1$) or dopamine$_2$ (D$_2$) receptors.
    B. Its effects on γ-aminobutyric acid B (GABA$_B$) receptors.
    C. Inhibition of glutamine-induced burst firing and decreased release of glutamate.
    D. Its effects on histamine$_1$ (H$_1$) receptors.
    E. All of the above.

39.2 The side effects most commonly associated with lamotrigine include

    A. Tremor, headache, and rash.
    B. Dizziness, headache, diplopia, nausea, and ataxia.
    C. Extrapyramidal symptoms, nausea, diarrhea, and rash.
    D. All of the above.
    E. None of the above.

39.3 Which of the following dosing strategies would best minimize the risk of lamotrigine-associated rash?

    A. Rapid escalation of dosage.
    B. 25 mg daily for 2 weeks if coadministered with valproic acid.
    C. Starting at dosages above 25 mg/day.
    D. 25 mg every other day for 2 weeks if coadministered with valproic acid.
    E. 50 mg daily for 14 days if coadministered with valproic acid.

39.4 Which of the following best describes the currently recommended clinical management strategy for lamotrigine-associated rash?

    A. Hold the next dose and seek immediate medical attention.
    B. Revert to the previous lower dose and monitor via telephone daily.
    C. Double the dose to "shoot through" the rash-inducing dosage.
    D. Hold the current dosage for 2 weeks before resuming dosage escalation.
    E. None of the above.

39.5 Drug interaction warnings for lamotrigine include which of the following?

    A. Reduced plasma concentration of lamotrigine when coadministered with carbamazepine.
    B. Reduced plasma concentration of lamotrigine when coadministered with oral contraceptives.
    C. Increased plasma concentration of lamotrigine when coadministered with valproic acid.
    D. All of the above.
    E. None of the above.

CHAPTER 40

Topiramate

Select the single best response for each question.

40.1 Topiramate has been approved by the U.S. Food and Drug Administration (FDA) for use in which of the following psychiatric disorders?

    A. Bipolar disorder in adolescents only.
    B. Bipolar disorder in adults only.
    C. Bipolar disorder in adolescents and adults.
    D. Rapid-cycling bipolar disorder.
    E. None of the above.

40.2 In a placebo-controlled study of topiramate in acute bipolar mania, the drug's efficacy was demonstrated in adolescent patients taking topiramate who completed the study. This study was prematurely discontinued for which of the following reasons?

    A. Patients lost too much weight.
    B. A high proportion of patients developed acidosis.
    C. Topiramate demonstrated no benefit in the adult cohort of this study.
    D. Common side effects, such as dizziness, were too difficult to manage, causing most patients to drop out of the study.
    E. There were ethical concerns about research on adolescents.

40.3 In an 8-week comparison of topiramate and sustained-release bupropion in 36 patients with bipolar depression (McIntyre et al. 2002), mean weight loss with bupropion was 1.2 kg. What was the mean weight loss for topiramate-treated patients?

    A. 7.6 kg.
    B. 6.6 kg.
    C. 8.6 kg.
    D. 5.6 kg.
    E. 3.6 kg.

40.4 Regarding findings from the first controlled study of topiramate monotherapy in acute bipolar disorder, which of the following statements about side effects is *true*?

    A. Significant dropout due to side effects was found in the topiramate-treated group compared with the placebo-treated group.
    B. Discontinuation due to side effects was no different with topiramate than it was with placebo.
    C. Discontinuation was higher in the placebo-treated group than the topiramate-treated group.
    D. Dyspepsia was the most common side effect in topiramate-treated patients.
    E. None of the above.

40.5   Two uncommon but potentially serious side effects of topiramate are

    A. Reversible metabolic acidosis and weight loss.
    B. Nephrolithiasis and secondary angle-closure glaucoma.
    C. Nephrolithiasis and weight loss.
    D. Myopia and breakthrough bleeding in females on birth control pills.
    E. Secondary angle-closure glaucoma and reversible metabolic acidosis.

CHAPTER 41

Cognitive Enhancers

Select the single best response for each question.

41.1 Evidence of cholinergic system involvement in the pathophysiology of Alzheimer's disease (AD) includes all of the following *except*

A. Greater reactivity to cholinergic blockade demonstrated by patients with AD compared with age-matched control subjects.

B. Reduced ChAT cell bodies in the basal forebrain at autopsy in patients with AD.

C. Deficits in attention and learning in animals with cholinergic system lesions.

D. Precipitation of age-dependent learning impairments in humans through blockade of the central cholinergic system with anticholinergic drugs such as scopolamine.

E. Increased choline acetyltransferase (ChAT) activity in the hippocampus and cerebral cortex in patients with AD.

41.2 Regarding shared characteristics of the acetylcholinesterase inhibitors (AChEIs) donepezil, rivastigmine, and galantamine, all of the following statements are correct *except*

A. They are all approved by the U.S. Food and Drug Administration for use in Alzheimer's disease.

B. They are all reversible AChEIs.

C. They are all naturally occurring substances derived from herbs or plants.

D. They have not been demonstrated to differ from one another in efficacy.

E. All of the above are correct.

41.3 All of the following cholinergic-active substances have been shown to improve cognitive functioning in Alzheimer's disease *except*

A. Nicotine.

B. Huperzine-α.

C. Tacrine.

D. Rivastigmine.

E. Physostigmine.

41.4 Which of the following statements regarding studies using nonsteroidal anti-inflammatory drugs (NSAIDs) in Alzheimer's disease (AD) is *true*?

A. Retrospective studies have indicated that NSAIDs could delay the onset of AD, but prospective studies did not find such an effect.

B. Meta-analysis of studies in patients taking NSAIDs for rheumatoid arthritis indicated a substantially decreased risk of developing AD.

C. In one prospective study, AD patients treated with indomethacin showed no differences compared with placebo-treated patients after 6 months.

D. There is only indirect evidence for inflammatory and immunological abnormalities in the AD brain.

E. All of the above.

41.5 *Ginkgo biloba*'s mechanism of action in preserving cognitive function is due to

    A. Its acetylcholinesterase activity.
    B. Its antioxidant activity.
    C. It ability to reduce cholesterol.
    D. Its activity with *N*-methyl-D-aspartate (NMDA) receptors.
    E. Its effects on estrogen hormone.

41.6 Memantine has been shown to improve cognition and/or reduce deterioration in which of the following?

    A. Alzheimer's disease only.
    B. Vascular dementia only.
    C. Both Alzheimer's disease and vascular dementia.
    D. Alzheimer's disease only, when used in combination with acetylcholinesterase inhibitors.
    E. None of the above.

CHAPTER 42

Sedative-Hypnotics

Select the single best response for each question.

42.1 Regarding the pharmacological profile of benzodiazepines, which of the following statements is *true?*

   A. They alter GABAergic (γ-aminobutyric acid [GABA]) receptors directly.
   B. They chemically bind to and permanently alter GABA receptors.
   C. They influence the influx of chloride ions into the cell.
   D. They do not have specific receptors in the central nervous system.
   E. None of the above.

42.2 All of the following statements regarding the GABA$_A$ receptor are true *except*

   A. It consists of five subunits, which form a rosette surrounding an ion channel pore for chloride ions.
   B. When activated by conformational changes due to the presence of a benzodiazepine, chloride ions exit the cell.
   C. Activation causes neuronal inhibition.
   D. The GABAergic system is widespread throughout the central nervous system.
   E. All of the above statements are true.

42.3 Which of the following statements about desmethyldiazepam is *true?*

   A. As a metabolite, it has a short half-life, and it is quickly excreted from the body.
   B. It is a metabolite only of diazepam.
   C. It has a long half-life and is ultimately oxidized to other compounds that are then conjugated and excreted.
   D. It has a long half-life, but it is directly conjugated and excreted.
   E. It undergoes oxidation to clorazepate and is then excreted.

42.4 Which of the following statements concerning the effects of most benzodiazepines on sleep architecture is *true?*

   A. Decrease sleep latency, increase the time in stage 2 sleep, and increase rapid eye movement (REM) latency.
   B. Decrease sleep latency, decrease the time in stage 2 sleep, and decrease REM latency.
   C. Suppress stage 3 and 4 sleep and decrease REM latency.
   D. Increase stage 3 and 4 sleep and increase REM latency.
   E. Lengthen slow-wave sleep and decrease REM latency.

42.5 Which of the following represents a contraindication to the use of a benzodiazepine for insomnia?

 A. Multiple sclerosis.
 B. Asthma.
 C. Anxiety disorders.
 D. Jet lag.
 E. Myasthenia gravis.

42.6 Which of the following statements concerning benzodiazepines is *false*?

 A. Overdose of benzodiazepines is usually not fatal.
 B. Benzodiazepines are safe for use during early pregnancy.
 C. Mental/cognitive impairment is clearly shown when using benzodiazepines.
 D. Benzodiazepine use can improve mental/cognitive function in very anxious patients.
 E. None of the above.

42.7 Reasons that benzodiazepines are preferred to barbiturates include all of the following *except*

 A. Barbiturates can depress respiration.
 B. Barbiturates cause patients to feel more "drugged" the next day.
 C. Barbiturates do not decrease sleep latency.
 D. Barbiturates are less safe in overdose compared with benzodiazepines.
 E. All of the above reasons are correct.

42.8 The most common reason/presentation for insomnia is

 A. Insomnia associated with psychiatric disorders.
 B. Insomnia associated with psychological factors and/or physiological tension/arousal.
 C. Insomnia associated with sleep-induced respiratory impairment.
 D. Insomnia perceived by a patient but not demonstrated by objective polysomnography.
 E. Insomnia associated with alcohol and/or drug use.

CHAPTER 43

Psychostimulants in Psychiatry: Amphetamine, Methylphenidate, and Modafinil

Select the single best response for each question.

43.1   The action of which molecular structure provides the rate-limiting step in the clinical effects of amphetamines?

  A. *N*-Methyl-D-aspartate (NMDA) receptors.
  B. Dopamine transporter (DAT).
  C. G-protein complex.
  D. γ-Aminobutyric acid B (GABA$_B$) receptors.
  E. Norepinephrine transporter (NET).

43.2   What is a known neurotoxic effect of methamphetamine and its potential consequences?

  A. The drug destroys acetylcholine neurons and increases the risk of cortical dementia.
  B. The drug destroys γ-aminobutyric acid B (GABA$_B$) receptors and increases the risk of panic disorder.
  C. The drug destroys dopaminergic neurons and may increase the risk of Parkinson's disease.
  D. All of the above.
  E. None of the above.

43.3   Amphetamine is partially metabolized by which of the following cytochrome P450 enzymes?

  A. 1A2.
  B. 2C9 and 2C19.
  C. 2D6.
  D. 2E1.
  E. 3A4/5.

43.4   Potential adverse effects associated with methylphenidate use include which of the following?

  A. Nervousness and insomnia.
  B. Growth impairment.
  C. Worsened tics.
  D. All of the above.
  E. None of the above.

43.5   Which of the following statements best describes modafinil's cytochrome P450 metabolism?

   A. Modafinil's metabolism occurs primarily via cytochrome P450 3A4/5.
   B. Modafinil induces metabolism at cytochrome P450 3A4/5, which can reduce the effectiveness of medications such as triazolam.
   C. Modafinil increases levels of medications metabolized at cytochrome P450 2C19, such as tricyclic antidepressants, phenytoin, and propranolol.
   D. All of the above.
   E. None of the above.

C H A P T E R   4 4

Electroconvulsive Therapy

Select the single best response for each question.

44.1 Electroconvulsive therapy (ECT) has been found to be effective in which of the following conditions?

A. Atypical depression, hypomania, and schizoaffective disorder.
B. Depression, mania, and drug-related psychosis.
C. Depression, mania, and schizotypal personality disorder.
D. Depression, mania, and schizoid personality disorder.
E. Depression, mania, and schizophrenia.

44.2 Electroconvulsive therapy (ECT) has been found to be effective in treating what percentage of individuals with treatment-resistant unipolar or bipolar depression?

A. 20%.
B. 40%.
C. 60%.
D. 80%.
E. 100%.

44.3 Electroconvulsive therapy (ECT) is effective in treating which of the following?

A. Acute psychotic break.
B. Catatonic schizophrenia.
C. Neuroleptic malignant syndrome.
D. All of the above.
E. None of the above.

44.4 Which of the following medical conditions increases the risk of complications from electroconvulsive therapy (ECT)?

A. Increased intracranial pressure.
B. Recent myocardial infarction.
C. Severe chronic obstructive pulmonary disease.
D. Recent cerebral infarction.
E. All of the above.

44.5 Which of the following statements best characterizes the memory loss attributed to ECT?

A. Anterograde memory loss can be temporary and retrograde memory loss can be permanent.
B. Anterograde memory loss can be permanent and retrograde memory loss can be temporary.
C. Both anterograde and retrograde memory loss can be temporary.
D. Both anterograde and retrograde memory loss can be permanent.
E. Anterograde memory loss can be permanent.

CHAPTER 45

Biology of Mood Disorders

Select the single best response for each question.

45.1 Which of the following statements best describes the state of current knowledge about genetic markers for bipolar disorder?

   A. Chromosome 21 has definitely been implicated.
   B. Chromosome 21 and the Y chromosome have definitely been implicated.
   C. After studies implicating chromosome 11 and the X chromosome were published, further studies have not supported these findings.
   D. After studies implicating chromosome 11 and the Y chromosome were published, further studies have not supported these findings.
   E. Chromosome 21 and the X chromosome have definitely been implicated.

45.2 Which of the following clinical findings has been demonstrated in patients with bipolar disorder?

   A. Decreased plasma cortisol concentration.
   B. Decreased cortisol in cerebrospinal fluid.
   C. Suppression of plasma glucocorticoid concentration after dexamethasone administration.
   D. Nonsuppression of plasma glucocorticoid concentration after dexamethasone administration.
   E. Increased diurnal variation of plasma cortisol concentrations.

45.3 Clinical response of depressed patients to antidepressant treatment has been associated with which of the following physiological measures?

   A. Increased metabolic activity in the rostral cingulate cortex.
   B. Decreased metabolic activity in the rostral cingulate cortex.
   C. Increased ventral prefrontal cortical activity.
   D. Increased metabolic activity in the left posterior cingulate cortex.
   E. None of the above.

45.4 Which of the following changes in the serotonergic system has been associated with depression?

   A. Decreased postsynaptic serotonin$_2$ (5-hydroxytryptamine [5-HT]$_2$) receptors.
   B. Increased plasma tryptophan concentrations.
   C. Increased prolactin response to fenfluramine.
   D. Increased postsynaptic 5-HT$_2$ receptors.
   E. Increased serotonin transporter (5-HTT) binding in midbrain.

45.5   Which of the following statements best describes the dexamethasone suppression test (DST)?

   A. The rate of cortisol nonsuppression correlates best with a diagnosis of atypical depression.
   B. The rate of cortisol nonsuppression correlates best with a diagnosis of nonpsychotic depression.
   C. The rate of cortisol nonsuppression correlates best with a diagnosis of psychotic depression.
   D. The rate of cortisol nonsuppression correlates best with a diagnosis of depression not otherwise specified (NOS).
   E. The rate of cortisol nonsuppression correlates best with a diagnosis of seasonal affective disorder.

CHAPTER 46

Neurobiology of Schizophrenia

Select the single best response for each question.

46.1 Which of the following sensory modalities is consistently impaired in individuals with schizophrenia?

A. Sight.
B. Hearing.
C. Touch.
D. Taste.
E. Smell.

46.2 Reduced volume of anterior, posterior, and (less consistently) total superior temporal gyrus has been correlated with which of the following clinical measures?

A. Persistence of negative symptoms.
B. Severity of auditory hallucinations and thought disorder.
C. Deficits in working memory.
D. Impaired processing of auditory evoked potentials.
E. Magnitude of comorbid mood dysregulation.

46.3 In 1991, McCarley et al. found the greatest P300 amplitude separation between persons with schizophrenia and controls for which of the following electrode sites?

A. Nondominant parietal lobe.
B. Left occipital lobe.
C. Left temporal lobe.
D. Dominant frontal lobe.
E. Nondominant frontal lobe.

46.4 The developmental histories of individuals with schizophrenia reveal higher rates of all of the following *except*

A. Heavy maternal alcohol use during the first trimester.
B. Maternal starvation during the first trimester.
C. Maternal influenza infection during the second trimester.
D. Rhesus and ABO blood-type incompatibility.
E. Perinatal anoxic birth injuries.

46.5 One of the most consistent neuroanatomic findings in schizophrenia has been

    A. Enlarged hippocampal volumes.
    B. Underdevelopment of the corpus callosum.
    C. Enlarged amygdala.
    D. Enlarged lateral ventricles.
    E. Pituitary hyperplasia.

46.6 The genetic contributions to schizophrenia may be best described as

    A. Sex-linked.
    B. Multifactorial.
    C. Mendelian.
    D. Mutations.
    E. Iatrogenic.

CHAPTER 47

Neurobiology of Anxiety Disorders

Select the single best response for each question.

47.1 The involvement of noradrenergic systems in enhanced memory consolidation of emotional material is evidenced by the blocking of this effect by

A. Clonidine.
B. Guanfacine.
C. Propranolol.
D. Yohimbine.
E. Bupropion.

47.2 Fear- or anxiety-inducing stimuli in which sensory modality are transmitted to the amygdala rather than to the dorsal thalamus?

A. Sight.
B. Hearing.
C. Touch.
D. Smell.
E. Taste.

47.3 Each of the following agents has been used to provoke panic attacks in experimental protocols *except*

A. Disulfiram.
B. Carbon dioxide (CO_2).
C. Cholecystokinin-4 (CCK-4).
D. Yohimbine.
E. Lactate.

47.4 Fear and anxiety states activate noradrenergic neurons in which of the following brain structures?

A. Amygdala.
B. Ventromedial hypothalamus.
C. Thalamus.
D. Hippocampus.
E. Locus coeruleus.

47.5 Early and chronic exposures to stressors may be associated with hippocampal damage, mediated through elevated levels of

A. Testosterone.
B. Corticotropin-releasing hormone (CRH).
C. Growth hormone.
D. Prolactin.
E. Substance P.

47.6 Dysregulation of dopaminergic release in which of the following brain structures is associated with helplessness behaviors and delayed extinction of conditioned fear responses?

A. Amygdala.
B. Nucleus accumbens.
C. Medial prefrontal cortex.
D. Tuberoinfundibular tract.
E. Cingulate gyrus.

47.7 Stimulation of which of the following neurotransmitter receptors is anxiolytic?

A. Corticotropin-releasing hormone receptor 1 (CRHR1).
B. Serotonin (5-hydroxytryptamine)$_{1A}$ (5-HT$_{1A}$).
C. 5-HT$_{2A}$.
D. Dopamine$_2$ (D$_2$).
E. α_1-Adrenergic.

CHAPTER 48

Biology of Alzheimer's Disease

Select the single best response for each question.

48.1   Of all the pathological alterations seen in Alzheimer's disease (AD), which of the following best correlates with cognitive deficits?

   A. Number of neurofibrillary tangles.
   B. Number of neuritic plaques.
   C. Location of amyloid deposition.
   D. Amount of cortical cellular loss.
   E. Loss of cortical synapses.

48.2   All of the following point to failed neurotransmission at cholinergic synapses in the neocortex and hippocampus in Alzheimer's disease (AD) *except*

   A. Acetylcholinesterase (AChE) inhibitors achieve a high degree (over 80%) of AChE inhibition, which explains their efficacy in AD.
   B. Presynaptic cholinergic markers are decreased in AD.
   C. Basal forebrain neurons degenerate in AD.
   D. Pharmacological blockage of basal forebrain muscarinic acetylcholine receptors impairs learning and memory.
   E. AChE inhibitors improve cognitive and behavioral problems associated with AD.

48.3   Which of the following statements regarding muscarinic and nicotinic receptors is *true*?

   A. Muscarinic$_4$ (M_4) receptors are decreased in Alzheimer's disease (AD).
   B . A muscarinic$_1$ (M_1) agonist has been shown to reduce hallucinations and agitation in AD.
   C. M_4 is the most abundant receptor in the cortex and hippocampus.
   D. M_1 is primarily an autoreceptor on cholinergic terminals.
   E. Nicotinic receptors have a very well-defined role in cholinergic transmission in AD.

48.4   The biggest risk factor for Alzheimer's disease (AD) is

   A. Presence of the apolipoprotein-E (APOE) ε4 allele.
   B. Poor linguistic abilities in early life.
   C. Age.
   D. Mutations in the amyloid precursor protein (*APP*) gene on chromosome 21, the presenilin 1 (*PS1*) gene on chromosome 4, and the presenilin 2 (*PS2*) gene on chromosome 1.
   E. None of the above.

48.5 Regarding prospective clinical trials of nonsteroidal anti-inflammatory drugs (NSAIDs) in Alzheimer's disease (AD), which of the following statements is *true*?

    A. NSAIDs have been found to reduce the risk of developing AD by 30%–80%.
    B. NSAIDs have shown no benefit in patients with AD.
    C. No prospective studies have been conducted, only retrospective studies.
    D. NSAID use has proven too risky, because of these agents' side effects.
    E. Studies have yielded mixed results, with some showing benefit for NSAIDs in AD and others not.

48.6 Which of the following is the primary focus of the leading theory of Alzheimer's disease (AD) pathogenesis?

    A. Inflammation.
    B. Oxidative injury.
    C. Mitochondrial dysfunction.
    D. Amyloid cascade.
    E. None of the above.

CHAPTER 49

Neurobiology of Substance Abuse Disorders

Select the single best response for each question.

49.1   The neural substrates of drug reward and reinforcement include which of the following?

    A. Extrapyramidal system.
    B. Dorsal raphe nuclei.
    C. Tegmental fields.
    D. Mesolimbic projections to the nucleus accumbens.
    E. All of the above.

49.2   The primary receptor site of action of cocaine is

    A. Dopamine transporter (DAT).
    B. Vesicular monoamine transporter (VMAT).
    C. Nicotinic acetylcholine (ACh) receptors.
    D. γ-Aminobutyric acid (GABA) receptors.
    E. *N*-Methyl-D-aspartate (NMDA) receptors.

49.3   The primary receptor site of action of ethanol is

    A. Dopamine transporter (DAT).
    B. Vesicular monoamine transporter (VMAT).
    C. Nicotinic acetylcholine (ACh) receptors.
    D. γ-Aminobutyric acid (GABA) and *N*-methyl-D-aspartate (NMDA) receptors.
    E. G proteins.

49.4   Functional neuroimaging studies have implicated which of the following mechanisms in opiate and nicotine dependence?

    A. Lack of reward-related striatal activation and lack of reinforcement-related activation of brain areas involved in reward processes.
    B. Significant reward-related striatal activation and lack of reinforcement-related activation of brain areas involved in reward processes.
    C. Significant reward-related striatal activation and significant reinforcement-related activation of brain areas involved in reward processing.
    D. Lack of reward-related striatal activation and significant reinforcement-related activation of brain areas involved in reward processing.
    E. None of the above.

49.5 Positron emission tomography (PET) imaging has been used to assess the effects of cocaine craving in cocaine-dependent subjects. Conditioned cocaine cues were found to be associated with activation of which of the following brain structures?

A. Amygdala.
B. Prefrontal cortex.
C. Anterior cingulate cortex.
D. All of the above.
E. None of the above.

CHAPTER 50

Biology of Eating Disorders

Select the single best response for each question.

50.1   Individuals with the binge-eating/purging subtype of anorexia nervosa are more likely than those with the restricting subtype to have a history of which of the following?

A. Behavioral dyscontrol.
B. Substance abuse.
C. Overt family conflict.
D. All of the above.
E. None of the above.

50.2   Which of the following statements concerning anorexia nervosa is *true*?

A. When at normal weight, patients with anorexia nervosa have increased plasma cortisol secretion.
B. Once increased, plasma and cerebrospinal fluid (CSF) levels of corticotropin-releasing hormone (CRH) never return to normal.
C. Intracerebroventricular CRH administration in experimental animals fails to produce physiological and behavioral changes similar to anorexia nervosa in humans.
D. The hypothalamic-pituitary-thyroid axis is activated by weight gain.
E. When underweight, patients with anorexia nervosa have increased plasma cortisol secretion.

50.3   Which of the following statements about patients with bulimia nervosa is *true*?

A. In comparison with control subjects, patients with bulimia nervosa have diminished release of cholecystokinin (CCK) following ingestion of a standardized test meal.
B. In comparison with control subjects, patients with bulimia nervosa have excessive release of CCK following ingestion of a standardized test meal.
C. In comparison with control subjects, patients with bulimia nervosa have no release of CCK following ingestion of a standardized test meal.
D. Standardized test meals have no effect on CCK levels in patients with bulimia nervosa.
E. None of the above.

50.4   In patients who achieve sustained recovery from bulimia nervosa, serum levels of leptin

A. Gradually increase over time.
B. Remain decreased.
C. Are associated with increased metabolic rate.
D. Are associated with reduced metabolic rate.
E. None of the above.

50.5   Which of the following statements regarding serotonin metabolism in anorexia nervosa is *true?*

   A. Cerebrospinal fluid (CSF) concentrations of 5-hydroxyindoleacetic acid (5-HIAA) are decreased in individuals with long-term weight recovery.
   B. When underweight, women with anorexia nervosa show significant elevations in basal CSF concentrations of 5-HIAA.
   C. Resumption of normal eating may unmask intrinsic abnormalities in serotonergic systems that mediate certain core behavioral or temperamental underpinnings of risk and vulnerability.
   D. All of the above.
   E. None of the above.

CHAPTER 51

Biology of
Personality Disorders

Select the single best response for each question.

51.1 Which of the following diagnoses is found at increased prevalence among the first-degree relatives of patients with schizophrenia?

   A. Antisocial personality disorder.
   B. Generalized anxiety disorder.
   C. Borderline personality disorder.
   D. Schizotypal personality disorder.
   E. Attention-deficit/hyperactivity disorder.

51.2 In response to amphetamine challenge, individuals with which of the following diagnoses are more likely than control subjects to become psychotic?

   A. Antisocial personality disorder.
   B. Generalized anxiety disorder.
   C. Borderline personality disorder.
   D. Avoidant personality disorder.
   E. Attention-deficit/hyperactivity disorder.

51.3 There is substantial comorbidity between which of the following diagnoses?

   A. Generalized social phobia and avoidant personality disorder.
   B. Panic disorder and avoidant personality disorder.
   C. Generalized social phobia and schizotypal personality disorder.
   D. Generalized social phobia and borderline personality disorder.
   E. Generalized anxiety disorder and avoidant personality disorder.

51.4 Structural magnetic resonance imaging (MRI) studies of subjects with schizotypal personality disorder have shown which of the following?

   A. Larger left and right caudate nucleus volumes compared with non–schizotypal personality disorder subjects.
   B. Larger relative size of putamen compared with schizophrenic or control subjects.
   C. Higher regional glucose metabolic rate in caudate compared with control subjects.
   D. Ventricular enlargement intermediate between that in control subjects and schizophrenic subjects.
   E. Smaller hippocampal volumes compared with control subjects.

51.5 Borderline personality disorder is associated with which of the following cognitive and perceptual disturbances?

    A. Odd thinking and speech.
    B. Ideas of reference.
    C. Odd beliefs.
    D. Transient, stress-related paranoid ideation.
    E. Superstitiousness.

CHAPTER 52

Treatment of Depression

Select the single best response for each question.

52.1   Hypotension is a common side effect of all of the following antidepressants *except*

   A. Trazodone.
   B. Mirtazapine.
   C. Venlafaxine.
   D. Imipramine.
   E. Maprotiline.

52.2   The two best predictors of antidepressant response are

   A. Side-effect profile and comorbid psychiatric symptoms.
   B. Gender and sedating versus activating properties.
   C. Family history of response and cost.
   D. A history of prior response to an agent and a family history of preferential response.
   E. None of the above.

52.3   The greatest threat to treatment response to a particular antidepressant agent is

   A. Common side effects.
   B. Nonadherence.
   C. Suicidal ideation.
   D. Comorbid conditions.
   E. Idiopathic side effects.

52.4   The two most troublesome antidepressant side effects, which can lead to drug discontinuation despite efficacy, are

   A. Weight gain and sexual side effects.
   B. Weight gain and orthostasis.
   C. Weight gain and sedation.
   D. Sexual side effects and nausea.
   E. Sexual side effects and anorexia.

52.5   Which of the following statements regarding possible pro-suicide effects of antidepressants is *true*?

   A. The phenomenon is likely not unique to any one antidepressant.
   B. Tricyclic antidepressants (TCAs) are pro-suicidal only at doses three to five times the therapeutic dose.
   C. Bupropion is the safest of the second- and third-generation antidepressants when taken in overdose.
   D. Selective serotonin reuptake inhibitors (SSRIs) have a narrow margin of safety.
   E. None of the above.

52.6 In the event of treatment nonresponse to a first antidepressive agent, the best strategy is to

    A. Augment with lithium.
    B. Augment with a stimulant.
    C. Augment with thyroid hormone.
    D. Increase the dosage past the manufacturer's recommendations.
    E. Change to an alternative agent in a different chemical/mechanism class.

CHAPTER 53

Treatment of
Bipolar Disorder

Select the single best response for each question.

53.1 What percentage of patients treated for apparent major depression in the outpatient setting subsequently receive a diagnosis of bipolar I or II disorder?

    A. 5%–10%.
    B. 15%–30%.
    C. >40%.
    D. <5%.
    E. Unknown.

53.2 All of the following drugs have shown efficacy in the treatment of acute mania in randomized, placebo-controlled trials *except*

    A. Olanzapine.
    B. Chlorpromazine.
    C. Carbamazepine.
    D. Lamotrigine.
    E. Divalproex.

53.3 All of the following are associated with better response rates to lithium in the treatment of acute mania *except*

    A. Few lifetime manic episodes.
    B. Classic manic or elated symptoms.
    C. Rapid-cycling symptoms.
    D. Presentation with psychotic symptoms.
    E. Presentation with no psychotic symptoms.

53.4 In comparing lithium to divalproex in the treatment of acute mania, which of the following statements is *false*?

    A. Divalproex works better in patients with depressive symptoms.
    B. Divalproex works better in patients with previous multiple mood episodes.
    C. Both lithium and divalproex can help with psychotic symptoms in acute mania.
    D. Both are efficacious for acute mania in comparison with placebo, but lithium is generally superior to divalproex in head-to-head trials.
    E. Both agents have better long-term efficacy in the treatment of acute mania in combination with other medications.

53.5 All of the following medications have been shown to have little to no efficacy in the treatment of acute mania *except*

A. Gabapentin.
B. Topiramate.
C. Clonazepam.
D. Carbamazepine.
E. Lamotrigine.

53.6 Recent studies suggest that the antidepressant-associated switch rate—the proportion of bipolar disorder patients who switch to manic symptoms in response to antidepressant treatment—is lower than previously believed (earlier estimated rates were as high as 70%). Which of the following best represents the current estimate of this rate?

A. 20%.
B. 30%.
C. 5%–15%.
D. <2%.
E. 50%.

53.7 Which of the following statements regarding the use of antidepressants in bipolar disorder is *true*?

A. Antidepressants should never be used in bipolar disorder.
B. Newer antidepressants should be considered over tricyclic antidepressants (TCAs) because of lower switch rates.
C. Lamotrigine may have effectiveness as an antidepressant and antimanic agent.
D. Olanzapine does not have antidepressant activity in acute bipolar depression.
E. None of the above.

CHAPTER 54

Treatment of Schizophrenia

Select the single best response for each question.

54.1   All of the following statements regarding positive symptoms of schizophrenia are correct *except*

   A.   Studies show that a high degree of positive symptoms correlates with a worse long-term prognosis.
   B.   Positive symptoms include hallucinations.
   C.   Positive symptoms respond to antipsychotic medications.
   D.   Positive symptoms are not the first set of symptoms that typically present in schizophrenia.
   E.   Positive symptoms are traditionally the focus of medication treatment.

54.2   Which of the following statements about gender differences in schizophrenia is *true*?

   A.   The onset of illness tends to be more acute in males than in females.
   B.   Men tend to have a higher level of premorbid functioning than women.
   C.   Women generally have a more favorable outcome than men.
   D.   The age at onset is, on average, 5 years younger in women than in men.
   E.   There are no differences between men and women in onset, tempo of onset, and level of premorbid functioning.

54.3   Regarding choice of an antipsychotic for a patient with acute psychosis in schizophrenia, all of the following statements are true *except*

   A.   Generally, second-generation (atypical) agents are preferred.
   B.   All of the second-generation (atypical) agents are more effective than the first-generation (typical) agents in the treatment of positive and negative symptoms.
   C.   It is acceptable to use a first-generation agent if a particular patient has responded to that agent in the past.
   D.   The main advantage of second-generation agents is their overall lower risk of causing extrapyramidal symptoms and tardive dyskinesia.
   E.   Clozapine may be therapeutically superior to any other antipsychotic medications.

54.4   According to findings from a meta-analysis of 15 studies, patients who are taking second-generation antipsychotics appear to demonstrate

   A.   Improved memory.
   B.   Less weight gain than with first-generation antipsychotics.
   C.   Better verbal fluency.
   D.   Better overall clinical outcome.
   E.   All of the above.

54.5 The leading cause of medical morbidity in patients with schizophrenia is

    A. Obesity.
    B. Diabetes.
    C. Human immunodeficiency virus–associated hepatitis.
    D. Cigarette smoking.
    E. Lack of exercise.

54.6 The leading cause of premature death in patients with schizophrenia is

    A. Comorbidities associated with obesity.
    B. Alcohol and drug use.
    C. Comorbidities associated with cigarette smoking.
    D. Risky sexual behaviors.
    E. Suicide.

54.7 Which of the following statements best describes the usual course of illness in schizophrenia?

    A. After the acute onset, the first 2–5 years are marked by little change in severity.
    B. Negative symptoms usually respond to medication treatment better than positive symptoms.
    C. Positive symptoms usually respond to medication treatment better than negative symptoms.
    D. Positive symptoms usually become increasingly prominent during the course of illness.
    E. All of the above statements are accurate.

54.8 Which of the following second-generation antipsychotics is most effective for treatment-resistant schizophrenia?

    A. Clozapine.
    B. Risperidone.
    C. Olanzapine.
    D. Quetiapine.
    E. Ziprasidone.

54.9 For severe tardive dyskinesia, which of the following medications may be useful?

    A. Pimozide.
    B. Clozapine.
    C. Haloperidol.
    D. L-Serine.
    E. L-Carnitine.

CHAPTER 55

Treatment of Anxiety Disorders

Select the single best response for each question.

55.1   Which of the following augmentation strategies has been found to be effective in treatment-resistant obsessive-compulsive disorder (OCD)?

A. Addition of venlafaxine to buspirone.
B. Addition of lithium to risperidone.
C. Addition of risperidone to a selective serotonin reuptake inhibitor (SSRI).
D. Addition of valproate to clomipramine.
E. Addition of gabapentin to an SSRI.

55.2   A patient with panic disorder develops agitation, insomnia, and nausea while taking fluoxetine. Which of the following agents might be useful in reducing these symptoms?

A. Mirtazapine.
B. Buspirone.
C. Lithium.
D. Venlafaxine.
E. Valproate.

55.3   A 19-year-old woman experiences panic attack symptoms when she eats, writes, or speaks in public. Which of the following agents has been found to be effective in treating these symptoms?

A. Atenolol.
B. Ondansetron.
C. Clonazepam.
D. Buspirone.
E. Olanzapine.

55.4   A 27-year-old man reports lifelong intermittent symptoms of worry, muscle tension, irritability, and difficulty falling asleep. Which of the following statements about possible pharmacological interventions is *true*?

A. If a benzodiazepine is prescribed, psychic symptoms will be more effectively treated than somatic ones.
B. If a benzodiazepine is prescribed, long-term use may be associated with development of tolerance, physiological dependence, and withdrawal.
C. If buspirone is prescribed, alleviation of anxiety symptoms will likely occur within the first week.
D. If venlafaxine is prescribed, alleviation of anxiety symptoms will likely occur only after the fifth week.
E. If a tricyclic antidepressant (TCA) is prescribed, only depressive symptoms will remit.

C H A P T E R   5 6

Management of Noncognitive Symptoms of Dementia: Behavioral and Psychological Symptoms of Dementia

Select the single best response for each question.

56.1   An 87-year-old man with Alzheimer's disease develops chronic symptoms of depression. Which of the following treatment strategies would be the best choice for this patient?

    A. Treat the patient with imipramine.
    B. Treat the patient with haloperidol.
    C. Treat the patient with maprotiline.
    D. Treat the patient with citalopram.
    E. Discontinue antidementia drugs.

56.2   A 93-year-old woman with Alzheimer's disease becomes acutely combative and agitated. Which of the following potential circumstances might explain these symptoms?

    A. The patient may have an underlying medical illness such as a urinary tract infection.
    B. The patient may be responding to a change in caregivers.
    C. The patient may be responding to a recent change in medication.
    D. The patient may be responding to a recent change in roommate.
    E. All of the above.

56.3   Which of the following drugs has been shown to be effective in the treatment of agitation and aggression in patients with dementia?

    A. Lamotrigine.
    B. Levetiracetam.
    C. Gabapentin.
    D. Valproate.
    E. Phenytoin.

56.4 Regarding benzodiazepine treatment of behavioral disturbances in dementia, which of the following statements is *true*?

A. Benzodiazepines are the treatment of choice for all dementia patients with behavioral disturbances.
B. Many clinical studies clearly show the efficacy of benzodiazepines for the treatment of behavioral disturbances in patients with dementia.
C. Benzodiazepines can be used for short-term treatment of behavioral disturbances associated with disruptions to routines or adjustments to changes.
D. Benzodiazepines should never be used as short-term treatment.
E. Benzodiazepines should be given only with antipsychotics.

C H A P T E R 5 7

Treatment of Childhood and Adolescent Disorders

Select the single best response for each question.

57.1 Which of the following agents or drug classes, in comparison with placebo, has demonstrated efficacy in the treatment of major depressive disorder in children and adolescents?

A. Tricyclic antidepressants (TCAs).
B. Fluoxetine.
C. Venlafaxine.
D. Mirtazapine.
E. None of the above.

57.2 Which of the following is the only medication to have been demonstrated, in a double-blind, placebo-controlled study, to be effective in the treatment of bipolar disorder in adolescents?

A. Lithium.
B. Divalproex.
C. Carbamazepine.
D. Olanzapine.
E. Lamotrigine.

57.3 Published open-label treatment studies in children and adolescents with posttraumatic stress disorder (PTSD) have supported the efficacy of all of the following agents *except*

A. Citalopram.
B. Clonidine.
C. Carbamazepine.
D. Propranolol.
E. Alprazolam.

57.4 The evidence base is *least* supportive of which of the following agents for treatment of child and adolescent attention-deficit/hyperactivity disorder (ADHD)?

A. Psychostimulants.
B. Tricyclic antidepressants (TCAs).
C. Selective serotonin reuptake inhibitors (SSRIs).
D. Atomoxetine.
E. Bupropion.

57.5 Aside from pimozide, the only other agent that has received U.S. Food and Drug Administration (FDA) approval as a treatment for Tourette's syndrome is

A. Risperidone.
B. Fluphenazine.
C. Clonidine.
D. Haloperidol.
E. Fluoxetine.

57.6 The incidence of serious rashes, including Stevens-Johnson syndrome, in pediatric patients taking lamotrigine is reported to be approximately

A. 10%.
B. 5%.
C. 1%.
D. 0.1%.
E. 0.01%.

CHAPTER 58

Treatment of Substance-Related Disorders

Select the single best response for each question.

58.1   In patients with hepatic impairment that has diminished their ability to metabolize medications, which of the following agents would be the best choice for prophylaxis of delirium tremens?

    A. Diazepam.
    B. Clonazepam.
    C. Alprazolam.
    D. Triazolam.
    E. Oxazepam.

58.2   When a person taking disulfiram drinks alcohol, the subsequent toxic reaction is due to accumulation of which of the following?

    A. Acetone.
    B. Alcohol.
    C. Acetaldehyde.
    D. Glutamate.
    E. Dopamine.

58.3   Although no medication has been clearly identified as effective in preventing relapse to cocaine abuse, double-blind studies have supported moderate benefit for which of the following?

    A. Desipramine.
    B. Bupropion.
    C. Fluoxetine.
    D. Amantadine.
    E. Pergolide.

58.4   Which of the following agents used in the treatment of opioid dependence is itself a partial agonist of the μ opioid receptor?

    A. Naltrexone.
    B. Buprenorphine.
    C. Methadone.
    D. Clonidine.
    E. Hydromorphone.

58.5 The hallucinogen methylenedioxymethamphetamine (MDMA; Ecstasy) is related to what class of drugs?

    A. Amphetamines.
    B. Opioids.
    C. Dissociative anesthetics.
    D. Cannabinoids.
    E. Benzodiazepine reverse agonists.

58.6 Efficacy in smoking cessation has been demonstrated by all of the following *except*

    A. Transdermal nicotine.
    B. Bupropion.
    C. Nortriptyline.
    D. Propranolol.
    E. Clonidine.

CHAPTER 59

Treatment of Eating Disorders

Select the single best response for each question.

59.1   Which of the following antidepressants is relatively contraindicated in the treatment of bulimia nervosa?

A. Bupropion.
B. Fluoxetine.
C. Imipramine.
D. Desipramine.
E. Trazodone.

59.2   Studies support the effectiveness in binge-eating disorder of all of the following interventions *except*

A. Fluvoxamine.
B. Phentermine + fluoxetine + cognitive-behavioral therapy (CBT).
C. Imipramine.
D. Topiramate.
E. Sibutramine.

59.3   Which of the following medications has demonstrated possible benefit in reducing relapse in weight-restored patients with anorexia nervosa?

A. Pimozide.
B. Escitalopram.
C. Naltrexone.
D. Olanzapine.
E. Fluoxetine.

59.4   Complications of bulimia nervosa include all of the following *except*

A. Dental caries.
B. Pulmonary hypertension.
C. Potassium depletion.
D. Salivary gland enlargement.
E. Exercise injuries.

59.5   Which of the following statements about anorexia nervosa is *true*?

    A. Diagnostic criteria require that a patient's weight be at least 75% below ideal body weight.

    B. Amenorrhea is uncommon in anorexia nervosa.

    C. Anorexia nervosa is the most lethal psychiatric disorder.

    D. Fluoxetine has proven effective in treating hospitalized patients with anorexia.

    E. Patients with anorexia tend to be especially cooperative with treatment.

CHAPTER 60

Treatment of Agitation and Aggression in the Elderly

Select the single best response for each question.

60.1   Which of the following statements regarding tardive dyskinesia in elderly patients is *true*?

   A. It may develop more rapidly and at lower doses than with younger patients.
   B. It is more common in patients with cortical atrophy.
   C. It is less likely to disappear when neuroleptics are discontinued.
   D. All of the above.
   E. None of the above.

60.2   Which group of elderly patients is at increased risk for neuroleptic malignant syndrome from conventional antipsychotics?

   A. Patients with cardiac disease.
   B. Patients with Parkinson's disease.
   C. Patients with cerebrovascular disease.
   D. Patients with hypertension.
   E. Patients with diabetes.

60.3   Side effects associated with clozapine use include which of the following?

   A. Agranulocytosis.
   C. Orthostasis.
   D. Anticholinergic symptoms.
   E. All of the above.
   E. None of the above.

60.4   Which of the following atypical antipsychotics has been found to effectively and safely treat agitation in the elderly?

   A. Ziprasidone.
   B. Quetiapine.
   C. Olanzapine.
   D. Aripiprazole.
   E. Risperidone.

60.5   Which of the following agents has been found to rapidly and safely treat sexual acting-out behavior in elderly men with dementia?

A. Lithium.
B. Buspirone.
C. Trazodone.
D. Medroxyprogesterone.
E. Lorazepam.

CHAPTER 61

Treatment of Personality Disorders

Select the single best response for each question.

61.1 Regarding use of antidepressants in treating borderline personality disorder patients, which of the following statements is *true*?

A. Tricyclic antidepressants (TCAs) and monoamine oxidase inhibitors (MAOIs) pose serious risks of overdose and dangerous adverse effects that are of particular concern in an unstable and an impulsive population.

B. Selective serotonin reuptake inhibitors (SSRIs) lose efficacy for aggression and irritability after 2 months of treatment.

C. SSRIs have not been found to decrease suicidality and self-injury in borderline personality disorder patients.

D. Phenelzine is far more effective than placebo in the treatment of borderline personality disorder patients in all behavioral and mood-sphere domains studied.

E. All of the above.

61.2 The three most useful classes of medications in the treatment of borderline personality disorder are

A. Benzodiazepines, azapirones, and serotonergic and noradrenergic reuptake inhibitors (SNRIs).

B. Selective serotonin reuptake inhibitors (SSRIs), mood stabilizers, and atypical antipsychotics.

C. Mood stabilizers, SSRIs, and stimulants.

D. Benzodiazepines, stimulants, and azapirones.

E. Benzodiazepines, nonbenzodiazepine hypnotics, and conventional antipsychotics.

61.3 Which of the following statements regarding comorbid personality disorders and Axis I disorders is *true*?

A. In one community survey, most patients (approximately 80%) with personality disorders who were deemed in need of treatment of Axis I disorders were not receiving such treatment.

B. Personality disorder comorbidity is strongly associated with poor medication compliance in bipolar patients.

C. In a large study, anxiety disorder patients with comorbid borderline personality disorder were more likely than those without a personality disorder diagnosis to be receiving multiple medications.

D. All of the above.

E. None of the above.

61.4   Conventional antipsychotics may be helpful in borderline personality disorder for which of the following problems?

    A. Suicidality.
    B. Ideas of reference.
    C. Social functioning.
    D. All of the above.
    E. None of the above.

61.5   Which of the following is the main indication for use of medications in the treatment of personality disorders?

    A. During periods of acute decompensation.
    B. For longer-term management of symptom clusters that are maladaptive and that may be responsive to medication.
    C. To treat reappearance or worsening of comorbid Axis I conditions.
    D. All of the above.
    E. None of the above.

CHAPTER 62

Psychiatric Emergencies

Select the single best response for each question.

62.1 Psychiatric emergencies can be divided into 1) those that do not require pharmacological intervention, 2) those in which pharmacological interventions are adjunctive, and 3) those in which medications are required. An example of the second class of psychiatric emergency would be

A. Assaultive or aggressive behavior.
B. Acute grief or trauma.
C. Neuroleptic-induced dystonia.
D. Ethanol withdrawal.
E. Anticholinergic delirium from tricyclic antidepressants.

62.2 Which of the following groupings represent psychotropic medications available for intravenous administration?

A. Buspirone, nefazodone, diazepam.
B. Trazodone, buspirone, lithium.
C. Lorazepam, diazepam, haloperidol.
D. Pimozide, lorazepam, sertraline.
E. Midazolam, venlafaxine, haloperidol.

62.3 Which of the following groupings represent psychotropic medications available for intramuscular administration?

A. Lorazepam, haloperidol, olanzapine.
B. Ziprasidone, diazepam, nefazodone.
C. Haloperidol, bupropion, lorazepam.
D. Clonazepam, lithium, amitriptyline.
E. Pimozide, paroxetine, ziprasidone.

62.4 Acute *severe* dystonic reactions (e.g., oculogyric crisis or laryngospasm) should be treated with

A. Intramuscular thiamine.
B. Intravenous diphenhydramine.
C. Oral benztropine.
D. Intravenous β-blockers.
E. Oral buspirone.

62.5   Which of the following symptoms is present in neuroleptic malignant syndrome (NMS)?

    A. Autonomic instability.
    B. Altered consciousness.
    C. Lead-pipe rigidity.
    D. Elevated creatine phosphokinase (CPK).
    E. All of the above.

62.6   The serotonin syndrome is a delirium characterized by which of the following?

    A. Neuromuscular abnormalities and autonomic instability.
    B. Sedation and hyporeflexia.
    C. Altered consciousness and flaccidity.
    D. Agitation and hyporeflexia.
    E. None of the above.

CHAPTER 63

Treatment During Late Life

Select the single best response for each question.

63.1 Which of the following pharmacokinetic functions do not change with age?

  A. Absorption.
  B. Distribution.
  C. Metabolism.
  D. Excretion.
  E. None of the above.

63.2 Which of the following brain imaging findings is associated with late-onset (after age 60 years) depression?

  A. Enlarged ventricles.
  B. Significant cerebrovascular disease.
  C. Cortical atrophy.
  D. Frontal lobe lesions.
  E. Central pontine myelinolysis.

63.3 Regarding use of tricyclic antidepressants (TCAs) versus selective serotonin reuptake inhibitors (SSRIs) in the treatment of late-life depression, which of the following statements is *true*?

  A. TCAs are the most prescribed class of antidepressants in the elderly population.
  B. SSRIs can be safely used in post–myocardial infarction patients.
  C. In elderly subjects, dropout rates with paroxetine have been found to be higher than rates with nortriptyline.
  D. SSRIs pose a significant risk of urinary retention and confusion.
  E. None of the above.

63.4 Regarding use of atypical antipsychotic drugs in the elderly, which of the following statements is *true*?

  A. Diabetic ketoacidosis is less common with clozapine and olanzapine compared with other atypicals.
  B. Fasting lipid levels have been reported to rise more with olanzapine than with risperidone.
  C. Higher doses of atypical antipsychotics are necessary to treat elderly patients.
  D. Extrapyramidal symptoms and tardive dyskinesia are less common in the elderly.
  E. All of the above.

63.5 Which antipsychotic drug is best tolerated by Parkinson's disease patients with psychosis?

  A. Haloperidol.
  B. Olanzapine.
  C. Clozapine.
  D. Thioridazine.
  E. Quetiapine.

CHAPTER 64

Psychopharmacology During Pregnancy and Lactation

Select the single best response for each question.

64.1   Which of the following antidepressants has received a Category B use-in-pregnancy rating?

    A. Sertraline.
    B. Fluoxetine.
    C. Nortriptyline.
    D. Desipramine.
    E. Bupropion.

64.2   Which selective serotonin reuptake inhibitor (SSRI) has the largest evidence base demonstrating safety during breastfeeding?

    A. Fluoxetine.
    B. Sertraline.
    C. Paroxetine.
    D. Fluvoxamine.
    E. Citalopram.

64.3   Which tricyclic antidepressant (TCA) has been found to be present at considerably higher levels in breastfeeding infants than other TCAs and is thus relatively contraindicated during breastfeeding?

    A. Clomipramine.
    B. Imipramine.
    C. Amitriptyline.
    D. Doxepin.
    E. Desipramine.

64.4   If valproate must be used during pregnancy, which of the following nutritional supplements is strongly recommended?

    A. Vitamin B_6 (pyridoxine).
    B. Vitamin B_1 (thiamine).
    C. Folate.
    D. Vitamin E (tocopherol).
    E. Vitamin C (ascorbic acid).

64.5 Clonazepam has received which of the following use-in-pregnancy category ratings?

A. Category A.
B. Category B.
C. Category C.
D. Category D.
E. Category X.

64.6 Which of the following statements about fluctuations of medication levels during pregnancy is *true*?

A. Nortriptyline doses are likely to require increases in order to maintain stable maternal blood levels as pregnancy progresses.
B. Maternal–fetal lithium concentration ratios at delivery are roughly 10 to 1.
C. Maternal valproate concentrations increase as pregnancy progresses.
D. Lamotrigine clearance decreases as pregnancy progresses.
E. None of the above.

CHAPTER 65

Treatment of Insomnia

Select the single best response for each question.

65.1   Which of the following treatments may relieve high-altitude insomnia?

    A. Continuous positive airway pressure.
    B. Acetazolamide.
    C. Tricyclic antidepressants.
    D. Benzodiazepines.
    E. Shifting of the sleep-cycle schedule.

65.2   Which of the following antidepressive agents increases rapid eye movement (REM) sleep?

    A. Bupropion.
    B. Clomipramine.
    C. Phenelzine.
    D. Venlafaxine.
    E. Sertraline.

65.3   Which of the following agents is considered the first-line treatment for periodic limb movements in sleep (PLMS) and restless legs syndrome (RLS)?

    A. Lorazepam.
    B. Clomipramine.
    C. Zolpidem.
    D. Ropinirole.
    E. Selective serotonin reuptake inhibitors.

65.4   Which of the following sleep-related disorders increases in frequency with increasing age?

    A. Sleep-related breathing disturbances.
    B. Depression.
    C. Periodic limb movements in sleep (PLMS).
    D. Insomnia due to a medical condition.
    E. All of the above.

65.5   Which of the following antidepressive agents reduces rapid eye movement (REM) sleep yet causes little or no sedation?

    A. Amitriptyline.
    B. Bupropion.
    C. Phenelzine.
    D. Nefazodone.
    E. Trazodone.

C H A P T E R   1

Neurotransmitters, Receptors, Signal Transduction, and Second Messengers in Psychiatric Disorders

Select the single best response for each question.

1.1   Which of the following compounds is able to rapidly penetrate lipid bilayer membranes and directly interact with cytoplasmic receptors inside cells to regulate gene transcription?

    A. Salts such as lithium.
    B. Hormones such as glucocorticosteroids.
    C. Amino acids such as L-tryptophan.
    D. All of the above.
    E. None of the above.

The correct response is option **B.**

Nuclear receptors are transcription factors that regulate the expression of target genes in response to steroid hormones and other ligands. Many hormones (including glucocorticoids, gonadal steroids, and thyroid hormones) are able to rapidly penetrate into the lipid bilayer membrane, because of their lipophilic composition, and thereby directly interact with these cytoplasmic receptors inside the cell. Upon activation by a hormone, the nuclear receptor–ligand complex translocates to the nucleus, where it binds to specific DNA sequences (termed *hormone-responsive elements*) and regulates gene transcription. **(p. 5)**

1.2   Where are the majority (>50%) of the serotonin (5-hydroxytryptamine [5-HT])–producing cell bodies located in the brain?

    A. Dorsal raphe nucleus.
    B. Tuberoinfundibular system.
    C. Nucleus basalis of Meynert.
    D. Throughout the cerebral cortex.
    E. Medial raphe nucleus.

The correct response is option **A.**

The dorsal raphe, the largest brain stem 5-HT nucleus, contains approximately 50% of the total 5-HT neurons in the mammalian central nervous system (Descarries et al. 1982). **(p. 9)**

1.3   Which of the following is the only low-molecular-weight neurotransmitter substance that is not derived from an amino acid?

A. Dopamine.
B. Serotonin.
C. Norepinephrine.
D. Glutamate.
E. Acetylcholine.

The correct response is option **E.**

Acetylcholine is the only major low-molecular-weight neurotransmitter substance that is not derived from an amino acid (Kandel et al. 2000). **(p. 18)**

1.4   How do benzodiazepines function?

A. By binding to a potentiator site on the γ-aminobutyric acid A (GABA$_A$) receptor, increasing the amplitude and duration of inhibiting postsynaptic currents in response to GABA binding.
B. By limiting production of GABA α-oxoglutarate transaminase.
C. By antagonistic binding of the GABA$_B$ receptor, decreasing the amplitude and duration of excitatory postsynaptic currents in response to GABA binding.
D. By inhibiting potentiation of γ subunits of GABA receptors.
E. None of the above.

The correct response is option **A.**

It is now well established that benzodiazepines function by binding to a potentiator site on the GABA$_A$ receptor, increasing the amplitude and duration of inhibitory postsynaptic currents in response to GABA binding. **(p. 25)**

1.5   Which of the following peptides are regulated by lithium?

A. Vasoactive intestinal peptide and corticotropin-releasing factor.
B. Leptin and cholecystokinin.
C. Neuromedin N and calcitonin gene–related peptide.
D. Vasopressin and gastrin.
E. Dynorphin and melanocyte-stimulating hormone.

The correct response is option **C.**

Neuromedin N is regulated by lithium. Calcitonin gene–related peptide is regulated by lithium and by electroconvulsive therapy. **(p. 29; see Table 1–2)**

References

Descarries L, Watkins KC, Garcia S, et al: The serotonin neurons in nucleus raphe dorsalis of adult rat: a light and electron microscope radioautographic study. J Comp Neurol 207:239–254, 1982

Kandel ER, Schwartz JH, Jessell TM: Principles of Neural Science. New York, McGraw-Hill, 2000

CHAPTER 2

Basic Principles of Molecular Biology and Genomics

Select the single best response for each question.

2.1   What is the function of chromatin?

    A. Provides structure to chromosomes.
    B. Represses gene expression by inhibiting the ability of transcription factors to access DNA.
    C. Ensures that enzyme genes are inactive until their expression is commanded.
    D. All of the above.
    E. None of the above.

The correct response is option **D.**

Although chromatin provides structure to the chromosomes, it also plays a critical role in transcriptional regulation in eukaryotes because it can repress gene expression by inhibiting the ability of transcription factors to access DNA. In fact, chromatin ensures that genes remain inactive until their expression is commanded. **(p. 56)**

2.2   *Transcription* is best described as

    A. The process of making proteins from mRNA codons.
    B. The process of synthesizing, in a 5′ to 3′ direction, an RNA molecule that is complementary to one strand of a gene's DNA and that becomes a template for translation.
    C. The process of synthesizing, in a 3′ to 5′ direction, an RNA molecule that is complementary to one strand of a gene's DNA.
    D. The process of making cloverleaf tRNA in ribosomes.
    E. None of the above.

The correct response is option **B.**

Only a fraction of all the genes in a genome can be expressed. These genes undergo the process of transcription, in which an RNA molecule complementary to one of the gene's DNA strands is synthesized in a 5′ to 3′ direction, using nucleotide triphosphates. Transcription can be classified into three discrete steps: initiation, mRNA chain elongation, and chain termination. **(p. 55)**

2.3   Which of the following statements about polymerase chain reaction (PCR) is *true?*

    A. PCR is a rapid procedure for replicating segments of DNA, utilizing bacteriophages.
    B. PCR is a procedure for cloning DNA, utilizing *Escherichia coli.*
    C. PCR is a linkage analysis procedure for localizing genes via examining cosegregation of phenotypes, using genetic markers.

D. PCR is an in vitro procedure, generally requiring heat, that allows for enzymatic amplification of specific segments of DNA without using living organisms.

E. None of the above.

The correct response is option **D**.

PCR is a rapid procedure for in vitro enzymatic amplification of specific segments of DNA. **(p. 59)**

2.4   Which of the following statements about antisense oligonucleotides (AOs) is *false*?

A. AOs are useful in studying gene and protein function because of their irreversibility.

B. AOs are short sequences of DNA that are complementary to regions of mRNA and block specific protein production when taken up by cells.

C. AOs are useful in studying gene and protein function because they are specific, effective, and reversible.

D. AOs have been injected into mice to limit overexpression of amyloid β to reverse deficits in learning and memory that are similar to those seen in Alzheimer's disease.

E. Unmodified AOs are rapidly degraded.

The correct response is option **A**.

When cells take up the short DNA molecules, synthesis of the protein from the specific mRNA is inhibited. The mechanism by which antisense oligonucleotides block the specific protein production remains unclear. Interfering with the selected mRNA stability or its translation may be one potential mechanism (Phillips et al. 1996). Because of the specificity, effectiveness, and reversibility of AOs, cell-based antisense experiments have proven useful in studying gene and protein function. **(p. 62)**

2.5   The term *knockout* in transgenic studies in mice refers to

A. Mice euthanized for use in antisense oligonucleotide studies.

B. The use of viral vectors with low toxicity and high infection rates to deliver gene sequences to mice.

C. The study of allelic variations (polymorphisms) by comparing wild type to "diseased" genotype in mice.

D. The use of bacteriophage techniques to study "blank" stretches of DNA in mice.

E. Mice in which an existing gene is inactivated or "knocked out" by replacing it or disrupting it with a "construct sequence" or artificial piece of DNA.

The correct response is option **E**.

Gene targeting refers to the homologous recombination that occurs between a specifically designed targeting construct and the chromosomal target of interest, in which recombination at the target locus leads to replacement of the native target sequence with the construct sequence. The method enables the precise introduction of a mutant into one of many murine genes and has proven invaluable in examining the roles of gene functions in complex biological processes. Most of the target constructs are used to disrupt a target and to eliminate gene function (conventional gene disruption, or "knockout"). Generally, a gene-targeting construct that contains positive–negative selection markers is prepared such that the target gene is interrupted by the gene for neomycin resistance. **(pp. 63–64)**

Reference

Phillips MI, Ambuhl P, Gyurko R: Antisense oligonucleotides for in vivo studies of angiotensin receptors. Adv Exp Med Biol 396:79–92, 1996

CHAPTER 3

Chemical Neuroanatomy of the Primate Brain

Select the single best response for each question.

3.1   Which of the following statements about the dopaminergic system is *false*?

    A. Dopamine neurotransmission is terminated through the actions of the dopamine transporter (DAT).

    B. The mediodorsal nucleus of the thalamus and the posterior vermis of the cerebellum (areas reported to be dysfunctional in schizophrenia) contain low densities of dopamine axons.

    C. The majority of dopamine cells, which synthesize approximately three-fourths of all the dopamine in the brain, are located in the anterior midbrain (mesencephalon).

    D. Primary sensory cortices (e.g., the visual cortex) generally have low densities of dopamine axons, and these are present only in layers 1 and 6.

    E. The major projection target of dopamine neurons in the substantia nigra is the striatum.

The correct response is option **B**.

Dopamine axons have been identified in the primate thalamus and cerebellum (Melchitzky and Lewis 2000, 2001), two brain regions traditionally thought not to receive dopamine innervation (Moore and Bloom 1978; Steriade et al. 1997). Identification of dopamine axons in these brain regions may be of importance to the pathophysiology and treatment of certain psychiatric disorders. **(pp. 70–71, 73)**

3.2   Which of the following statements about the noradrenergic system is *false*?

    A. Primary somatosensory and visual cortices have a very low density of norepinephrine neurons.

    B. Norepinephrine-containing neurons in the central nervous system are located predominantly in the medulla and pons.

    C. In the hypothalamus, the paraventricular nucleus contains the highest density of norepinephrine axons.

    D. In the amygdala, the basolateral nuclei contain the highest density of norepinephrine axons.

    E. Norepinephrine elicits responses in the postsynaptic cell via G-protein–mediated second-messenger systems.

The correct response is option **A**.

All areas of the cerebral cortex receive noradrenergic projections (Gatter and Powell 1977; Porrino and Goldman-Rakic 1982); however, certain areas have higher densities of norepinephrine axons than do other areas. For example, primary somatosensory and visual cortices have a very high density of norepinephrine axons (Lewis and Morrison 1989; Morrison et al. 1982). Within the hypothalamus and amygdala, the paraventricular and basolateral nuclei, respectively, contain the highest density of norepinephrine axons in these structures. **(pp. 75–76)**

3.3   What percentage of serotonin (5-hydroxytryptamine [5-HT]) in the body is found in the brain?

    A. 95%.

    B. 70%.

    C. 25%–40%.

    D. 10%.

    E. 2%.

The correct response is option **E**.

Only 2% of the body's 5-HT is found in the brain. **(p. 76)**

3.4   Of the serotonin (5-hydroxytryptamine [5-HT]) receptors, 5-HT$_3$ is the only 5-HT subtype that does not belong to the G-protein receptor superfamily. To which receptor family does this subtype belong?

    A. G-protein subfamily.

    B. Ligand-gated ion channels.

    C. Nuclear receptors.

    D. Ionotropic receptors.

    E. Hormone-responsive elements.

The correct response is option **B**.

The 5-HT$_3$ receptor belongs to the ligand-gated ion channel family. **(p. 78)**

3.5   Which of the following statements about neuropeptide Y is *true*?

    A. Neuropeptide Y has a role in regulating eating behaviors.

    B. Cerebrospinal fluid (CSF) levels of neuropeptide Y are higher in patients with depression.

    C. Plasma levels of neuropeptide Y are higher in patients with depression.

    D. CSF and plasma levels of neuropeptide Y decrease after electroconvulsive therapy.

    E. All of the above.

The correct response is option **A**.

In addition to having a role in the regulation of eating behavior, neuropeptide Y has been implicated in affective disorders. For example, CSF and plasma levels of neuropeptide Y are lower in patients with depression than in control groups (Nilsson et al. 1996; Westrin et al. 1999), and these levels increase after electroconvulsive treatment (Mathé et al. 1996). **(p. 83)**

References

Gatter KC, Powell TPS: The projection of the locus ceruleus upon the neocortex in the macaque monkey. Neuroscience 2:441–445, 1977

Lewis DA, Morrison JH: The noradrenergic innervation of monkey prefrontal cortex: a dopamine-beta-hydroxylase immunohistochemical study. J Comp Neurol 282:317–330, 1989

Mathé AA, Rudorfer W, Stenfors C, et al: Effects of electroconvulsive treatment on somatostatin, neuropeptide Y, endothelin, and neurokinin A concentrations in cerebrospinal fluid of depressed patients. Depression 3:250–256, 1996

Melchitzky DS, Lewis DA: Tyrosine hydroxylase- and dopamine transporter-immunoreactive axons in the primate cerebellum: evidence for a lobular- and laminar-specific dopamine innervation. Neuropsychopharmacology 22:466–472, 2000

Melchitzky DS, Lewis DA: Dopamine transporter-immunoreactive axons in the mediodorsal thalamic nucleus of the macaque monkey. Neuroscience 103/104:1035–1044, 2001

Moore RY, Bloom FE: Central catecholamine neuron systems: anatomy and physiology of the dopamine systems. Annu Rev Neurosci 1:129–169, 1978

Morrison JH, Foote SL, O'Connor D, et al: Laminar, tangential and regional organization of the noradrenergic innervation of monkey cortex: dopamine-beta-hydroxylase immunohistochemistry. Brain Res Bull 9:309–319, 1982

Nilsson C, Karlsson G, Blennow K, et al: Differences in neuropeptide Y-like immunoreactivity of the plasma and platelets of human volunteers and depressed patients. Peptides 17:359–362, 1996

Porrino LJ, Goldman-Rakic PS: Brainstem innervation of prefrontal and anterior cingulate cortex in the rhesus monkey revealed by retrograde transport of HRP. J Comp Neurol 205:63–76, 1982

Steriade M, Jones EG, McCormick DA: Thalamus: Organisation and Function. Amsterdam, Elsevier Science, 1997

Westrin Å, Ekman R, Träskman-Bendz L: Alterations of corticotropin-releasing hormone (CRH) and neuropeptide Y (NPY) plasma levels in mood disorder patients with a recent suicide attempt. Eur Neuropsychopharmacol 9:205–211, 1999

C H A P T E R   4

Electrophysiology

Select the single best response for each question.

4.1   Regarding the opening of chloride ion channels in a neuron, which of the following statements is *false*?

   A. Neuronal activity decreases.
   B. Chloride ions leave the neuron.
   C. The neuron becomes hyperpolarized.
   D. Chloride ions enter the neuron.
   E. γ-Aminobutyric acid (GABA) is often the neurotransmitter involved in opening neuronal chloride channels.

The correct response is option **B**.

Because chloride ions are negatively charged, an electrical gradient prevents them from entering the cell. However, the concentration of chloride is so much higher in the extracellular fluid than it is within the cell that the chemical gradient predominates. As a result, the opening of chloride ion channels causes chloride to flow into the cell, hyperpolarizing the membrane. In fact, the opening of chloride ion channels is the mechanism through which GABA, the primary inhibitory neurotransmitter in the brain, decreases neuronal activity. **(p. 91; see Figure 4–1)**

4.2   Which of the following statements regarding extracellular/neuronal ion concentrations is *true*?

   A. Calcium exists in equal concentrations both intra- and extracellularly.
   B. Calcium's concentration gradient is less extreme than sodium's gradient.
   C. Calcium ion concentrations are very low within the cell in order to use the ion for specialized purposes.
   D. Calcium ion concentrations are very high within the cell in order to use the ion for specialized purposes.
   E. The extracellular fluid contains much more calcium than sodium.

The correct response is option **C**.

Like sodium, calcium exists at higher concentrations outside the cell than within the cell; however, because of calcium's extremely low intracellular concentration, its concentration gradient is more extreme than sodium's. The neuron maintains this low intracellular concentration of calcium in order to use the ion for specialized purposes. Thus, calcium influx causes neurotransmitter release, activates calcium-gated ion channels, and triggers second-messenger systems. After entering the neuron, calcium is rapidly sequestered into intracellular organelles to terminate its action and to reset the neuron before the next event. **(p. 91)**

4.3   An ion channel that opens in response to a neurotransmitter is referred to as a

A. Ligand-gated channel.
B. Voltage-gated channel.
C. Ion-gated channel.
D. Voltage-dependent channel.
E. Neurotransmitter-gated channel.

The correct response is option **A.**

A neurotransmitter that activates an ion channel is referred to as a *ligand-gated channel.* Voltage-gated or voltage-dependent channels open in response to depolarization. Options C and E represent incorrect use of the nomenclature. **(pp. 90–91)**

4.4   In research examining actual neuronal response to stimuli, such as from a drug, the least invasive method is

A. Field potential recordings.
B. Electroencephalograms.
C. Single-unit extracellular recordings.
D. Patch clamp recordings.
E. Whole-cell recordings.

The correct response is option **B.**

Electroencephalograms are the least invasive of the procedures available for measuring neuronal response, but they have the disadvantage of being unable to measure small groups of neurons or individual neurons. All of the other methods listed are in vivo or in vitro techniques for measuring groups of neurons (field potential recordings) or individual neurons. **(pp. 91–97)**

4.5   The most complete model of a neuronal system's functioning or of its response to drug application can be derived by

A. Using in vitro findings.
B. Using only in vivo findings.
C. Using the best in vitro findings that correlate with in vivo findings.
D. Comparing the results obtained in vitro with those obtained from the intact organism.
E. Examining the intact organism and ignoring the in vitro findings.

The correct response is option **D.**

The most complete model of a neuronal system's functioning or of its response to drug application can be derived by comparing the results obtained in vitro with those in the intact organism. In vitro findings are valid and can usefully supplement in vivo and intact animal results of experimentation. No single electrophysiological technique has an overwhelming advantage in psychopharmacological research. **(pp. 98–101)**

4.6   Electrophysiological measurements of drug response are best used for detecting

    A. Neurotransmitter release over long periods of time.
    B. Transient electrophysiological events.
    C. Neurotransmitter release over both short and long periods of time.
    D. Both transient and sustained electrophysiological events.
    E. None of the above.

The correct response is option **B.**

Actions of transmitters at presynaptic terminals can dramatically alter the amount of neurotransmitter they release, independent of neuronal discharge, over time (Grace 1991). Therefore, electrophysiological measurements are better for measuring and detecting transient events. **(p. 102)**

Reference

Grace AA: Phasic versus tonic dopamine release and the modulation of dopamine system responsivity: a hypothesis for the etiology of schizophrenia. Neuroscience 41:1–24, 1991

CHAPTER 5

Animal Models

Select the single best response for each question.

5.1   Learned helplessness was one of the earliest studied animal models for depression. Animal models exposed to uncontrollable stress have been shown to exhibit all of the following *except*

    A. Changes in noradrenergic and serotonergic brain systems.
    B. Altered sleep patterns.
    C. Ability to learn avoidance–escape behavior.
    D. Diminished consumption of food and water.
    E. Social impairments.

The correct response is option **C.**

Uncontrollable stress in animal models has been shown to actually reduce the ability to learn appropriate avoidance behaviors (Maier 2001; Weiss and Kilts 1998). Animals exposed to uncontrollable stress, but not those exposed to controllable stress, also exhibit diminished consumption of food and water, loss of responding to rewarding brain stimulation, altered sleep patterns and early morning awakening, and social impairments. In addition, uncontrollable stress induces significant changes in noradrenergic (Weiss 1991), serotonergic (Maier et al. 1995), γ-aminobutyric acid (GABA)–ergic (Petty and Sherman 1981), and adenosinergic (Minor et al. 1994) brain systems that conceivably could mediate the behavioral abnormalities observed in animal models of learned helplessness. **(p. 106)**

5.2   Avoidance–escape deficits in rats are reversed by subchronic administration of which of the following drug classes?

    A. Neuroleptics.
    B. Anxiolytics.
    C. Stimulants.
    D. Antidepressants.
    E. Sedatives.

The correct response is option **D.**

Avoidance–escape deficits in rats can be reversed by subchronic treatment with many antidepressant drugs, but not by stimulants, neuroleptics, sedatives, or anxiolytics (Weiss and Kilts 1998). **(p. 106)**

5.3   Which of the following statements regarding chronic stress models in rats is *true*?

A. Behavioral measures of anhedonia are restored to normal by administration of antidepressants.
B. Chronic stress levels of glucocorticoids in rodents are easy to maintain.
C. There is evidence that antidepressants work by decreasing dopamine potentiation in the nucleus accumbens.
D. Glucocorticoid levels always decrease.
E. None of the above.

The correct response is option **A.**

The effects of antidepressants in rats exposed to chronic mild stress are apparently mediated by an *increase* in the sensitivity or density of reward-related dopamine receptors in the nucleus accumbens. Evidence that antidepressant drugs reverse the stress-induced anhedonia by potentiating dopamine neurotransmission comes from a series of studies in which the therapeutic responses to tricyclic antidepressants were reversed by dopamine receptor antagonists (see Willner 1997 for review). Whereas patients with major depression often show elevated levels of plasma cortisol (the principal glucocorticoid in humans), chronic stress levels of glucocorticoids in rodents are extraordinarily difficult to maintain (Rivier and Vale 1987; Young and Akil 1985). For this reason, most rodent models rely on repetitive stressors that bear little resemblance to the social-psychological experiences that trigger or aggravate depression in humans. **(p. 107)**

5.4   Regarding animal and human studies on hypercortisolism, cognition, and depression, which of the following statements is *true*?

A. Chronic administration of hydrocortisone in humans improves prefrontal cognitive performance.
B. Drugs that block glucocorticoids at the receptor level are being tested as possible antidepressants.
C. Hypercortisolism enhances cognition.
D. Hypercortisolism improves stress-induced depression in squirrel monkeys.
E. None of the above.

The correct response is option **B.**

Generally, chronic stress in animal models and in humans has been shown to increase cortisol levels and, in some instances, certain cognitive deficits. In humans with stress-related psychiatric disorders, those with psychotic depression present most consistently with chronic endogenous hypercortisolism (Nelson and Davis 1997) and impairments on tests of prefrontal-dependent functions (Schatzberg et al. 2000). On the basis of these findings, drugs that block glucocorticoid effects at the receptor level are being tested as novel medications for patients with psychotic depression (Belanoff et al. 2001). **(p. 108)**

5.5   Mice genetically engineered to lack serotonin$_{1A}$ (5-hydroxytryptamine [5-HT$_{1A}$]) receptors throughout the brain demonstrate

A. Decreased food and water consumption.
B. Increased anxiety-like behaviors on a variety of tests.
C. Improved inhibitory control of the line-of-sight response.
D. Decreased anxiety-like behaviors on a variety of tests.
E. Reduced inhibitory control of the line-of-sight response.

The correct response is option **B.**

Mice genetically engineered to lack 5-HT$_{1A}$ receptors throughout the brain normally show increased anxiety-like behaviors on a variety of tests (Gross et al. 2002). Inhibitory control of the line-of-sight response is a test of cognition used in studies of hypercortisolism. Decreased food and water consumption is often seen in learned helplessness models (Maier 2001; Weiss and Kilts 1998). (pp. 106, 108, 110)

5.6　An advantage of using animal models to study psychiatric disorders is that

　　A. Animals are very similar genetically and behaviorally to humans.
　　B. Humans are often too difficult to study.
　　C. Animal life spans are generally shorter than human life spans, thereby facilitating longitudinal research.
　　D. Animals are simpler to study.
　　E. There are no advantages to using animals to better understand human psychiatric disorders.

The correct response is option **C**.

Humans and animals have genetic and behavioral differences as well as similarities (see Weiss and Kilts 1998). Both groups can be difficult to study, but the shorter life span of animals allows for longitudinal research and neurodevelopmental studies that would be much more difficult and much slower with humans. (p. 111)

References

Belanoff JK, Flores BH, Kalezhan M, et al: Rapid reversal of psychotic depression using mifepristone. J Clin Psychopharmacol 21:516–521, 2001

Gross C, Zhuang X, Stark K, et al: Serotonin$_{1A}$ receptor acts during development to establish normal anxiety-like behaviour in the adult. Nature 416:396–400, 2002

Maier SF: Exposure to the stressor environment prevents the temporal dissipation of behavioral depression/learned helplessness. Biol Psychiatry 49:763–773, 2001

Maier SF, Grahn RE, Watkins LR: 8-OH-DPAT microinjected in the region of the dorsal raphe nucleus blocks and reverses the enhancement of fear conditioning and interference with escape produced by exposure to inescapable shock. Behav Neurosci 109:404–412, 1995

Minor TR, Winslow JL, Chang WC: Stress and adenosine, II: adenosine analogs mimic the effect of inescapable shock on shuttle-escape performance in rats. Behav Neurosci 108:265–276, 1994

Nelson JC, Davis JM: DST studies in psychotic depression: a meta-analysis. Am J Psychiatry 154:1497–1503, 1997

Petty F, Sherman AD: GABAergic modulation of learned helplessness. Pharmacol Biochem Behav 15:567–570, 1981

Rivier C, Vale W: Diminished responsiveness of the hypothalamic-pituitary-adrenal axis of the rat during exposure to prolonged stress: a pituitary-mediated mechanism. Endocrinology 121:1320–1328, 1987

Schatzberg AF, Posener JA, DeBattista C, et al: Neuropsychological deficits in psychotic versus nonpsychotic major depression and no mental illness. Am J Psychiatry 157:1095–1100, 2000

Weiss JM: Stress-induced depression: critical neurochemical and electrophysiological changes, in Neurobiology of Learning, Emotion and Affect. Edited by Madden J. New York, Raven, 1991, pp 123–154

Weiss JM, Kilts CD: Animal models of depression and schizophrenia, in The American Psychiatric Press Textbook of Psychopharmacology, 2nd Edition. Edited by Schatzberg AF, Nemeroff CB. Washington, DC, American Psychiatric Press, 1998, pp 89–131

Willner P: Validity, reliability and utility of the chronic mild stress model of depression: a 10-year review and evaluation. Psychopharmacology (Berl) 134:319–329, 1997

Young EA, Akil H: Corticotropin-releasing factor stimulation of adrenocorticotropin and beta-endorphin release: effects of acute and chronic stress. Endocrinology 117:23–30, 1985

CHAPTER 6

Psychoneuroendocrinology

Select the single best response for each question.

6.1   The anterior pituitary gland secretes all of the following hormones *except*

    A. Adrenocorticotropic hormone (ACTH).
    B. Follicle-stimulating hormone (FSH).
    C. Thyrotropin-releasing hormone (TRH).
    D. Prolactin.
    E. Growth hormone.

The correct response is option **C**.

TRH is found in the hypothalamus and is responsible for stimulating the anterior pituitary hormone thyrotropin (also called thyroid-stimulating hormone [TSH]) (Sarapura et al. 2002). **(pp. 115, 119)**

6.2   In depression, increased hypothalamic-pituitary-adrenal (HPA) axis activity has been shown to be

    A. Initially mediated by increased secretion of adrenal cortisol.
    B. Found in only a handful of studies and difficult to replicate.
    C. Associated with increased hypothalamic-pituitary drive that is primarily mediated by hypersecretion of corticotropin-releasing hormone (CRH).
    D. Continuous throughout a depressed person's life span and unchanged by treatment.
    E. None of the above.

The correct response is option **C**.

Increased HPA axis activity in depression has been one of the most frequently replicated biological abnormalities in depression (Holsboer 1995; Peteranderl et al. 2002; Rubin et al. 2001). A body of evidence points toward increased hypothalamic-pituitary drive that is mediated by hypersecretion of CRH. A number of studies indicate that abnormal HPA axis activity is related to treatment response as well as to long-term outcome of depression (Hatzinger et al. 2002), although the dysregulation may also reflect a "trait-like" component (Krieg et al. 2001). **(p. 118)**

6.3   Evidence that increased endogenous hypothalamic-pituitary-adrenal (HPA) axis activity is associated with alterations in emotions includes all of the following *except*

    A. Exogenous corticosteroids cause alterations in emotions.
    B. Patients with severe depression show elevated serum cortisol concentrations over a 24-hour period.
    C. Depressed patients have a blunted response on the dexamethasone suppression test (DST).
    D. Depressed patients show a blunted adrenocorticotropic hormone (ACTH) response to corticotropin-releasing hormone (CRH).
    E. Depressed patients have high evening cortisol levels.

The correct response is option **A.**

Although exogenous steroids often alter emotions (Steckler et al. 1999; Tsigos and Chrousos 2002), this effect is not a consistent finding and does not explain why the HPA axis activity is associated with endogenous depression. Sachar et al. (1970) reported elevated serum cortisol concentrations over a 24-hour period in patients with severe depression. The cortisol concentrations were particularly elevated in the evening and during the night, when the activity of the axis is usually low, suggesting that the depressed patients were highly stressed. Along with increased circulating cortisol concentrations, patients with depression show resistance to feedback suppression of the HPA axis by cortisol and dexamethasone. A blunted ACTH response to CRH, but a relatively normal cortisol response, suggests that the hypercortisolism in depression reflects a defect at or above the hypothalamus, coupled with adrenal hypertrophy and hyperresponsiveness (Steckler et al. 1999). **(p. 118)**

6.4   Antidepressants may exert their action in part by

  A. Upregulating the hypothalamic-pituitary-adrenal (HPA) axis.
  B. Downregulating the HPA axis.
  C. Increasing mRNA synthesis of hypothalamic corticotropin-releasing hormone (CRH).
  D. Increasing adrenocorticotropic hormone (ACTH).
  E. Increasing cortisol.

The correct response is option **B.**

Evidence has accumulated that normalization of the HPA system might be the final necessary step for stable remission of depression (Hatzinger et al. 2002; Shelton 2000). Antidepressants can downregulate the HPA axis in humans, and animal studies show that antidepressants can reduce hypothalamic CRH mRNA expression. Accordingly, an increase in ACTH, upregulation of the HPA axis, or an increase in cortisol would have the opposite effect. **(p. 119)**

6.5   Regarding the finding that most patients with depression show some alterations in thyroid function, which of the following is *true*?

  A. Changes include decreased levels of thyroxine (T_4).
  B. Changes include increased levels of triiodothyronine (T_3).
  C. Changes include a more pronounced nocturnal rise in thyroid-stimulating hormone (TSH).
  D. An enhanced response of TSH secretion to thyrotropin-releasing hormone (TRH) stimulation is seen in 25% of patients with depression.
  E. A blunted response of TSH secretion to TRH stimulation is seen in 25% of patients with depression.

The correct response is option **E.**

About 25% of depressed patients show a blunted TSH response to TRH stimulation (Hendrick et al. 1998), which is the opposite of what one would expect to see in primary hypothyroidism. Other changes include increased levels of T_4, decreased levels of T_3, a loss of the nocturnal rise of TSH, and a predisposition to autoimmune thyroiditis (Foltyn et al. 2002; Jackson 1998). **(p. 120)**

6.6   Regarding the thyrotropin-releasing hormone (TRH) stimulation test in depression, which of the following statements is *true*?

   A. The thyroid-stimulating hormone (TSH) response to TRH stimulation in depressed patients does not change after a course of treatment.
   B. Successful treatment of depression is always predicated on normalization of the TSH response to TRH stimulation.
   C. Relapse rates following successful treatment of depression are independent of the posttreatment results of the TRH stimulation test.
   D. A higher rate of relapse is seen after a successful course of depression treatment in those patients whose TRH stimulation of TSH does not normalize.
   E. None of the above.

The correct response is option **D**.

Following treatment of depression, TSH response to TRH and to thyroxine (T_4) levels tends to normalize (Jackson 1998), and a higher rate of relapse has been noted in patients whose blunted TSH response to TRH fails to normalize after a successful course of antidepressant or electroconvulsive therapy (ECT) (Hendrick et al. 1998). **(p. 120)**

6.7   Blunting of growth hormone (GH) in response to challenge agents has been found in all of the following psychiatric disorders *except*

   A. Schizophrenia.
   B. Obsessive-compulsive disorder.
   C. Bipolar disorder/mania.
   D. Panic disorder.
   E. Depression.

The correct response is option **C**.

There is evidence of a blunted response of GH to numerous challenge agents in many psychiatric disorders (Cooney et al. 1997a, 1997b; Corrêa et al. 2001; Meltzer et al. 2001; O'Keane et al. 1994; Tandon and Halbreich 2003). However, in patients with mania, GH secretion in response to baclofen, a γ-aminobutyric acid (GABA) agonist, is enhanced (Davis et al. 1997; Shiah et al. 1999). **(p. 121)**

6.8   In depression, altered levels or blunted responses to various challenge agents have been found for all of the following *except*

   A. Prolactin.
   B. Thyroid-stimulating hormone (TSH).
   C. Luteinizing hormone (LH).
   D. Growth hormone.
   E. Adrenocorticotropic hormone (ACTH).

The correct response is option **C**.

No differences in the gonadotropins LH and follicle-stimulating hormone (FSH) have been found in depressed women compared with control subjects (Young et al. 2000). **(p. 122)**

References

Cooney JM, Lucey JV, Dinan TB: Enhanced growth hormone responses to pyridostigmine challenge in patients with panic disorder. Br J Psychiatry 170:159–161, 1997a

Cooney JM, Lucey JV, O'Keane V, et al: Specificity of the pyridostigmine/growth hormone challenge in the diagnosis of depression. Biol Psychiatry 42:827–833, 1997b

Corrêa H, Duval F, Claude MM, et al: Noradrenergic dysfunction and antidepressant treatment response. Eur Neuropsychopharmacol 11:163–168, 2001

Davis LL, Trivedi M, Choate A, et al: Growth hormone response to the GABA-B agonist baclofen in major depressive disorder. Psychoneuroendocrinology 22:129–140, 1997

Foltyn W, Nowakowska-Zajdel E, Danikiewicz A, et al: Hypothalamic-pituitary-thyroid axis in depression. Psychiatr Pol 36:281–292, 2002

Hatzinger M, Hemmeter UM, Baumann K, et al: The combined DEX-CRH test in treatment course and long-term outcome of major depression. J Psychiatr Res 36:287–297, 2002

Hendrick V, Altshuler L, Whybrow P: Psychoneuroendocrinology of mood disorders: the hypothalamic-pituitary-adrenal axis. Psychiatr Clin North Am 21:277–293, 1998

Holsboer F: Neuroendocrinology of mood disorders, in Psychopharmacology: The Fourth Generation of Progress. Edited by Bloom FE, Kupfer DJ. New York, Raven, 1995, pp 957–969

Jackson IM: The thyroid axis and depression. Thyroid 8:951–956, 1998

Krieg J-C, Lauer CJ, Schreiber W, et al: Neuroendocrine, polysomnographic and psychometric observations in healthy subjects at high familial risk for affective disorders: the current state of the "Munich vulnerability study." J Affect Disord 62:33–37, 2001

Meltzer HY, Lee MA, Jayathilake K: The blunted plasma cortisol response to apomorphine and its relationship to treatment response in patients with schizophrenia. Neuropsychopharmacology 24:278–290, 2001

O'Keane V, Abel K, Murray RM: Growth hormone responses to pyridostigmine in schizophrenia: evidence for cholinergic dysfunction. Biol Psychiatry 36:582–588, 1994

Peteranderl C, Antonijevic IA, Steiger A, et al: Nocturnal secretion of TSH and ACTH in male patients with depression and healthy controls. J Psychiatr Res 36:189–196, 2002

Rubin R, Dinan TG, Scott LV: The neuroendocrinology of affective disorders, in Hormones, Brain and Behavior. Edited by Pfaff D, Arnold AP, Etgen AM, et al. New York, Academic Press, 2001, pp 230–245

Sachar EJ, Hellman L, Fukushima DK, et al: Cortisol production in depressive illness. Arch Gen Psychiatry 23:289–298, 1970

Sarapura VD, Samuels MH, Ridgway EC: Thyroid-stimulating hormone, in The Pituitary. Edited by Melmed S. London, Blackwell Scientific, 2002, pp 172–216

Shelton RC: Cellular mechanisms in the vulnerability to depression and response to antidepressants. Psychiatr Clin North Am 23:1–15, 2000

Shiah IS, Yatham LN, Lam RW, et al: Growth hormone response to baclofen in patients with mania: a pilot study. Psychopharmacology (Berl) 147:280–284, 1999

Steckler T, Holsboer F, Reul JMHM: Glucocorticoids and depression. Baillieres Best Pract Res Clin Endocrinol Metab 13:597–614, 1999

Tandon R, Halbreich U: The second-generation 'atypical' antipsychotics: similar improved efficacy but different neuroendocrine side effects. Psychoneuroendocrinology 28:1–7, 2003

Tsigos C, Chrousos GP: Hypothalamic-pituitary-adrenal axis, neuroendocrine factors and stress. J Psychosom Res 53:865–871, 2002

Young EA, Midgley AR, Carlson NE, et al: Alterations in the hypothalamic-pituitary-ovarian axis in depressed women. Arch Gen Psychiatry 57:1157–1162, 2000

CHAPTER 7

Principles of Pharmacokinetics and Pharmacodynamics

Select the single best response for each question.

7.1   Which of the following statements about presystemic elimination is *true*?

A. A first-pass or presystemic elimination effect is indicated by an increased amount of parent drug reaching the systemic circulation after oral administration.
B. A first-pass effect is indicated by a reduced quantity of metabolites after oral administration.
C. Presystemic metabolism of drugs is minimally accomplished by cytochrome P450 enzymes in the luminal epithelium of the small intestine.
D. Cytochrome P450 3A4 has a profound effect on presystemic drug metabolism.
E. First-pass metabolism is not associated with P-glycoproteins.

The correct response is option **D.**

Intestinal cytochrome P450 3A4 has a profound effect on presystemic drug metabolism. Up to 43% of orally administered midazolam, for example, is metabolized as it passes through the intestinal mucosa (Paine et al. 1996). **(p. 132)**

7.2   Which of the following statements about protein binding is *false*?

A. Drug binding in the tissues cannot be directly measured in vivo.
B. Displacement of drug from plasma protein binding sites may result from drug–drug interactions.
C. Plasma protein binding displacement interactions are a major source of variability in psychopharmacology.
D. Compensatory change occurs in the body to buffer the impact of drug-binding interactions.
E. None of the above.

The correct response is option **C.**

Plasma protein binding displacement interactions are rarely a major source of variability in psychopharmacology (Sellers 1979; see DeVane 2002 for review). **(p. 134)**

7.3   The time required from the first administered dose to the point at which approximate steady state occurs is equivalent to

A. 9–10 half-lives.
B. 1–2 half-lives.
C. 2 weeks.
D. 2 days.
E. 4–5 half-lives.

The correct response is option **E.**

The time required from the first administered dose to the point at which an approximate steady state occurs is equivalent to a total of 4–5 elimination half-lives. **(p. 135)**

7.4   The time course of tolerance to psychoactive drug effects varies from minutes to weeks. The operative elements in the development of tolerance include which of the following?

A. Homeostatic changes in receptor sensitivity from blockade of various transporters.
B. Acute depletion of a neurotransmitter or cofactor.
C. Receptor agonist or antagonist effects.
D. All of the above.
E. None of the above.

The correct response is option **D.**

The time course of tolerance to psychoactive drug effects varies from minutes to weeks. Acute tolerance to some euphoric effects of cocaine can occur following a single dose (Foltin and Fischman 1991). Tolerance to the sedative effects of various drugs may take weeks. The mechanisms operative in the development of tolerance include acute depletion of a neurotransmitter or cofactor, homeostatic changes in receptor sensitivity from blockade of various transporters, or receptor agonist or antagonist effects. **(p. 137)**

7.5   Which of the following statements concerning the metabolic consequences of genetic polymorphisms is *false*?

A. Genetic polymorphism in a drug-metabolizing enzyme results in a subpopulation of individuals who are poor or rapid metabolizers of substrates of the affected enzyme.
B. When an active drug is administered to a person who is a poor metabolizer of the enzyme responsible for the drug's metabolism, higher drug concentrations can be expected, leading to an exaggerated response or potential toxicity.
C. When a drug whose therapeutic effect depends on formation of an active metabolite is administered to a person who is a poor metabolizer of the enzyme responsible for the drug's metabolism, high concentrations of the metabolite can be expected, leading to an exaggerated response or potential toxicity.
D. The most serious consequences of genetic polymorphisms occur in poor metabolizers who are administered active drugs with narrow therapeutic windows.
E. For cytochrome P450 2D6, poor metabolizer status is inherited as an autosomal recessive trait.

The correct response is option **C.**

The potential clinical consequences of being a poor metabolizer will vary according to the activity of the administered drug and of any active metabolites. When the drug is active and a pathway is affected—a situation that usually produces an inactive metabolite—higher drug concentrations can be expected. This result can lead to an exaggerated response and potential toxicity. The most serious consequences would be expected from drugs with a narrow therapeutic window. For example, when perphenazine (a drug with a narrow therapeutic window) was given to elderly patients who were poor metabolizers of cytochrome P450 2D6, extrapyramidal side effects were exaggerated (Pollock et al. 1995). If the therapeutic effects depend on the formation of an active metabolite, diminished response can be expected from a lower concentration of metabolite in individuals who are poor metabolizers. For example, normal doses of codeine, which is partially metabolized to the more potent morphine, may provide an inadequate analgesic effect. For cytochrome P450 2D6, poor metabolizer status is inherited as an autosomal recessive trait. At least 70 different alleles have been defined for the 2D6 gene, and many types of null mutations result in impaired 2D6 activity (Gonzalez and Idle 1994). A goal of current research in pharmacogenetics is to apply phenotyping and genotyping as an aid in the initial selection of drugs and drug doses to achieve a plasma concentration that is both safe and effective (Pollock et al. 1995). **(pp. 139–140)**

References

DeVane CL: Clinical significance of drug binding, protein binding and binding displacement drug interactions. Psychopharmacol Bull 36:5–21, 2002

Foltin RW, Fischman MW: Smoked and intravenous cocaine in humans: acute tolerance, cardiovascular and subjective effects. J Pharmacol Exp Ther 257:247–261, 1991

Gonzalez FJ, Idle JR: Pharmacogenetic phenotyping and genotyping: present status and future potential. Clin Pharmacokinet 26:59–70, 1994

Paine MF, Shen DD, Kunze KL, et al: First-pass metabolism of midazolam by the human intestine. Clin Pharmacol Ther 60:14–24, 1996

Pollock BG, Mulsant BH, Sweet RA, et al: Prospective cytochrome P450 phenotyping for neuroleptic treatment in dementia. Psychopharmacol Bull 31:327–331, 1995

Sellers EM: Plasma protein displacement interactions are rarely of clinical significance. Pharmacology 18:225–227, 1979

CHAPTER 8

Brain–Immune System Interactions: Relevance to the Pathophysiology and Treatment of Neuropsychiatric Disorders

Select the single best response for each question.

8.1 Examples of the innate immunity response include all of the following *except*

   A. Phagocytes.
   B. Complement C3.
   C. Tumor necrosis factor–α (TNF-α).
   D. T lymphocytes.
   E. Acute-phase reactants.

The correct response is option **D.**

Innate immunity provides a first line of defense by attacking foreign substances rapidly in a nonspecific manner, without requiring that a specific antigen (or antibody-generating molecule) be recognized. Innate immune response is provided by effector cells, such as phagocytes (macrophages, neutrophils) and natural killer cells; soluble mediators, such as complement C3 and acute-phase reactants; and representative cytokines, such as TNF-α, interleukin-1α and β, and interleukin-6. **(pp. 148, 149; see Table 8–1)**

8.2 Which of the following immune system changes are seen in major depression?

   A. Decreased white blood cells.
   B. Decreased interleukin-6.
   C. Increased natural killer (NK) cell activity.
   D. Decreased haptoglobin.
   E. Decreased lymphocyte percentage.

The correct response is option **E.**

Besides decreased lymphocyte percentage, immune system alterations in major depression also include *increased* white blood cells, increased neutrophil percentage, increased CD4-to-CD8 ratio, *decreased* NK cell activity, decreased mitogen-induced lymphocyte proliferation, *increased* interleukin-6, *increased* haptoglobin, and increased prostaglandin E2. **(p. 151; see Table 8–2)**

8.3   Which of the following statements about how glucocorticoids modulate immune functioning is *true*?

    A. They increase cytokine production and function.
    B. They inhibit cytokine production and function.
    C. They facilitate arachidonic acid pathways.
    D. They increase production of T cells.
    E. They inhibit production of haptoglobin.

The correct response is option **B**.

Identified effects of glucocorticoids on the immune (and inflammatory) system (see Raison et al. 2002 for review) include modulation of immune cell trafficking throughout the body; modulation of cell death pathways (i.e., apoptosis); inhibition of arachidonic acid pathway products (e.g., prostaglandins) that mediate inflammation and sickness symptoms (e.g., fever); modulation of Th1/Th2 cellular immune response patterns in a manner that inhibits Th1 (cell-mediated) responses and promotes Th2 (antibody) responses; inhibition of T-cell– and NK-cell–mediated cytotoxicity; and inhibition of cytokine production and function through interaction of glucocorticoid receptors with transcription factors (nuclear factor kappa B, in particular). **(p. 152)**

8.4   Which of the following statements best describes the effect of antidepressants on immune responsiveness?

    A. Antidepressants increase immune responsiveness.
    B. Antidepressants have no effect on immune responsiveness.
    C. Antidepressants decrease immune responsiveness.
    D. Antidepressants of different types either increase or decrease immune responsiveness.
    E. Only antidepressants of the selective serotonin class increase immune responsiveness.

The correct response is option **C**.

In general, antidepressants have been found to *decrease* immune responsiveness. **(p. 157)**

8.5   Which of the following statements is *true*?

    A. The increased prevalence of major depression in the United States may be caused in part by the increased consumption of omega-3 fatty acids.
    B. The increased prevalence of bipolar disorder in the United States may be caused in part by the increased consumption of omega-3 fatty acids, which have anti-inflammatory effects.
    C. The decreased prevalence of bipolar disorder in the United States may be caused in part by the increased consumption of omega-3 fatty acids, which increase prostaglandins and proinflammatory cytokines.
    D. The increased prevalence of major depression in the United States may be caused in part by the decreased consumption of omega-3 fatty acids, which increase prostaglandins and proinflammatory cytokines.
    E. The increased prevalence of major depression in the United States may be caused in part by the decreased consumption of omega-3 fatty acids, which inhibit prostaglandins and proinflammatory cytokines.

The correct response is option **E**.

It has been suggested that the increased prevalence of major depression observed in the Western world over the last half century may be caused, at least in part, by a decrease in the consumption of omega-3 fatty acids (Maes et al. 1999), which are well known to have anti-inflammatory effects via the inhibition of prostaglandins and proinflammatory cytokines. Consistent with this, populations that consume diets high in omega-3 fatty acids (found especially in fish) appear to have diminished rates of major depression (Tanskanen et al. 2001). Conversely, patients with major depression have been reported to have decreased serum concentrations of omega-3 fatty acids (Maes et al. 1999). These observations suggest that the administration of omega-3 fatty acids might be beneficial to patients with mood disorders. In one study, it was reported that the administration of omega-3 fatty acids to patients with bipolar disorder under double-blind, placebo-controlled conditions significantly decreased disease relapse (Stoll et al. 1999). **(pp. 158–159)**

References

Maes M, Christophe A, Delanghe J, et al: Lowered omega 3 polyunsaturated fatty acids in serum phospholipids and cholesteryl esters of depressed patients. Psychiatry Res 85:275–291, 1999

Raison CL, Gumnick JF, Miller AH: Neuroendocrine-immune interactions: implications for health and behavior, in Hormones, Brain and Behavior, Vol 5. San Diego, CA, Academic Press, 2002, pp 209–261

Stoll AL, Severus WE, Freeman MP, et al: Omega 3 fatty acids in bipolar disorder: a preliminary double-blind, placebo-controlled trial (comments). Arch Gen Psychiatry 56:407–412, 1999

Tanskanen A, Hibbeln JR, Tuomilehto J, et al: Fish consumption and depressive symptoms in the general population in Finland. Psychiatr Serv 52:529–531, 2001

CHAPTER 9

Brain Imaging in Psychopharmacology

Select the single best response for each question.

9.1   Regarding brain imaging technologies now in common use, which of the following statements is *true*?

   A. Positron emission tomography (PET) has gained rapid acceptance because of the widespread availability of tomography units.
   B. PET has gained rapid acceptance because it does not involve radioactive exposure.
   C. Functional magnetic resonance imaging (fMRI) has gained rapid acceptance because of the lack of radioactive exposure and the availability of MRI units.
   D. PET has gained rapid acceptance because it can be repeated within a short time on the same subject.
   E. PET has gained acceptance because it does not employ injectable substances.

The correct response is option **C.**

PET and fMRI are the two technologies most commonly used today to study the human brain "in action." The past decade's explosion of information about human brain function has resulted in large part from these two techniques. In particular, fMRI has gained rapid acceptance because of the widespread availability of MRI scanners and the lack of radioactive exposure. PET, by contrast, employs radioactive tracers that limit its repeated use on the same subject, and the limited availability of PET equipment means that PET scans are expensive. **(pp. 163, 166; see Table 9–1)**

9.2   Which of the following statements best describes an advantage of positron emission tomography (PET) over functional magnetic resonance imaging (fMRI)?

   A. PET is less expensive than MRI.
   B. PET allows for event-related design experiments.
   C. PET allows for longitudinal studies of the same subject.
   D. PET allows for metabolic and receptor mapping.
   E. PET is easier to perform and can be conducted by one person.

The correct response is option **D.**

A major advantage of PET over fMRI is that PET allows for metabolic and receptor mapping. Among PET's disadvantages, however, are its invasiveness (injection of a radioactive isotope prevents the use of PET for longitudinal studies in which the same subjects are scanned repeatedly over an extended period of time); its expense (availability of PET equipment is limited, resulting in higher utilization costs); and its lengthier temporal resolution (because of the lifetime of the isotope), which prevents use of the sophisticated, event-related designs possible with fMRI. Finally, the PET acquisition procedure is time-consuming and resource-intensive, unlike the MRI experimental setup, which is easy to manipulate and can be operated by just one person. **(p. 166; see Table 9–1)**

9.3   Which of the following statements best characterizes a major difference between electroencephalography (EEG) and magnetoencephalography (MEG)?

A. MEG uses relatively simple equipment.
B. MEG requires cutting-edge technology.
C. EEG requires cutting-edge technology.
D. EEG requires a higher density of scale electrodes.
E. Only MEG is a surface technology.

The correct response is option **B.**

EEG and MEG have very different technical requirements. Whereas EEG uses relatively simple equipment—basically a multielectrode helmet, an amplifying and filtering device, and a computer— MEG employs cutting-edge technology, because the detection of a magnetic field intensity as weak as the one produced by the brain (~20,00 billion times weaker than the intensity of the earth's magnetic field) requires the use of superconducting coil units based on superconducting quantum interference device technology. **(p. 170)**

9.4   Which of the following statements best describes the limitations of functional brain imaging techniques for diagnosis?

A. Functional brain imaging has a high rate of false negatives.
B. Functional brain imaging is relatively insensitive, because there are few ways a brain scan may appear to be abnormal.
C. Functional brain imaging has a high rate of false positives.
D. Functional brain imaging studies in clinical populations have been characterized by excessively large sample sizes.
E. None of the above.

The correct response is option **C.**

For a brain imaging task to be useful diagnostically, it must meet the same requirements as any medical test—namely, sensitivity and specificity. *Sensitivity*, which measures the ability of a test to detect the presence of a disorder, is usually characterized by a low rate of false negatives. Sensitivity, however, is not generally a problem with functional brain imaging. If anything, functional magnetic resonance imaging (fMRI) is *too* sensitive, because there are so many possible ways in which a brain scan might appear "abnormal." *Specificity*, which measures the ability of a test to exclude the presence of a disorder when it is truly not present, is usually characterized by a low rate of false positives. fMRI has a high rate of false positives, and this lack of specificity is the main limitation of functional brain imaging for diagnosis. Like any diagnostic test, brain imaging differences depend on the demonstration that a specific cohort of patients differs statistically from a control group. Until recently, the majority of brain imaging studies in clinical populations have been limited by small sample sizes. Cohorts of 10– 20 subjects per group are typical, and sizes larger than this are the exception. The result is that the majority of functional studies of particular disorders have found statistically different activations in specific brain regions; however, because of the small sample sizes, it has not been possible to determine appropriate parameters of "normality." **(p. 171)**

9.5   The isotopes most commonly used in positron emission tomography (PET) are

A. Carbon-11, chlorine-18, and nitrogen-14.
B. Carbon-11, oxygen-15, fluorine-18, and nitrogen-13.
C. Carbon-12, oxygen-14, fluorine-18, and nitrogen-13.
D. Carbon-11 and oxygen-14.
E. Carbon-12, oxygen-15, and lithium-18.

The correct response is option **B**.

Positrons are produced indirectly by the radioactive decay of particular isotopes. The most commonly used isotopes—carbon-11 (^{11}C), oxygen-15 (^{15}O), fluorine-18 (^{18}F), and nitrogen-13 (^{13}N)—are produced in a cyclotron by the bombardment of targets with high-energy protons. **(p. 168)**

CHAPTER 10

Statistics and Clinical Trial Design in Psychopharmacology

Select the single best response for each question.

10.1 "Statistical significance" is an indicator of

A. The validity of a study.
B. The clinical relevance of a study.
C. The quality of a study.
D. A double-blind, placebo-controlled study design.
E. An odds ratio greater than one.

The correct response is option **C.**

A statement that an effect is statistically significant is often interpreted as an indication that the effect is large, important, or exciting. However, "statistically significant" is more a comment on the quality of the study than on the size of the treatment's effect. Statistical significance is *necessary*, but not *sufficient*, to consider a treatment clinically significant. **(p. 175)**

10.2 A "negative study" is a study in which

A. The study drug produces a negative outcome.
B. It is demonstrated that the study drug produces no significant effect compared with the control (i.e., placebo).
C. The study findings generate *P* values greater than 0.05.
D. Bias has been introduced into the study design.
E. The study produces a negative NNT (number needed to treat) value.

The correct response is option **B.**

A statement that an effect is "not statistically significant" is often mistakenly taken as a demonstration that the treatment and the control or comparison are equivalent. In reality, such a statement means that the study design was not adequate to detect any effect size: it was a "failed study," not a "negative study." **(p. 175)**

10.3   A "failed study" is a study in which

A. The study fails to get published in a peer-reviewed journal.
B. A high dropout rate requires modification of the study design.
C. Investigators fail to maintain the blind.
D. The results are eventually discovered to have been fabricated.
E. The effects of a study drug are not "statistically significant."

The correct response is option E.

A "failed study" is one in which the study design is not adequate to detect an effect size. The effect may actually have been quite large and clinically significant, but the sample size may have been too small, the outcome measures poorly measured, and/or the design and analysis poorly chosen. (p. 175)

10.4   *Number needed to treat* (NNT) is defined as

A. The number of subjects that need to be exposed to a treatment in order to average one more response than would be achieved with the control drug.
B. The number of subjects that need to be treated in order to ensure an odds ratio greater than one.
C. The number of subjects that need to be exposed to a treatment in order to achieve a *P* value of less than 0.05.
D. Equal to 1 minus the risk difference.
E. The ratio of sensitivity to specificity.

The correct response is option A.

NNT, equal to 1 divided by the risk difference, is the average number of subjects that would need to be treated with treatment *T* in order for one additional subject to benefit than would have benefited from control condition C. (p. 176; see also Table 10–1)

10.5   Which of the following is a necessary feature of a "clinically significant effect"?

A. An effect size greater than 20% of baseline measures.
B. An odds ratio greater than 1.
C. The demonstration of statistical significance.
D. The ability of this statistic to alter the practice patterns of clinicians who are made aware of these study results.
E. A number needed to treat (NNT) of less than 100.

The correct response is option C.

A clinically significant effect is an effect that is statistically significant and large enough that clinicians might reasonably be motivated to use the treatment (*T*) rather than the control agent/condition (C) for patients in their practice who are similar to those patients specified by the inclusion/exclusion criteria of the study. (p. 175)

C H A P T E R   1 1

Pharmacoeconomics

Select the single best response for each question.

11.1   Cost comparison of two or more treatment strategies of equal efficacy is termed

    A.   Cost-effectiveness analysis.
    B.   Cost minimization analysis.
    C.   Cost utility analysis.
    D.   Cost–benefit analysis.
    E.   Cost correlation analysis.

The correct response is option **B.**

There are four basic models of pharmacoeconomic analysis, each of which addresses a somewhat different question: cost minimization, cost-effectiveness, cost–benefit, and cost utility. *Cost minimization analysis,* the simplest of these pharmacoeconomic models, involves a cost comparison of two or more treatment strategies in which there is equal efficacy. Because the efficacy of each comparator is assumed to be equal, studies based on such an analysis assume that outcomes are similar. **(p. 186)**

11.2   According to a British study by Guest and Cookson (1999), which of the following accounted for the largest portion of costs attributable to schizophrenia in the 5 years following initial diagnosis?

    A.   Inpatient hospitalization costs.
    B.   Medication costs.
    C.   Property damage caused during acute exacerbations of illness.
    D.   Lost productivity.
    E.   Treatment of iatrogenic complications.

The correct response is option **D.**

In a cost-of-illness simulation conducted by Guest and Cookson (1999) in England, government health expenditures and lost productivity costs were the largest components of the cost of illness of schizophrenia in the 5 years following initial diagnosis. Lost productivity accounted for nearly 50% of the cost of the illness. Direct treatment costs accounted for nearly 40% of the total costs, the bulk of which was the result of inpatient costs. Medication costs accounted for only 2% of the total cost. The authors concluded that treatment strategies that reduce hospitalization and foster return to work are the most successful in reducing the cost of illness of schizophrenia. **(p. 188)**

11.3 Factors that contribute to the superior cost-effectiveness of atypical versus typical antipsychotic agents include all of the following *except*

A. More benign side-effect profiles.
B. Reduced levels of acute extrapyramidal side effects (EPS) and tardive dyskinesia.
C. Improved medication compliance.
D. Reduction in inpatient hospitalization days.
E. Less weight gain.

The correct response is option **E.**

Typical antipsychotic medications caused many side effects, including EPS and tardive dyskinesia. The development of newer medications, the atypical antipsychotics, heralded a new treatment era. Atypical antipsychotics are significantly more expensive than traditional antipsychotics; however, increased compliance and reductions in inpatient days support a pharmacoeconomic argument for their use. These newer medications have, in general, much more benign side-effect profiles, as well as substantially reduced levels of EPS and tardive dyskinesia. **(p. 188)**

11.4 According to pharmacoeconomic studies, which of the following antidepressants is the *least* cost-effective?

A. Imipramine.
B. Fluoxetine.
C. Mirtazapine.
D. Venlafaxine.
E. Bupropion.

The correct response is option **A.**

There is overwhelming evidence that the more tolerable antidepressants, including selective serotonin reuptake inhibitors (such as fluoxetine), mirtazapine, venlafaxine, and bupropion, are more cost-effective treatments for depression than are the tricyclic antidepressants (such as imipramine). **(p. 196; see also pp. 194–195)**

11.5 According to a pharmacoeconomic analysis by Greenberg et al. (1999), which of the following accounted for the largest portion of costs attributable to anxiety disorders?

A. Lost productivity.
B. Psychiatric treatment costs.
C. Nonpsychiatric medical treatment costs.
D. Prescription medication costs.
E. Mortality costs.

The correct response is option **C.**

Greenberg et al. (1999) estimated the total economic burden of anxiety disorders at $42.3 billion per year in 1990, or $1,542 per patient. This included $23 billion (54%) in nonpsychiatric medical treatment costs, $13.3 billion (31%) in psychiatric treatment costs, $4.1 billion (10%) in indirect workplace costs, $1.2 billion (3%) in mortality costs, and $0.8 billion (2%) in prescription pharmaceutical costs. These data demonstrated the high use of general medical services by patients with anxiety disorders. **(p. 197)**

11.6   According to various pharmacoeconomic studies, the class of illnesses with the highest associated total costs in the United States is

A. Schizophrenia spectrum disorders.
B. Dissociative disorders.
C. Anxiety disorders.
D. Depressive disorders.
E. Bipolar spectrum disorders.

The correct response is option **D.**

Greenberg et al. (2001) estimated that in 2000, the annual total cost of depression in the United States was between $71 billion and $86 billion. In 1985, the estimated total cost of schizophrenia in the United States was $22.7 billion, of which 45% was direct costs and 55% was indirect costs. The total economic burden of bipolar disorder is estimated at $45 billion per year, of which $7 billion is for direct treatment (Wyatt and Henter 1995). The total economic burden of anxiety disorders was estimated at $42.3 billion per year in 1990, or $1,542 per patient (Greenberg et al. 1999). This includes $23 billion (54%) in nonpsychiatric medical treatment costs. **(pp. 187, 192, 196)**

References

Greenberg PE, Sisitsky T, Kessler RC, et al: The economic burden of anxiety disorders in the 1990s. J Clin Psychiatry 60:427–435, 1999

Greenberg P, Leong S, Birnbaum H: Cost of depression: current assessment and future directions. Expert Review of Pharmacoeconomics and Outcomes Research 1:69–76, 2001

Guest JF, Cookson RF: Cost of schizophrenia to UK society. An incidence-based cost-of-illness model for the first 5 years following diagnosis. Pharmacoeconomics 15:597–610, 1999

Wyatt RJ, Henter I: An economic evaluation of manic-depressive illness—1991. Soc Psychiatry Psychiatr Epidemiol 30:213–219, 1995

CHAPTER 12

Tricyclic and Tetracyclic Drugs

Select the single best response for each question.

12.1   Which of the following is a secondary-amine tricyclic antidepressant (TCA)?

A. Amitriptyline.
B. Maprotiline.
C. Protriptyline.
D. Clomipramine.
E. Doxepin.

The correct response is option **C.**

The three secondary-amine TCA compounds are desipramine (Norpramin), nortriptyline (Aventyl, Pamelor), and protriptyline (Vivactil). Amitriptyline, clomipramine, and doxepin are tertiary amines. Maprotiline is a tetracyclic compound. **(p. 208)**

12.2   Tertiary-amine tricyclic antidepressants (TCAs), as distinguished from their secondary-amine TCA metabolites, are more potent in blocking the reuptake of which of the following neurotransmitters?

A. Serotonin.
B. Norepinephrine.
C. Dopamine.
D. Acetylcholine.
E. Glutamate.

The correct response is option **A.**

The tertiary-amine tricyclics—amitriptyline, imipramine, and clomipramine—are more potent in blocking the serotonin transporter (5-HTT). The secondary-amine TCAs—desipramine, nortriptyline, and protriptyline—are much more potent in blocking the norepinephrine transporter (NET). The tertiary amines have greater affinity for the 5-HTT, whereas the secondary amines are relatively more potent at the NET (Bolden-Watson and Richelson 1993; Richelson and Nelson 1984; Tatsumi et al. 1997). **(pp. 208, 209; see also Table 12–1)**

12.3   The least anticholinergic of the tricyclic antidepressants (TCAs) is

A. Protriptyline.
B. Nortriptyline.
C. Doxepin.
D. Desipramine.
E. Imipramine.

The correct response is option **D.**

Desipramine is the least anticholinergic among the TCAs (Richelson and Nelson 1984). Amitriptyline is the most anticholinergic, not only of the TCAs but of all antidepressants. Doxepin is the most potent histamine$_1$ antagonist among the TCAs (although one of the newer antidepressants, mirtazapine, is even more potent). **(p. 210)**

12.4   The tricyclic antidepressant (TCA) least likely to cause orthostatic hypotension is

A. Desipramine.
B. Nortriptyline.
C. Trimipramine.
D. Clomipramine.
E. Amitriptyline.

The correct response is option **B.**

Orthostatic hypotension is one of the most common reasons for discontinuation of TCA treatment (Glassman et al. 1979). It can occur with all of the tricyclics but appears to be less pronounced with nortriptyline (Roose et al. 1981; Thayssen et al. 1981). **(p. 221)**

12.5   The cytochrome P450 enzyme chiefly responsible for hydroxylation of nortriptyline and desipramine is

A. 1A2.
B. 2C9.
C. 2C19.
D. 2D6.
E. 3A4.

The correct response is option **D.**

The cytochrome P450 2D6 pathway appears responsible for hydroxylation of desipramine and nortriptyline (Brosen et al. 1991). In fact, desipramine has been considered the prototypic substrate for 2D6 because it has no other major metabolic pathways. **(p. 212)**

12.6   Which of the following cytochrome P450 enzymes is involved in the demethylation of tertiary-amine tricyclic antidepressants (TCAs) to secondary-amine TCAs?

A. 2B6.
B. 2C9.
C. 2C19.
D. 2D6.
E. 2E1.

The correct response is option **C.**

Demethylation of the tertiary-amine compounds appears to involve a number of cytochrome P450 enzymes, including 1A2, 3A4, and 2C19. **(p. 212)**

12.7   Which of the tricyclic antidepressants (TCAs) is most effective in the treatment of obsessive-compulsive disorder (OCD)?

   A. Imipramine.
   B. Amitriptyline.
   C. Doxepin.
   D. Desipramine.
   E. Clomipramine.

The correct response is option **E.**

Unlike depression, which responds to a variety of antidepressant agents, OCD appears to require treatment with a serotonergic agent. Clomipramine, the most serotonergic of the TCAs, is approved by the U.S. Food and Drug Administration for use in OCD, and its efficacy in this disorder is well established (Greist et al. 1995). Studies comparing its effectiveness with that of noradrenergic agents such as desipramine found that clomipramine was substantially superior (Leonard et al. 1989). Although the selective serotonin reuptake inhibitors are effective in treating OCD, there is a suggestion that clomipramine may be superior to them as well (Greist et al. 1995). **(p. 218)**

12.8   The most potent histamine$_1$ (H$_1$) receptor blocker among the tricyclic antidepressants (TCAs) is

   A. Amitriptyline.
   B. Clomipramine.
   C. Doxepin.
   D. Imipramine.
   E. Trimipramine.

The correct response is option **C.**

Several of the tricyclic compounds and the tetracyclic maprotiline have clinically significant antihistamine effects. Doxepin is the most potent H$_1$ receptor blocker among the TCAs. It is more potent that the commonly administered antihistamine diphenhydramine. More recently, however, doxepin has been overtaken by the new-generation antidepressant mirtazapine and the atypical antipsychotic olanzapine, which are even more potent antihistamines. **(p. 220)**

12.9   The principal cause of death following tricyclic antidepressant (TCA) overdose is

   A. Cardiac arrhythmia.
   B. Status epilepticus.
   C. Aspiration leading to adult respiratory distress syndrome.
   D. Hemorrhagic cerebrovascular accident.
   E. Hepatorenal syndrome.

The correct response is option **A.**

Death from TCA overdose most commonly occurs as a result of cardiac arrhythmia. **(p. 223)**

References

Bolden-Watson C, Richelson E: Blockade of newly developed antidepressants of biogenic amine uptake into rat brain synaptosomes. Life Sci 52:1023–1029, 1993

Brosen K, Zeugin T, Meyer UA: Role of P450IID6, the target of the sparteine-debrisoquin oxidation polymorphism, in the metabolism of imipramine. Clin Pharmacol Ther 49:609–617, 1991

Glassman AH, Bigger JT Jr, Giardina EV, et al: Clinical characteristics of imipramine induced orthostatic hypotension. Lancet 1:468–472, 1979

Greist JH, Jefferson JW, Kobak KA, et al: Efficacy and tolerability of serotonin transport inhibitors in obsessive-compulsive disorder: a meta-analysis. Arch Gen Psychiatry 52:53–60, 1995

Leonard HL, Swedo S, Rapoport JL, et al: Treatment of obsessive compulsive disorder in children and adolescents with clomipramine and desipramine: a double-blind crossover comparison. Arch Gen Psychiatry 46:1088–1092, 1989

Richelson E, Nelson A: Antagonism by antidepressants of neurotransmitter receptors of normal human brain in vitro. J Pharmacol Exp Ther 230:94–102, 1984

Roose SP, Glassman AH, Siris SG, et al: Comparison of imipramine and nortriptyline-induced orthostatic hypotension: a meaningful difference. J Clin Psychopharmacol 1:316–319, 1981

Tatsumi M, Groshan K, Blakely RD, et al: Pharmacological profile of antidepressants and related compounds at human monoamine transporters. Eur J Pharmacol 340:249–258, 1997

Thayssen P, Bjerre M, Kragh-Sorenson P, et al: Cardiovascular effects of imipramine and nortriptyline in elderly patients. Psychopharmacology (Berl) 74:360–364, 1981

CHAPTER 13

Fluoxetine

Select the single best response for each question.

13.1   The selective serotonin reuptake inhibitor with active metabolites and the longest half-life is

  A. Paroxetine.
  B. Sertraline.
  C. Citalopram.
  D. Escitalopram.
  E. Fluoxetine.

The correct response is option **E.**

Fluoxetine is principally metabolized to norfluoxetine, which has activity similar to that of fluoxetine on serotonin reuptake. The elimination half-life of norfluoxetine is longer (4–15 days) than that of fluoxetine (4–6 days). **(p. 235; see also Table 13–2)**

13.2   What is the washout period for fluoxetine before a monoamine oxidase inhibitor (MAOI) may be safely administered?

  A. 1 day.
  B. 5 days.
  C. 30 days.
  D. 5 weeks.
  E. 3 months.

The correct response is option **D.**

A 5-week washout from fluoxetine is recommended before initiating treatment with an MAOI (Ciraulo and Shader 1990). **(p. 235)**

13.3   Which cytochrome P450 enzyme(s) does fluoxetine inhibit to any degree?

  A. 2C9 and 2C19.
  B. 2D6.
  C. 3A3/4.
  D. All of the above.
  E. None of the above.

The correct response is option **D.**

Through inhibition of cytochrome P450 2D6, fluoxetine may elevate the concentration of concomitantly administered drugs that rely on this enzyme for metabolism. The data with respect to fluoxetine's inhibition of other cytochrome P450 enzymes, such as 3A3/4, 2C9, and 2C19, are less consistent, but the potential for interaction exists. **(p. 241)**

13.4 Acute treatment of fluoxetine overdose includes which of the following?

　　A. Hemodialysis.
　　B. Supportive care only.
　　C. Ipecac and charcoal.
　　D. Alkalinization of the urine.
　　E. Naltrexone.

The correct response is option **B.**

Borys et al. (1992), in a prospective multicenter study, concluded that the emergent symptoms of fluoxetine overdose are minor and of short duration; thus, aggressive supportive care is the only intervention necessary. **(p. 241)**

13.5 Fluoxetine does not generally require a taper to avoid a withdrawal syndrome, because

　　A. It has active metabolites with long half-lives.
　　B. It has no active metabolites.
　　C. It is rapidly and fully metabolized, leading to fewer adverse events.
　　D. All of the above.
　　E. None of the above.

The correct response is option **A.**

Rosenbaum et al. (1998) compared the effects of a 5- to 8-day abrupt discontinuation from fluoxetine, paroxetine, or sertraline in three groups of patients with depression receiving maintenance therapy. Patients from the paroxetine and sertraline groups had a significant increase in adverse events, whereas patients in the fluoxetine group experienced no increase in adverse events. SSRIs with short half-lives (e.g., paroxetine) should be tapered. Because of its extended half-life, fluoxetine does not require tapering. **(p. 241)**

References

Borys DJ, Setzer SC, Ling LJ, et al: Acute fluoxetine overdose: a report of 234 cases. Am J Emerg Med 10:115–120, 1992

Ciraulo DA, Shader RI: Fluoxetine drug-drug interactions, I: antidepressants and antipsychotics. J Clin Psychopharmacol 10:48–50, 1990

Rosenbaum JF, Fava M, Hoog SL, et al: Selective serotonin reuptake inhibitor discontinuation syndrome: a randomized clinical trial. Biol Psychiatry 44:77–87, 1998

CHAPTER 14

Sertraline

Select the single best response for each question.

14.1 Sertraline has been approved by the U.S. Food and Drug Administration (FDA) for which of the following indications?

A. Major depressive disorder.
B. Obsessive-compulsive disorder (OCD).
C. Posttraumatic stress disorder.
D. Premenstrual dysphoric disorder.
E. All of the above.

The correct response is option **E.**

Sertraline is currently approved by the FDA for the treatment of major depressive disorder, OCD and pediatric OCD, posttraumatic stress disorder, panic disorder, premenstrual dysphoric disorder, and, most recently, social anxiety disorder. **(p. 249)**

14.2 The most common adverse effect of sertraline is

A. Tinnitus.
B. Gastrointestinal disturbances.
C. Sexual dysfunction.
D. Weight gain.
E. Acne.

The correct response is option **B.**

Sertraline was associated with a number of adverse effects in premarketing evaluations, the most common of which were gastrointestinal disturbances ("Zoloft" 2001). **(p. 253)**

14.3 The elimination half-life of sertraline is

A. 2 weeks.
B. 5 weeks.
C. 125 hours.
D. 26–32 hours.
E. 5–10 hours.

The correct response is option **D.**

The elimination half-life of sertraline is 26–32 hours, and steady-state levels are achieved after 7 days. **(p. 248)**

14.4   Which of the following cytochrome P450 enzymes is responsible for the metabolism of sertraline?

A. 1A2.
B. 2C9, 2C19, 2D6, and 3A4.
C. 1A2 and 2E1.
D. 2E1.
E. 2D6.

The correct response is option **B**.

The enzymes involved in metabolism of sertraline to desmethylsertraline remain unclear (Greenblatt et al. 1999). Although six different cytochrome P450 enzymes have the capacity to catalyze this reaction, none accounts for more than 25% of sertraline's clearance. The contribution of each cytochrome P450 enzyme is dependent on not only the protein's activity on the substrate, as evidenced through in vitro models, but also the abundance of the enzyme. Given these properties, one computer model found that the greatest contribution to the demethylation of sertraline is from 2C9 (about 23%), with 3A4 and 2C19 each contributing about 15%, 2D6 adding 5%, and 2B6 contributing 2% to the process (Greenblatt et al. 1999; Lee et al. 1999). **(pp. 248–249)**

14.5   Sertraline's metabolite, desmethylsertraline, has which of the following characteristics?

A. It is an inactive compound.
B. It has greater activity and potency than sertraline in blocking reuptake of serotonin (5-hydroxytryptamine [5-HT]).
C. It is one-tenth as active as sertraline in blocking reuptake of 5-HT.
D. It is a prodrug.
E. None of the above.

The correct response is option **C**.

Sertraline is metabolized to desmethylsertraline. This compound is approximately one-tenth as active in blocking the reuptake of 5-HT; it also lacks antidepressant activity in animal models (Heym and Koe 1988). **(p. 247)**

References

Greenblatt D, von Moltke L, Harmatz J, et al: Human cytochromes mediating sertraline biotransformation: seeking attribution. J Clin Psychopharmacol 19:489–493, 1999

Heym J, Koe BK: Pharmacology of sertraline: a review. J Clin Psychiatry 49:40–45, 1988

Lee A, Chan W, Harralson A, et al: The effects of grapefruit juice on sertraline metabolism: an in vitro and in vivo study. Clin Ther 21:1890–1899, 1999

Zoloft (sertraline hydrochloride) tablets and oral concentrate (package insert). New York, Pfizer, 2001

CHAPTER 15

Paroxetine

Select the single best response for each question.

15.1   Which selective serotonin reuptake inhibitor (SSRI) is the most potent inhibitor of the norepinephrine transporter (NET)?

    A. Fluoxetine.
    B. Sertraline.
    C. Citalopram.
    D. Escitalopram.
    E. Paroxetine.

The correct response is option **E.**

Data from both humans and rodents (e.g., Gilmor et al. 2002; Owens et al. 2000), using the transfected human norepinephrine transporter (NET), revealed that paroxetine is the most potent inhibitor of the NET among the SSRIs. **(p. 260; see also Figure 15–2)**

15.2   Which SSRI is the most anticholinergic (with anticholinergic effects similar to those of desipramine)?

    A. Fluoxetine.
    B. Sertraline.
    C. Citalopram.
    D. Escitalopram.
    E. Paroxetine.

The correct response is option **E.**

The affinity of paroxetine for the muscarinic cholinergic receptor is approximately 22 nmol, which is similar to that of desipramine, although paroxetine is used in lower doses than desipramine and is therefore less anticholinergic than that drug. This property may account for its mild anticholinergic side effects, including dry mouth, blurry vision, and constipation (Owens et al. 1997). However, compared with nortriptyline, paroxetine has virtually no measurable anticholinergic activity in geriatric patients treated for depression (Pollock et al. 1998). **(pp. 260–261; see also Table 15–1)**

15.3   In prescribing paroxetine for elderly patients, which of the following pharmacokinetic properties of this drug should be taken into consideration?

    A. Paroxetine is the least anticholinergic of the selective serotonin reuptake inhibitors (SSRIs).
    B. Paroxetine is the least potent inhibitor of cytochrome P450 2D6 among the SSRIs.
    C. There is a threefold increase in maximum plasma concentration in elderly subjects.
    D. The drug's half-life is reduced by 50% in elderly patients.
    E. Paroxetine is associated with type 2 diabetes.

The correct response is option **C.**

The pharmacokinetic properties of paroxetine appear to be affected by age. Bayer et al. (1989) reported a threefold increase in maximum plasma concentration in elderly subjects compared with younger subjects. **(p. 262)**

15.4   Which selective serotonin reuptake inhibitor (SSRI) is the most potent inhibitor of cytochrome P450 2D6?

A. Paroxetine.
B. Sertraline.
C. Citalopram.
D. Escitalopram.
E. Fluoxetine.

The correct response is option **A.**

Paroxetine is the most potent inhibitor of the 2D6 enzyme system of all the SSRIs (Crewe et al. 1992; Nemeroff et al. 1996). As both a substrate for and an inhibitor of its own metabolism, paroxetine has a nonlinear pharmacokinetic profile, such that higher doses produce disproportionately greater plasma drug concentrations as the enzyme becomes saturated and, therefore, less available for metabolic activity (Preskorn 1993). **(p. 262)**

15.5   For patients with obsessive-compulsive disorder (OCD), optimal treatment with paroxetine typically requires

A. 10 mg/day, 3–12 weeks until response.
B. ≥60 mg/day, 3–12 weeks until response.
C. 20 mg/day, 2–4 weeks until response.
D. 40 mg/day, less than 2 weeks until response.
E. None of the above.

The correct response is option **B.**

Typically, total daily doses of greater than or equal to 60 mg of paroxetine are required to optimally treat OCD. Although patients characteristically respond to treatment within 3–4 weeks, clinical improvement may not be discernible until 10–12 weeks; therefore, a standard drug trial of up to 12 weeks should be conducted before an alternative medication is considered (Rasmussen et al. 1993). **(p. 268)**

References

Bayer AJ, Roberts NA, Allen EA, et al: The pharmacokinetics of paroxetine in the elderly. Acta Psychiatr Scand Suppl 350:152–155, 1989

Crewe HK, Lennard MS, Tucker GT, et al: The effect of selective serotonin re-uptake inhibitors on cytochrome P450 2D6 (CYP2D6) activity in human liver microsomes. Br J Clin Pharmacol 34:262–265, 1992

Gilmor ML, Owens MJ, Nemeroff CB: Inhibition of norepinephrine uptake in patients with major depression treated with paroxetine. Am J Psychiatry 159:1702–1710, 2002

Nemeroff CB, DeVane CL, Pollock BG: Newer antidepressants and the cytochrome P450 system. Am J Psychiatry 153:311–320, 1996

Owens MJ, Morgan WN, Plott SJ, et al: Neurotransmitter receptor and transporter binding profiles of antidepressants and their metabolites. J Pharmacol Exp Ther 283:1305–1322, 1997

Owens MJ, Knight DJ, Nemeroff CB: Paroxetine binding to the rat norepinephrine transporter in vivo. Biol Psychiatry 47:842–845, 2000

Pollock GB, Mulsant BH, Nebes R, et al: Serum anticholinergicity in elderly depressed patients treated with paroxetine or nortriptyline. Am J Psychiatry 155:1110–1112, 1998

Preskorn SH: Pharmacokinetics of antidepressants: why and how they are relevant to treatment. J Clin Psychiatry 54 (suppl 9):14–34, 1993

Rasmussen SA, Eisen JL, Pato MT: Current issues in the pharmacologic management of obsessive compulsive disorder. J Clin Psychiatry 54 (suppl 6):4–9, 1993

CHAPTER 16

Fluvoxamine

Select the single best response for each question.

16.1   Fluvoxamine is approved by the U.S. Food and Drug Administration (FDA) for use in treating which of the following?

A.   Major depression.
B.   Panic disorder.
C.   Obsessive-compulsive disorder (OCD).
D.   Posttraumatic stress disorder.
E.   OCD in adults only.

The correct response is option **C.**

In 1994, the FDA approved fluvoxamine for treatment of OCD across all age groups. Although there is good research to support its use in the treatment of a variety of other psychiatric disorders across the life span, including major depression (Kasper et al. 1992), panic disorder (Figgitt and McClellan 2000), and posttraumatic stress disorder (Tucker et al. 2000), it has not received FDA approval for these other indications. **(pp. 284, 286–288)**

16.2   Which of the following statements accurately describes fluvoxamine's pharmacokinetic profile?

A.   Well absorbed orally, long half-life, high protein binding, metabolized to active metabolites.
B.   Well absorbed, moderate half-life, low protein binding, excreted unchanged by the renal system.
C.   Well absorbed, moderate half-life, low protein binding, metabolized to inactive metabolites.
D.   Poorly absorbed, short half-life, high protein binding, metabolized to inactive metabolites.
E.   Poorly absorbed, long half-life, low protein binding, metabolized to active metabolites.

The correct response is option **C.**

Fluvoxamine is well absorbed after oral intake (Van Harten 1993), with a mean plasma half-life reached 19 hours after single-dose administration (De Vries et al. 1992); has low protein binding compared with other selective serotonin reuptake inhibitors; and is metabolized extensively by oxidative metabolism in the liver to inactive metabolites. **(p. 285)**

16.3   Steady-state fluvoxamine levels are reported to be

A.   Two- to fourfold higher in children than in adolescents.
B.   Two- to fourfold lower in children than in adolescents.
C.   The same in children as in adolescents.
D.   Lower in female children compared with male children.
E.   None of the above.

The correct response is option **A.**

Steady-state fluvoxamine concentrations are reported to be two- to fourfold higher in children than in adolescents, with female children showing significantly higher concentrations compared with male children. **(p. 285)**

16.4   Fluvoxamine has been demonstrated in placebo-controlled studies to be efficacious in which of the following?

   A. Trichotillomania.
   B. Relapse of alcohol dependence.
   C. Anxiety disorders in the elderly.
   D. Social phobia.
   E. Pathological gambling.

The correct response is option **D.**

In a double-blind, placebo-controlled trial (Stein et al. 1999) and a randomized controlled trial ("Fluvoxamine for the Treatment of Anxiety Disorders in Children and Adolescents" 2001) of fluvoxamine for social phobia, fluvoxamine reduced scores on standard symptom scales compared with placebo. Fluvoxamine has shown limited results with trichotillomania (Stanley et al. 1997). No placebo-controlled studies of fluvoxamine in anxiety disorders have been reported, although fluvoxamine was found to be effective in an open trial of 12 older patients with a variety of anxiety disorders (Wylie et al. 2000). In one large study, patients taking fluvoxamine tended to do worse in maintaining abstinence from alcohol (Chick et al. 2004). Fluvoxamine's efficacy in pathological gambling has not been clearly demonstrated; fluvoxamine improved pathological gambling in males and younger patients, but not in the full sample (Hollander et al. 2000). **(pp. 287, 288)**

16.5   Which of the following statements about sexual side effects of fluvoxamine is *true*?

   A. Sexual side effects with fluvoxamine are similar in frequency to those with other selective serotonin reuptake inhibitors (SSRIs).
   B. Sexual side effects with fluvoxamine are fewer in frequency than with other SSRIs.
   C. Fluvoxamine provokes more delayed orgasm than does paroxetine.
   D. Investigators find an increased incidence of sexual dysfunction when spontaneous reporting rather than direct questioning is used.
   E. Sexual dysfunction may persist for a long period after discontinuation of fluvoxamine.

The correct response is option **A.**

Sexual dysfunction during fluvoxamine treatment appears to be the same as that during treatment with other SSRIs. Results of a prospective multicenter study of outpatients being treated with fluvoxamine, fluoxetine, paroxetine, or sertraline showed that paroxetine provokes more delay of orgasm or ejaculation and more impotence than does fluvoxamine, fluoxetine, or sertraline. Overall, a significant increase in the incidence of sexual dysfunction was seen when direct questioning (58%) versus spontaneous reporting by patients (14%) was used. Patients' sexual function improved when the dose of the SSRI was lowered or tapered (Montejo-Gonzalez et al. 1997). In general, it is important to reassure the patient that sexual difficulties are reversible after discontinuation of the drug. **(p. 288)**

16.6   Fluvoxamine shows potent inhibition of which cytochrome P450 enzyme?

   A. 2C19.
   B. 3A4.
   C. 2D6.
   D. 2E1.
   E. 1A2.

The correct response is option **E**.

Fluvoxamine is a weak inhibitor of cytochrome P450 2D6, a moderate inhibitor of cytochrome P450 enzymes 2C19 and 3A4, and a potent inhibitor of cytochrome P450 1A2. **(p. 289)**

References

Chick J, Aschauer H, Hornik K: Efficacy of fluvoxamine in preventing relapse in alcohol dependence: a one-year, double-blind, placebo-controlled multicentre study with analysis by typology. Drug Alcohol Depend 74:61–70, 2004

De Vries MH, Raghoebar M, Mathlener IS, et al: Single and multiple oral dose fluvoxamine kinetics in young and elderly subjects. Ther Drug Monit 14:493–498, 1992

Figgitt DP, McClellan KJ: Fluvoxamine: an updated review of its use in the management of adults with anxiety disorders. Drugs 60:925–954, 2000

Fluvoxamine for the treatment of anxiety disorders in children and adolescents. RUPP Anxiety Study Group. N Engl J Med 344:1279–1285, 2001

Hollander E, DeCaria CM, Finkell JN, et al: A randomized double-blind fluvoxamine/placebo crossover trial in pathologic gambling. Biol Psychiatry 47:813–817, 2000

Kasper S, Fuger J, Moller HJ: Comparative efficacy of antidepressants. Drugs 43 (suppl 2):11–23, 1992

Montejo-Gonzalez A, Liorca G, Izquierdo J, et al: SSRI-induced sexual dysfunction: fluoxetine, paroxetine, sertraline, and fluvoxamine in a prospective, multicenter, and descriptive clinical study of 344 patients. J Sex Marital Ther 23:176–194, 1997

Stanley MA, Breckenridge JK, Swann AC: Fluvoxamine treatment in trichotillomania. J Clin Psychopharmacol 17:278–283, 1997

Stein MB, Fyer AJ, Davidson JRT, et al: Fluvoxamine treatment of social phobia (social anxiety disorder): a double-blind, placebo-controlled study. Am J Psychiatry 156:756–760, 1999

Tucker P, Smith KL, Marx B, et al: Fluvoxamine reduces physiologic reactivity to trauma scripts in posttraumatic stress disorder. J Clin Psychopharmacol 20:367–372, 2000

Van Harten J: Clinical pharmacokinetics of selective serotonin reuptake inhibitors. Clin Pharmacokinet 24:203–220, 1993

Wylie ME, Miller MD, Shear MK: Fluvoxamine pharmacotherapy of anxiety disorders in later life: preliminary open-trial data. J Geriatr Psychiatry Neurol 13:43–48, 2000

CHAPTER 17

Citalopram and *S*-Citalopram

Select the single best response for each question.

17.1   Comparisons of *S*-citalopram and *R*-citalopram have revealed all of the following *except*

    A. *S*-Citalopram is 30-fold more potent than *R*-citalopram in inhibiting the serotonin transporter (5-HTT).

    B. *S*-Citalopram's half-life is the same as that of *R*-citalopram.

    C. *S*-Citalopram's half-life is shorter than that of *R*-citalopram.

    D. *S*-Citalopram may have less propensity to inhibit cytochrome P450 enzymes than does *R*-citalopram.

    E. *S*- and *R*-citalopram undergo similar metabolism by cytochrome P450 enzymes.

The correct response is option **B**.

Preclinical studies indicate that inhibition of 5-HTT activity resides in the *S*-enantiomer (Hyttel et al. 1992), with *S*-citalopram being 30-fold more potent than *R*-citalopram at inhibiting serotonin transport (Owens et al. 2001). *S*-Citalopram also appears to be more selective than *R*-citalopram both in terms of inhibition of monoamine reuptake and in terms of neurotransmitter receptor interactions (Owens et al. 2001). Additionally, some in vitro evidence indicates that *S*-citalopram has a slightly lower potential to interact with the liver cytochrome P450 system compared with *R*-citalopram, which decreases the likelihood for drug–drug interactions at the level of drug metabolism (von Moltke et al. 2001). The human cytochromes involved in the metabolism of *S*-citalopram are the same as those reported for *R*-citalopram (von Moltke et al. 2001). The average half-lives of the two enantiomers differ. In one study of five hospitalized depressed patients, the half-life of *S*-citalopram (42 ± 13 hours) was shorter than that of *R*-citalopram (66 ± 11 hours) (Voirol et al. 1999). **(pp. 291, 293)**

17.2   Citalopram has been shown in double-blind, placebo-controlled trials to have efficacy in the treatment of which of the following?

    A. Major depression, obsessive-compulsive disorder (OCD), and bulimia.

    B. Major depression, OCD, and trichotillomania.

    C. OCD, panic disorder, and poststroke depression.

    D. Panic disorder, poststroke depression, and pathological gambling.

    E. Major depression and panic disorder only.

The correct response is option **C**.

Citalopram's efficacy in the treatment of depression has been shown in at least 11 placebo-controlled clinical trials (for review, see Keller 2000). Although its use in other psychiatric conditions has not been as thoroughly studied, the few well-controlled trials that have been completed suggest that citalopram may have a significant role in treating a wide range of psychiatric illnesses, including OCD (Montgomery et al. 2001), panic disorder (Lepola et al. 1998), poststroke depression (Andersen et al. 1994), and anxiety associated with depression (Flicker and Hakkarainen 1998). **(pp. 295–297)**

17.3   The most common side effects of citalopram are

A. Nausea, increased sweating, and dry mouth.
B. Sexual side effects, tremor, and somnolence.
C. Nausea, headache, and diarrhea.
D. Sexual side effects.
E. Cardiac conduction effects, nausea, and dry mouth.

The correct response is option **A.**

In a meta-analysis of 746 depressed patients who took part in several short-term clinical trials, the most common adverse events associated with citalopram were nausea and vomiting (20%), increased sweating (18%), and dry mouth and headache (17%) (Baldwin and Johnson 1995). The incidence rates of these adverse events were less than 10% above those seen with placebo and were comparable to those seen with other selective serotonin reuptake inhibitors. At therapeutic doses, citalopram does not have significant cardiovascular effects. Analysis of electrocardiographic (ECG) data from prospective studies in healthy volunteers and patients, as well as retrospective ECG data from all clinical trials conducted from 1978 to 1996 (a total of 40 trials), concluded that citalopram is without significant effect on cardiac conduction and repolarization (Rasmussen et al. 1999). **(p. 298)**

17.4   Citalopram has a low likelihood of drug–drug interactions because

A. It is highly protein-bound.
B. It is metabolized mainly by cytochrome P450 2C19.
C. It is eliminated primarily via renal clearance.
D. It is a potent inhibitor of several cytochrome P450 enzymes; therefore, it increases the levels of coadministered drugs.
E. It is metabolized by three different cytochrome P450 enzymes; therefore, inhibition of any one of these enzymes by another drug is unlikely to significantly affect citalopram's metabolism.

The correct response is option **E.**

Because multiple cytochrome P450 enzymes (2C19, 3A4, and 2D6) contribute equally to the metabolism of citalopram, inhibition of any one of these enzymes by another drug is unlikely to significantly affect the overall metabolism of citalopram. In addition, citalopram is less strongly protein-bound than many other compounds and therefore is less susceptible to drug–drug interactions at the level of protein binding. Renal clearance is only a small part of citalopram's clearance; thus, reduced renal function does not have a major effect on the drug's kinetics (Joffe et al. 1998). Citalopram is not a potent inhibitor of enzymes; in vitro studies show that citalopram only weakly inhibits cytochrome P450 enzymes 1A2 and 2C19 and does not significantly inhibit 2C9, 2E1, and 3A (von Moltke et al. 1999). Citalopram is also a relatively weak inhibitor of 2D6. **(p. 298; see also pp. 292, 293)**

17.5   The side effects of *S*-citalopram differ from those of citalopram in which of the following ways?

A. *S*-Citalopram is associated with greater cardiovascular effects.
B. *S*-Citalopram is associated with fewer sexual side effects.
C. *S*-Citalopram is associated with greater gastrointestinal effects.
D. *S*-Citalopram and citalopram have similar side-effect profiles.
E. *S*-Citalopram is associated with greater weight gain.

The correct response is option **D.**

In general, the side effects associated with *S*-citalopram are similar to those observed with citalopram. **(p. 298)**

References

Andersen G, Vestergaard K, Lauritzen L: Effective treatment of poststroke depression with the selective serotonin reuptake inhibitor citalopram. Stroke 25:1099–1104, 1994

Baldwin D, Johnson FN: Tolerability and safety of citalopram. Reviews in Contemporary Pharmacotherapy 6:315–325, 1995

Flicker C, Hakkarainen H: Citalopram in anxious depression: anxiolytic effects and lack of activation. Biol Psychiatry 43:1S–133S, 1998

Hyttel J, Bogeso KP, Perregaard J, et al: The pharmacological effect of citalopram residues in the (S)-(+)-enantiomer. J Neural Transm Gen Sect 88:157–160, 1992

Joffe P, Larsen FS, Pedersen V, et al: Single-dose pharmacokinetics of citalopram in patients with moderate renal insufficiency or hepatic cirrhosis compared with healthy subjects. Eur J Clin Pharmacol 54:237–242, 1998

Keller MB: Citalopram therapy for depression: a review of 10 years of European experience and data from US clinical trials. J Clin Psychiatry 61:896–908, 2000

Lepola UM, Wade AG, Leinonen EV, et al: A controlled, prospective, 1-year trial of citalopram in the treatment of panic disorder. J Clin Psychiatry 59:528–534, 1998

Montgomery SA, Kasper S, Stein DJ, et al: Citalopram 20 mg, 40 mg and 60 mg are all effective and well tolerated compared with placebo in obsessive-compulsive disorder. Int Clin Psychopharmacol 16:75–86, 2001

Owens MJ, Knight DL, Nemeroff CB: Second-generation SSRIs: human monoamine transporter binding profile of escitalopram and R-fluoxetine. Biol Psychiatry 50:345–350, 2001

Rasmussen SL, Overo KF, Tanghoj P: Cardiac safety of citalopram: prospective trials and retrospective analyses. J Clin Psychopharmacol 19:407–415, 1999

Voirol P, Rubin C, Bryois C, et al: Pharmacokinetic consequences of a citalopram treatment discontinuation. Ther Drug Monit 21:263–266, 1999

von Moltke LL, Greenblatt DJ, Grassi JM, et al: Citalopram and desmethylcitalopram in vitro: human cytochromes mediating transformation, and cytochrome inhibitory effects. Biol Psychiatry 46:839–849, 1999

von Moltke LL, Greenblatt DJ, Giancarlo GM, et al: Escitalopram (S-citalopram) and its metabolites in vitro: cytochromes mediating biotransformation, inhibitory effects, and comparison to R-citalopram. Drug Metab Dispos 29:1102–1109, 2001

CHAPTER 18

Monoamine Oxidase Inhibitors

Select the single best response for each question.

18.1   Endogenous substrates for monoamine oxidase (MAO) isoenzymes include

    A. Acetylcholine, dopamine, and epinephrine.
    B. Tyramine, serotonin, and histamine.
    C. Epinephrine, dopamine, and serotonin.
    D. Histamine, acetylcholine, and serotonin.
    E. Tyramine, acetylcholine, and dopamine.

The correct response is option **C**.

The physiological functions of MAO's two isoenzymes—monoamine oxidase A (MAO-A) and monoamine oxidase B (MAO B)—have not been fully elucidated. The main substrates for MAO-A are epinephrine, norepinephrine, and serotonin. The main substrates for MAO-B are phenylethylamine, phenylethanolamine, tyramine, and benzylamine. Dopamine and tryptamine are metabolized by both MAO-A and MAO-B. **(p. 303)**

18.2   The therapeutic effect of monoamine oxidase inhibitors (MAOIs) is believed to be due to

    A. Amine accumulation in stored vesicles.
    B. Increases in amine levels at the synapse.
    C. Indirect norepinephrine and dopamine effects similar to those of stimulants.
    D. Amine accumulation in the cytoplasm, which leads to secondary adaptive mechanisms.
    E. Decreases in amine levels at the synapse.

The correct response is option **D**.

The target function of MAOIs is regulation of the monoamine content within the nervous system. Because MAO is bound to the outer surface of the plasma membrane of the mitochondria, in neurons, MAO is unable to deaminate amines that are present inside stored vesicles and can metabolize only amines that are present in the cytoplasm. As a result, MAO maintains a low cytoplasmic concentration of amines within the cells. Inhibition of neuronal MAO produces an increase in the amine content in the cytoplasm. Initially, it was believed that the therapeutic action of MAOIs was a result of this amine accumulation. More recently, it has been suggested that secondary adaptive mechanisms may be important for the antidepressant action of these agents. **(p. 304)**

18.3 Classic and irreversible monoamine oxidase inhibitors (MAOIs) have been shown in double-blind, placebo-controlled studies to be efficacious in all of the following *except*

A. Major depressive disorder.
B. Obsessive-compulsive disorder (OCD).
C. Panic disorder.
D. Dysthymia.
E. "Atypical" depression.

The correct response is option **B**.

Studies clearly indicate that MAOIs can be effective in major depression, "atypical" depression, panic disorder, and dysthymia. Although initial case reports suggested that MAOIs may be effective in OCD, no double-blind studies have confirmed efficacy. **(p. 305; see Table 18–2)**

18.4 Dietary restrictions with irreversible monoamine oxidase inhibitors (MAOIs) can be a challenge for patients. Which of the following groupings of foods/drinks can be ingested in moderation when taking an MAOI?

A. Cream cheese, coffee, chocolate, and beer.
B. Red wine, cheese, tea, and soy sauce.
C. Chicken liver, colas, cream cheese, and soy sauce.
D. Sherry, monosodium glutamate, and chocolate.
E. None of the above.

The correct response is option **A**.

All of the MAOI diets recommend restriction of cheese (with the exception of cream cheese and cottage cheese), red wine, sherry, liqueurs, pickled fish, overripe (aged) fruit, brewer's yeast, fava beans, beef and chicken liver, and fermented products. Other diets also recommend restriction of all alcoholic beverages, coffee, chocolate, colas, tea, yogurt, soy sauce, avocados, and bananas. The more restrictive the diet, the greater the risk of patient noncompliance. Furthermore, many of the compounds—for example, avocados and bananas—rarely cause hypertensive crisis. For example, an interaction may occur only if overripe fruit is eaten or, in the case of bananas, if the skin is eaten (which is an uncommon practice in the United States). Similarly, unless a person ingests large amounts of caffeine, the interaction is usually not clinically significant. **(p. 308; see Table 18–3)**

18.5 The most common and problematic side effect with phenelzine and isocarboxazid—both hydrazine-type, irreversible monoamine oxidase inhibitors (MAOIs)—is

A. Hypertensive crisis if tyramine is consumed.
B. Hepatitis.
C. Postural hypotension.
D. Headache.
E. Urinary hesitancy.

The correct response is option **C**.

For these two MAOIs, the most difficult side effect, often leading to discontinuation, is postural hypotension. Side effects similar to those of other MAOIs also occur. Although hepatitis secondary to phenelzine may occur, this effect is quite rare (<1 in 30,000). The other side effects listed also occur but are less frequent or are more easily managed. **(p. 310)**

18.6 All of the following statements regarding headaches with the use of monoamine oxidase inhibitors (MAOIs) are correct *except*

A. Headaches may occur with tyramine ingestion.
B. Headaches may be a result of a hypertensive crisis, in which case treatment with nifedipine is indicated.
C. Headaches may be due to low blood pressure (i.e., histamine headache).
D. Headaches are a common side effect of taking MAOIs and are not serious.
E. A severe headache after consuming food in someone taking an MAOI should receive prompt medical attention, given the potential risk of serious consequences such as cerebral hemorrhage.

The correct response is option **D.**

Headaches can be a common side effect of MAOIs. However, a severe headache can signal a hypertensive crisis precipitated by tyramine ingestion. The reaction usually develops within 20–60 minutes after ingestion of food. Occasionally, the reaction can be very severe and may lead to alteration of consciousness, hyperpyrexia, cerebral hemorrhage, and death. The classic treatment of the hypertensive reaction is phentolamine (5 mg) administered intravenously (Youdim et al. 1987; Zisook 1984). More recently, nifedipine, a calcium channel blocker, has been shown to be effective. It is important to differentiate a hypertensive reaction from histamine headache, which can also occur with an MAOI. Histamine headaches are usually accompanied by hypotension, colic, loose stools, salivation, and lacrimation (Cooper 1967). **(pp. 307–308)**

18.7 Drug–drug interactions are a potential drawback to use of irreversible monoamine oxidase inhibitors (MAOIs). Concomitant use with an MAOI must be avoided for all of the following drugs *except*

A. Carbamazepine.
B. Stimulants.
C. Selective serotonin reuptake inhibitors.
D. Meperidine.
E. L-Tryptophan.

The correct response is option **A.**

Carbamazepine, along with tricyclic antidepressants, can be used cautiously together with MAOIs in treating refractory depression. Stimulants, selective serotonin reuptake inhibitors, meperidine, and L-tryptophan are contraindicated in combination with MAOIs. **(p. 309, see Table 18–4)**

18.8 Regarding moclobemide, a reversible monoamine oxidase A (MAO-A) inhibitor, which of the following statements is *true*?

A. Moclobemide is effective as an adjunct treatment for Parkinson's disease.
B. Moclobemide has been shown to be effective for both endogenous and nonendogenous depression.
C. Dietary restrictions for moclobemide are similar to those for classic monoamine oxidase inhibitors (MAOIs).
D. Side effects of moclobemide are similar to those of classic MAOIs.
E. None of the above.

The correct response is option **B.**

Unlike the classic MAOIs, moclobemide has been shown to be effective in both endogenous and nonendogenous depression. It is selegiline (an MAO-B inhibitor), not moclobemide, that has been shown to be effective in Parkinson's disease. Intravenous tyramine pressor tests indicate that although a single dose of moclobemide increases tyramine sensitivity (Cusson et al. 1991), this increase is marginal compared with the increase associated with other MAOIs. Under most conditions, there appears to be limited drug–food interaction. Nausea is the only side effect noted to be greater in patients taking moclobemide than in patients taking placebo. Thus, the profile of moclobemide seems to be ideal in that the drug causes few or no major side effects. **(pp. 310–311, 312)**

References

Cooper AJ: MAO inhibitors and headache (letter). BMJ 2:420, 1967

Cusson JR, Goldenberg E, Larochelle P: Effect of a novel monoamine oxidase inhibitor, moclobemide, on the sensitivity to intravenous tyramine and norepinephrine in humans. J Clin Pharmacol 31:462–467, 1991

Youdim MBH, DaPrada M, Amrein R (eds): The cheese effect and new reversible MAO-A inhibitors. Proceedings of the Round Table of the International Conference on New Directions in Affective Disorders, Jerusalem, Israel, April 5–9, 1987

Zisook S: Side effects of isocarboxazid. J Clin Psychiatry 45 (7, part 2):53–58, 1984

CHAPTER 19

Trazodone and Nefazodone

Select the single best response for each question.

19.1   Which of the following statements best describes the receptor profile of trazodone?

  A. It is a mixed serotonin antagonist/agonist.
  B. It is a serotonin agonist.
  C. It is a serotonin antagonist.
  D. It is a serotonin, norepinephrine, and dopamine agonist.
  E. It is a serotonin, norepinephrine, and dopamine antagonist.

The correct response is option **A.**

Trazodone can be viewed as a mixed serotonergic agonist/antagonist, with the relative amount of *m*-chlorophenylpiperazine (mCPP) accumulation affecting the relative degree of the predominant agonist activity. **(p. 316)**

19.2   A 25-year-old man has been treated with trazodone 50 mg/day for sleep. If fluoxetine is added for the treatment of major depression, which of the following is likely to occur?

  A. Blood levels of trazodone's active metabolite will decrease.
  B. Blood levels of trazodone's active metabolite will increase.
  C. Blood levels of trazodone will decrease.
  D. Blood levels of both trazodone and its active metabolite will decrease.
  E. None of the above.

The correct response is option **B.**

Trazodone's active metabolite *m*-chlorophenylpiperazine (mCPP) is cleared more slowly than the parent compound and reaches higher concentrations in the brain than in plasma (Caccia et al. 1981). The cytochrome P450 2D6 and 3A microsomal enzyme systems also appear to play a role in trazodone metabolism. 3A inhibitors such as ketoconazole, ritonavir, and indinavir inhibit trazodone clearance (see Zalma et al. 2000), and ketoconazole inhibits mCPP formation (Rotzinger et al. 1998). The addition of fluoxetine to trazodone treatment can cause increases in plasma concentrations of both trazodone and mCPP (Maes et al. 1997). **(pp. 316, 318)**

19.3   In which of the following circumstances is the serotonin syndrome likely to develop?

  A. When a monoamine oxidase inhibitor (MAOI) is added to trazodone.
  B. When paroxetine is added to trazodone.
  C. When venlafaxine is added to trazodone.
  D. When duloxetine is added to trazodone.
  E. All of the above.

The correct response is option **E.**

The combination of trazodone with an MAOI, as with other antidepressants, should be handled with great caution, although there are case reports of the successful combination of trazodone with an MAOI (Zimmer et al. 1984). Development of the serotonin syndrome has been associated with the combination of trazodone with other proserotonergic agents, including MAOIs (Bodner et al. 1995). **(p. 318)**

19.4   A patient with major depression is prescribed nefazodone at a starting dosage of 200 mg twice a day. If the total daily dose is doubled, which of the following is likely to occur?

A.   Blood levels of nefazodone will be doubled.
B.   Plasma half-life will remain steady.
C.   Blood levels of nefazodone's four active metabolites will be decreased.
D.   Blood levels of nefazodone will be more than doubled.
E.   Blood levels of nefazodone will increase by 125%.

The correct response is option **D**.

Nefazodone has nonlinear kinetics, leading to greater-than-proportional mean plasma concentrations at higher dosages. Thus, if the dosage were doubled, blood levels of the drug would more than double. Nefazodone has three, not four, active metabolites: desethyl hydroxynefazodone (triazole dione), hydroxynefazodone, and *m*-chlorophenylpiperazine (mCPP). **(p. 319)**

References

Bodner RA, Lynch T, Lewis L, et al: Serotonin syndrome. Neurology 45:219–223, 1995

Caccia S, Ballabio M, Fanelli R, et al: Determination of plasma and brain concentrations of trazodone and its metabolite, 1-m-chlorophenylpiperazine, by gas-liquid chromatography. J Chromatogr 210:311–318, 1981

Maes M, Westenberg H, Vandoolaeghe E, et al: Effects of trazodone and fluoxetine in the treatment of major depression: therapeutic pharmacokinetic and pharmacodynamic interactions through formation of meta-chlorophenylpiperazine. J Clin Psychopharmacol 17:358–364, 1997

Rotzinger S, Fang J, Baker GB: Trazodone is metabolized to m-chlorophenylpiperazine by CYP3A4 from human sources. Drug Metab Dispos 26:572–575, 1998

Zalma A, von Moltke LL, Granda BW, et al: In vitro metabolism of trazodone by CYP3A: inhibition by ketoconazole and human immunodeficiency viral protease inhibitors. Biol Psychiatry 47:655–661, 2000

Zimmer B, Daly F, Benjamin L: More on combination antidepressant therapy. Arch Gen Psychiatry 41:527–528, 1984

CHAPTER 20

Bupropion

Select the single best response for each question.

20.1   Bupropion has been approved by the U.S. Food and Drug Administration (FDA) for which of the following indications?

    A. Major depression and panic disorder.
    B. Generalized anxiety disorder and smoking cessation.
    C. Major depression and smoking cessation.
    D. Panic disorder and smoking cessation.
    E. Obsessive-compulsive disorder and major depression.

The correct response is option **C**.

Bupropion's two FDA-approved indications are depression, for which bupropion is marketed under the names of Wellbutrin and Wellbutrin SR (sustained release), and smoking cessation, for which it is marketed under the name of Zyban. **(p. 330)**

20.2   A patient who is taking bupropion SR (sustained release) 300 mg daily for major depression develops rash, joint pain, fever, and lymphadenopathy. What is the likely diagnosis?

    A. An allergic reaction to the red dye in bupropion SR.
    B. A toxic drug interaction with caffeine.
    C. A toxic drug interaction with nicotine.
    D. Serum sickness.
    E. An unrelated medical illness.

The correct response is option **D**.

Allergic responses to bupropion, including Stevens-Johnson syndrome and a serum sickness–like reaction, which are characterized by arthralgias, fever, and rash, as well as lymphadenopathy, have been reported (Kanani et al. 2000; McCollom et al. 2000). Such responses are generally responsive to corticosteroid treatment. **(p. 334)**

20.3   Bupropion differs from the selective serotonin reuptake inhibitors (SSRIs) in which of the following ways?

    A. It has a higher incidence of sexual side effects and a lower incidence of sedation and weight gain.
    B. It has a lower incidence of sexual side effects and a lower incidence of sedation and weight gain.
    C. It has a lower incidence of sexual side effects and a higher incidence of sedation and weight gain.
    D. It has a lower incidence of sexual side effects and weight gain and a higher incidence of sedation.
    E. It has a higher incidence of sexual side effects and sedation and a lower incidence of weight gain.

The correct response is option **B**.

Bupropion sets itself apart from currently available antidepressants by its side-effect profile. In contrast to SSRIs, bupropion has been shown to be associated with lower rates of sexual dysfunction, less sedation, minimal effects on weight, and no discontinuation symptoms. **(p. 327)**

20.4   Which of the following statements about bupropion and attention-deficit/hyperactivity disorder (ADHD) is *true*?

   A. Bupropion is U.S. Food and Drug Administration approved for the treatment of ADHD in persons younger than 18 years.
   B. In clinical studies, bupropion has been found to be more effective than methylphenidate products for the treatment of ADHD.
   C. Bupropion is a second-line agent in the treatment of ADHD.
   D. Bupropion is less effective in the treatment of the inattentive form than of the combined form of ADHD.
   E. Bupropion is less effective in the treatment of girls than it is in boys with ADHD.

The correct response is option **C**.

Current recommendations suggest that bupropion is a useful second-line agent for uncomplicated ADHD and perhaps a first-line agent in patients with comorbid substance abuse or mood disorder (Cantwell 1998; Wilens et al. 2001). **(p. 333)**

20.5   Which of the following adverse effects of bupropion are clinically most common?

   A. Weight gain.
   B. Agitation, tremor, and insomnia.
   C. Dry mouth.
   D. Sexual dysfunction.
   E. All of the above.

The correct response is option **B.**

Clinically, the most common reason that adverse effects limit or prevent bupropion treatment tends to be the overstimulation effects of agitation, tremor, and insomnia (Settle 1998). **(p. 334)**

References

Cantwell DP: ADHD through the life span: the role of bupropion in treatment. J Clin Psychiatry 59:92–94, 1998

Kanani AS, Kalicinsky C, Warrington RJ, et al: Serum sickness–like reaction with bupropion sustained release. Canadian Journal of Allergy and Clinical Immunology 5:27–29, 2000

McCollom RA, Elbe DHT, Ritchie AH: Bupropion-induced serum sickness–like reaction. Ann Pharmacother 34:471–473, 2000

Settle E: Bupropion sustained release: side effect profile. J Clin Psychiatry 59 (suppl 4):32–36, 1998

Wilens TE, Spencer TJ, Biederman J, et al: A controlled clinical trial of bupropion for attention deficit hyperactivity disorder in adults. Am J Psychiatry 158:282–288, 2001

CHAPTER 21

Mirtazapine

Select the single best response for each question.

21.1 Mirtazapine is classified as…

A. A selective serotonin reuptake inhibitor (SSRI).
B. A noradrenergic and specific serotonergic antidepressant (NaSSA).
C. A serotonergic and noradrenergic reuptake inhibitor (SNRI).
D. A phenylpiperazine antidepressant.
E. A monoamine oxidase inhibitor (MAOI).

The correct response is option **B.**

Mirtazapine is described as a noradrenergic and specific serotonergic antidepressant (Holm and Markham 1999; Kent 2000; Nutt 1998). **(p. 341)**

21.2 A 27-year-old man who is taking mirtazapine for generalized anxiety disorder and major depression experiences significant sedation at a dosage of 7.5 mg/day. Which neurotransmitter receptor is most likely being affected?

A. Histamine$_1$ (H$_1$).
B. Serotonin$_2$ (5-hydroxytryptamine [5-HT]$_2$).
C. Dopamine$_2$ (D$_2$).
D. Serotonin$_3$ (5-HT$_3$).
E. None of the above.

The correct response is option **A.**

Mirtazapine has high affinity for H$_1$ receptors (De Boer 1996), blockade of which causes sedation and drowsiness. **(p. 341)**

21.3 Mirtazapine is primarily metabolized by which cytochrome P450 enzymes?

A. 2E1.
B. 3A5.
C. 1A2, 2D6, and 3A4.
D. 1A2 and 2E1.
E. 2C9 and 2C19.

The correct response is option **C.**

Mirtazapine is a substrate for cytochrome P450 1A2, 2D6, and 3A4 (Fawcett and Barkin 1998b; "Remeron" 2002). **(p. 342)**

21.4 A 49-year-old woman has major depression with a significant anxiety component. She is currently taking valproate for a seizure disorder. She has lost 8 kg in the past 2 months, and she reports great difficulty in falling asleep. Which of the following antidepressants would be the best choice for this patient?

A. Bupropion.
B. Fluoxetine.
C. Desipramine.
D. Selegiline.
E. Mirtazapine.

The correct response is option **E.**

Meta-analyses of placebo-controlled studies of patients with depression and associated symptoms of anxiety have demonstrated that mirtazapine-treated patients exhibit significant improvements in symptoms of anxiety (Fawcett and Barkin 1998a; Nutt 1998), beginning as early as the first week of treatment (Fawcett and Barkin 1998a). Mirtazapine appears to have no clinically significant effects on seizure threshold or on the cardiovascular system (Claghorn and Lesem 1995; Fawcett and Barkin 1998b; Kent 2000; Montgomery 1995). In addition, a trial of mirtazapine in patients with cancer revealed significant improvements in mood, anxiety, insomnia, appetite, weight, and pain symptoms by the study endpoint (Theobold et al. 2002). It has been suggested that mirtazapine could prove to be a safe and effective adjunct to cancer chemotherapy because of its ability to treat nausea via a serotonin$_3$ (5-hydroxytryptamine [5-HT]$_3$) receptor antagonism effect; insomnia, anorexia, and weight loss via histamine$_1$ (H$_1$) receptor antagonism; symptoms of depression via enhanced 5-HT and noradrenergic transmission by way of α_2-adrenergic, 5-HT$_2$, and 5-HT$_3$ receptor blockade; and symptoms of anxiety via 5-HT$_2$ and 5-HT$_3$ receptor antagonism (Kast 2001). **(pp. 343, 344, 345)**

21.5 A 19-year-old woman takes 150 mg of mirtazapine in a suicide attempt. Which of the following consequences is likely?

A. Stevens-Johnson syndrome.
B. Prolonged QTc.
C. Seizure.
D. Renal failure.
E. Disorientation and drowsiness, with tachycardia.

The correct response is option **E.**

Symptoms reported in cases of mirtazapine overdose include disorientation, drowsiness, impaired memory, and tachycardia (Fawcett and Barkin 1998b; Kent 2000; Montgomery 1995; Stimmel et al. 1997). **(p. 345)**

References

Claghorn JL, Lesem MD: A double-blind placebo-controlled study of Org 3770 in depressed outpatients. J Affect Disord 34:165–171, 1995

De Boer T: The pharmacologic profile of mirtazapine. J Clin Psychiatry 57 (suppl 4):19–25, 1996

Fawcett J, Barkin RL: A meta-analysis of eight randomized, double-blind controlled clinical trials of mirtazapine for the treatment of patients with major depression and symptoms of anxiety. J Clin Psychiatry 59:123–127, 1998a

Fawcett J, Barkin RL: Review of the results from clinical studies on the efficacy, safety and tolerability of mirtazapine for the treatment of patients with major depression. J Affect Disord 51:267–285, 1998b

Holm KJ, Markham A: Mirtazapine: a review of its use in major depression. Drugs 57:607–631, 1999

Kast RE: Mirtazapine may be useful in treating nausea and insomnia of cancer chemotherapy. Support Care Cancer 9:469–470, 2001

Kent JM: SNaRIs, NaSSAs, and NaRIs: new agents for the treatment of depression. Lancet 355:911–918, 2000

Montgomery SA: Safety of mirtazapine: a review. Int Clin Psychopharmacol 10 (suppl 4):37–45, 1995

Nutt DJ: Efficacy of mirtazapine in clinically relevant subgroups of depressed patients. Depress Anxiety 7 (suppl 1):7–10, 1998

Remeron (package insert). Physicians' Desk Reference, 56th Edition. Montvale, NJ, Medical Economics Company, 2002

Stimmel GL, Dopheide JA, Stahl SM: Mirtazapine: an antidepressant with noradrenergic and specific serotonergic effects. Pharmacotherapy 17:10–21, 1997

Theobold DE, Kirsh KE, Holtszclaw E, et al: An open-label, crossover trial of mirtazapine (15 and 30 mg) in cancer patients with pain and other distressing symptoms. J Pain Symptom Manage 23:442–447, 2002

CHAPTER 22

Venlafaxine

Select the single best response for each question.

22.1 Which of the following drugs is minimally protein-bound?

A. Olanzapine.
B. Fluoxetine.
C. Warfarin.
D. Venlafaxine.
E. All of the above.

The correct response is option **D**.

According to the manufacturer's package insert, both venlafaxine and its primary metabolite, O-desmethylvenlafaxine (ODV), are minimally bound to plasma albumin at therapeutic concentrations (27% and 30%, respectively). **(p. 350)**

22.2 What is venlafaxine's primary route of excretion?

A. Pulmonary.
B. Hepatic.
C. Renal.
D. None of the above.
E. Unknown.

The correct response is option **C**.

Renal elimination is the primary route of excretion for venlafaxine, its primary metabolite (O-desmethylvenlafaxine [ODV]), and its other minor metabolites (Howell et al. 1993). **(p. 350)**

22.3 Which of the following drugs may produce a greater antidepressant response than selective serotonin reuptake inhibitors (SSRIs)?

A. Venlafaxine.
B. Lithium.
C. St. John's wort.
D. Mirtazapine.
E. Trazodone.

The correct response is option **A**.

Results from meta-analyses of published and unpublished studies comparing venlafaxine with SSRIs have provided further evidence that venlafaxine may produce a significantly greater antidepressant response than fluoxetine and perhaps than SSRIs as a class (Einarson et al. 1999; Smith et al. 2002; Thase et al. 2001). **(p. 351)**

22.4 Which of the following statements regarding treatment-emergent adverse effects of venlafaxine is *true*?

    A. Nausea is the most frequent treatment-emergent side effect, but it diminishes markedly after the first few weeks of therapy.

    B. Nausea is rarely a side effect.

    C. Nausea is the most frequent treatment-emergent side effect and rarely diminishes over time.

    D. The incidence and intensity of nausea are greater with extended-release (XR) venlafaxine than with immediate-release (IR) venlafaxine.

    E. None of the above.

The correct response is option **A**.

Nausea is the most frequently reported treatment-emergent adverse effect associated with venlafaxine therapy, with an incidence of 35% in short-term placebo-controlled trials (Preskorn 1995). Because of its rapid absorption and low protein binding, venlafaxine may pass more quickly from the bloodstream to the central nervous system (when compared with other serotonin [5-hydroxytryptamine (5-HT)] reuptake inhibitors), which probably explains the higher incidence of nausea early in treatment. The severity of this side effect diminishes markedly after the first few weeks of therapy, presumably because of downregulation or desensitization of brain stem $5\text{-}HT_3$ receptors. Because patients treated with XR venlafaxine have lower peak plasma concentrations of the drug, the incidence and intensity of nausea early in treatment may be somewhat *lower* with the XR formulation than with the IR formulation (Cunningham 1997). **(p. 355)**

22.5 Which of the following statements regarding potential hypertensive adverse effects of venlafaxine is *true*?

    A. All patients develop transient hypertension.

    B. Sustained hypertension is dose related with the immediate-release (IR) formulation.

    C. All treatment-emergent hypertension requires the addition of antihypertensive agents.

    D. Treatment-emergent hypertension requires discontinuation of venlafaxine.

    E. None of the above.

The correct response is option **B**.

Treatment with venlafaxine will cause sustained increases in blood pressure in some patients. Experience with the IR formulation in studies of depressed patients indicated that sustained hypertension was dose related, increasing from 3% to 7% at dosages of 100–300 mg/day, and to 13% at dosages above 300 mg/day (Thase 1998). Because approximately 50% of cases of treatment-emergent high blood pressure remitted spontaneously with continued therapy (Thase 1998), watchful waiting is a reasonable first strategy when elevation is modest. When hypertension persists, dosage reduction, switching antidepressants, or symptomatic treatment with an antihypertensive should be considered. **(p. 355)**

References

Cunningham LA: Once-daily venlafaxine extended release (XR) and venlafaxine immediate release (IR) in outpatients with major depression. Venlafaxine XR 208 Study Group. Ann Clin Psychiatry 9:157–164, 1997

Einarson TR, Arikian SR, Casciano J, et al: Comparison of extended-release venlafaxine, selective serotonin reuptake inhibitors, and tricyclic antidepressants in the treatment of depression: a meta-analysis of randomized controlled trials. Clin Ther 21:296–308, 1999

Howell SR, Husbands GE, Scatina JA, et al: Metabolic disposition of ^{14}C-venlafaxine in mouse, rat, dog, rhesus monkey and man. Xenobiotica 23:349–359, 1993

Preskorn SH: Comparison of the tolerability of bupropion, fluoxetine, imipramine, nefazodone, paroxetine, sertraline, and venlafaxine. J Clin Psychiatry 56:12–21, 1995

Smith D, Dempster C, Glanville J, et al: Efficacy and tolerability of venlafaxine compared with selective serotonin reuptake inhibitors and other antidepressants: a meta-analysis. Br J Psychiatry 180:396–404, 2002

Thase ME: Effects of venlafaxine on blood pressure: a meta-analysis of original data from 3744 depressed patients. J Clin Psychiatry 59:502–508, 1998

Thase ME, Entsuah AR, Rudolph RL: Remission rates during treatment with venlafaxine or selective serotonin reuptake inhibitors. Br J Psychiatry 178:234–241, 2001

CHAPTER 23

Duloxetine and Milnacipran

Select the single best response for each question.

23.1 Duloxetine and milnacipran are classified as

A. Selective serotonin reuptake inhibitors (SSRIs).
B. Tricyclic antidepressants (TCAs).
C. Monoamine oxidase inhibitors (MAOIs).
D. α_2-Adrenergic antagonists.
E. Serotonergic and noradrenergic reuptake inhibitors (SNRIs).

The correct response is option **E.**

Duloxetine hydrochloride and milnacipran join venlafaxine as members of a class of antidepressants known as serotonergic and noradrenergic reuptake inhibitors (SNRIs). **(p. 361)**

23.2 Regarding potential drug interactions, blood levels of duloxetine are most likely to be increased when it is coadministered with drugs that potently inhibit which cytochrome P450 enzyme?

A. 1A2.
B. 2D6.
C. 3A4.
D. 2C9.
E. 2C19.

The correct response is option **A.**

Administration of cytochrome P450 1A2 inhibitors such as fluvoxamine may result in elevated duloxetine concentrations. **(pp. 367–368)**

23.3 Serious drug interactions can result if duloxetine or milnacipran is coadministered with which of the following?

A. Selective serotonin reuptake inhibitors (SSRIs).
B. Monoamine oxidase inhibitors (MAOIs).
C. St. John's wort.
D. All of the above.
E. None of the above.

The correct response is option **D.**

Both duloxetine and milnacipran should be considered likely to have potentially serious interactions if given concomitantly with monoamine oxidase inhibitors. Both could induce adverse interactions if given over a prolonged period with SSRIs and possibly even with herbals such as St. John's wort. **(p. 368)**

23.4   Conditions for which duloxetine may be beneficial include which of the following?

    A. Chronic pain.
    B. Stress urinary incontinence.
    C. Depression.
    D. All of the above.
    E. None of the above.

The correct response is option **D**.

Duloxetine's efficacy in treating major depressive disorder has been demonstrated in six double-blind, placebo-controlled or active-comparator studies (for a review, see Nemeroff et al. 2002). In addition, duloxetine has been shown to benefit anxiety spectrum symptoms and chronic pain, producing significant improvement on Ham-D$_{17}$ Anxiety/Somatization subscale and Visual Analog Scale of pain severity scores, respectively (Detke et al. 2002). Finally, initial results from an early evaluation of 553 women randomized to placebo or duloxetine indicated significant and dose-dependent decreases in episode frequency of incontinence among duloxetine-treated women (Norton et al. 2002). **(pp. 363–365, 366)**

References

Detke MJ, Lu Y, Goldstein DJ, et al: Duloxetine 60 mg once daily dosing versus placebo in the acute treatment of major depression. J Psychiatr Res 36:383–390, 2002

Nemeroff CB, Schatzberg AF, Goldstein DJ, et al: Duloxetine for the treatment of major depressive disorder. Psychopharmacol Bull 36:106–132, 2002

Norton P, Zinner N, Yalcin I, et al: Duloxetine Urinary Incontinence Study Group: duloxetine versus placebo in the treatment of stress urinary incontinence. Am J Obstet Gynecol 187:40–48, 2002

CHAPTER 24

Benzodiazepines

Select the single best response for each question.

24.1   When administered orally, the benzodiazepine that produces the most rapid onset of action is

A. Lorazepam.
B. Chlordiazepoxide.
C. Prazepam.
D. Diazepam.
E. None of the above.

The correct response is option **D**.

Diazepam is rapidly absorbed and acts quickly, chlordiazepoxide and lorazepam have intermediate rates of absorption and onset of action, and prazepam is slowly absorbed and has a slow onset of action. **(p. 372)**

24.2   When administered orally, the benzodiazepine with the longest elimination half-life is

A. Flurazepam.
B. Clonazepam.
C. Diazepam.
D. Prazepam.
E. Lorazepam.

The correct response is option **A**.

Of the benzodiazepines listed above, flurazepam, at 40–120 hours, has the longest elimination half-life. The half-lives of the remaining options are as follows: clonazepam, 24–56 hours; diazepam, 26–50 hours; prazepam, >21 hours; and lorazepam, 10–20 hours. **(p. 373; see Table 24–1)**

24.3   When administered orally, the benzodiazepine with the shortest elimination half-life is

A. Lorazepam.
B. Oxazepam.
C. Triazolam.
D. Temazepam.
E. Alprazolam.

The correct response is option **C**.

Of the benzodiazepines listed above, triazolam, at 2–4 hours, has the shortest elimination half-life. The half-lives of the remaining options are as follows: lorazepam, 10–20 hours; oxazepam, 5–15 hours; temazepam, 6–16 hours; and alprazolam, 10–15 hours. **(p. 373; see Table 24–1)**

24.4   The triazolobenzodiazepines (i.e., alprazolam and triazolam) undergo phase I metabolism almost exclusively through which of the following cytochrome P450 enzymes?

A. 1A2.
B. 2B6.
C. 2C19.
D. 2D6.
E. 3A4.

The correct response is option **E.**

The triazolobenzodiazepines are metabolized principally by the cytochrome P450 enzyme 3A4. **(p. 373; see Table 24–1)**

24.5   All of the following pharmacological properties have been described for the benzodiazepine receptor *except*

A. Anticonvulsant effects.
B. Negative ionotropic effects.
C. Muscle relaxation effects.
D. Anxiolytic effects.
E. Sedative-hypnotic effects.

The correct response is option **B.**

Four distinct pharmacological properties have been described for the benzodiazepine receptor: anxiolytic, hypnotic, anticonvulsant, and muscle relaxation effects. Anxiolytic and sedative-hypnotic actions are mainly mediated by the benzodiazepine ω_1 receptor, and muscle relaxation through the ω_2 receptor. Most benzodiazepines interact with both of these receptor subtypes. **(p. 375)**

24.6   Phenytoin and barbiturates can precipitate benzodiazepine withdrawal through which of the following mechanisms?

A. Delayed gastric emptying.
B. Inhibition of hepatic conjugation.
C. Hepatic enzyme induction.
D. Inhibition of hepatic glucuronidation.
E. None of the above.

The correct response is option **C.**

Phenytoin and barbiturates cause hepatic enzyme induction and thus can reduce benzodiazepine half-life (Scott et al. 1983). **(pp. 377–378)**

Reference

Scott AK, Kher AS, Steele WH, et al: Oxazepam pharmacokinetics in patients with epilepsy treated long term with phenytoin alone or in combination with phenobarbitone. Br J Clin Pharmacol 16:441–444, 1983

CHAPTER 25

Buspirone and Gepirone

Select the single best response for each question.

25.1   Buspirone is thought to exert its anxiolytic actions through agonism of which of the following neurotransmitter receptors?

A. Serotonin (5-hydroxytryptamine)$_{1A}$ (5-HT$_{1A}$).
B. 5-HT$_{2A}$.
C. 5-HT$_{2C}$.
D. α_1-Adrenergic.
E. α_2-Adrenergic.

The correct response is option **A**.

5-HT$_{1A}$ receptor agonists have been developed as anxiolytic and antidepressant medications. Buspirone and gepirone, two 5-HT$_{1A}$ agonists, may exert their anxiolytic and antidepressive effects by initiating long-term changes in 5-HT neurotransmission. **(p. 393)**

25.2   Buspirone is metabolized principally by which of the following cytochrome P450 enzymes?

A. 1A2.
B. 2C19.
C. 2D6.
D. 2E1.
E. 3A4.

The correct response is option **E**.

Buspirone is metabolized by the cytochrome P450 enzyme 3A4 in the liver; therefore, inhibitors of 3A4 potentially increase plasma levels of the drug. Buspirone is not known to inhibit any cytochrome P450 enzyme. **(p. 394)**

25.3   The existing evidence base most strongly supports the effectiveness of buspirone in the treatment of

A. Obsessive-compulsive disorder (OCD).
B. Posttraumatic stress disorder (PTSD).
C. Panic disorder.
D. Generalized anxiety disorder (GAD).
E. Social phobia.

The correct response is option **D**.

In a meta-analysis of eight placebo-controlled studies involving 520 patients with GAD, buspirone was significantly more effective than placebo (Gammans et al. 1992). Buspirone is superior to placebo in the treatment of GAD even when depressive symptoms are present (Gammans et al. 1992; Sramek et al. 1996). (pp. 395, 397)

25.4   All of the serotonin (5-hydroxytryptamine [5-HT]) receptors are members of the G protein–coupled superfamily *except*

   A. 5-HT_{1A}.
   B. 5-HT_{2A}.
   C. 5-HT_{2C}.
   D. 5-HT_{3}.
   E. 5-HT_{4}.

The correct response is option **D**.

All of the 5-HT receptors with the exception of 5-HT_3 are members of the G protein–coupled superfamily. These receptors have differential affinity for 5-HT (Uphouse 1997). (p. 391)

25.5   Buspirone's major metabolite, which lacks the parent drug's serotonergic effects, is

   A. *m*-Chlorophenylpiperazine (mCPP).
   B. 1-Pyrimidinyl-piperazine (1-PP).
   C. 5-Hydroxyindoleacetic acid (5-HIAA).
   D. 3-Hydroxy-4-methoxyphenylglycol (MHPG).
   E. Homovanillic acid (HVA).

The correct response is option **B**.

The primary metabolite of buspirone is 1-PP. Brain levels of 1-PP can be several times higher than blood levels. 1-PP lacks buspirone's serotonergic effects but may block α_2-noradrenergic receptors and cause an increase in MHPG production. This effect is of interest because one study found a strong correlation between 1-PP blood levels and buspirone's efficacy in alcoholic patients (Tollefson et al. 1991). (p. 394)

25.6   The side effect most frequently encountered with buspirone is

   A. Nausea.
   B. Headache.
   C. Dizziness.
   D. Night sweats.
   E. Agitation.

The correct response is option **C**.

Buspirone has few side effects, both absolutely and relative to placebo. The rates reported are 12% for dizziness, 6% for headache, 8% for nausea, 5% for nervousness, 3% for light-headedness, and 2% for agitation ("Buspirone: Seven-Year Update" 1994). (p. 396)

References

Buspirone: seven-year update. J Clin Psychiatry 55:222–229, 1994

Gammans RE, Stringfellow JC, Hvizdos AJ, et al: Use of buspirone in patients with generalized anxiety disorder and coexisting depressive symptoms: a meta-analysis of eight randomized, controlled trials. Neuropsychobiology 25:193–201, 1992

Sramek JJ, Tansman M, Suri A, et al: Efficacy of buspirone in generalized anxiety disorder with coexisting mild depressive symptoms. J Clin Psychiatry 57:287–291, 1996

Tollefson GD, Lancaster SP, Montague-Clouse J: The association of buspirone and its metabolite 1-pyrimidinylpiperazine in the remission of comorbid anxiety with depressive features and alcohol dependency. Psychopharmacol Bull 27:163–170, 1991

Uphouse L: Multiple serotonin receptors: too many, not enough, or just the right number? Neurosci Biobehav Rev 21:679–698, 1997

CHAPTER 26

Investigational Treatments for Mood and Anxiety Disorders: CRH Receptor Antagonists, NK-1 Receptor Antagonists, and Glucocorticoid Receptor Antagonists

Select the single best response for each question.

26.1 Substance P receptor (neurokinin-1 [NK-1] receptor) antagonists are currently being investigated in the treatment of

A. Psychosis.
B. Obsessive-compulsive symptoms.
C. Depression.
D. Intractable pain.
E. Mania.

The correct response is option **C.**

After the initial report of an NK-1 receptor antagonist (Snider et al. 1991), many such antagonists were synthesized and tested, but none proved effective in treating pain in humans. Barden et al. (1983) found that antidepressants decrease substance P biosynthesis and suggested that alterations in NK-1 signaling may contribute to the clinical effects of these agents. Hence, it came as somewhat of a surprise when, 15 years later, Kramer et al. (1998) reported that in a double-blind, controlled study in which the NK-1 receptor antagonist MK-869 (300 mg at night) was compared with paroxetine (20 mg at night) and placebo, the two active drugs showed equivalent antidepressant effects and were superior to placebo in patients with major depressive disorder. All of the major pharmaceutical companies have several NK-1 antagonists in early clinical development. **(p. 411)**

26.2   In animal models of depression, antidepressant response correlates with

A. Decreased transcription and translation of brain glucocorticoid receptors (GRs).
B. Increased activity of corticotropin-releasing hormone (CRH).
C. Enhancement of the activity of hypothalamic vasopressin.
D. Diminished mineralocorticoid receptor (MR) functioning.
E. Improved GR functioning.

The correct response is option **E.**

In a study using the combined dexamethasone/CRH test, increasing dosages of dexamethasone were given to patients with depression and to patients in the control group to establish a dose–response curve. The curve showed the decreased sensitivity of GRs, to which dexamethasone selectively binds, among patients with depression (Modell et al. 1997). This decreased functional sensitivity of GRs results in the insufficient suppression of hypothalamic vasopressin and of other GR-related adrenocorticotropic hormone (ACTH) secretagogues. This phenomenon gradually disappears under successful treatment, thus raising the possibility that reinstatement of adequate GR function is of potential use as a marker for antidepressant action. Recent animal models support this hypothesis (Keck et al. 2002, 2003). **(p. 414)**

26.3   The mechanism by which metyrapone and ketoconazole are thought to exert possible antidepressant activity is

A. Inhibition of corticosteroid synthesis.
B. Inhibition of cytochrome P450 3A4.
C. Corticotropin-releasing hormone (CRH) receptor antagonism.
D. Catecholamine reuptake blockade.
E. Antagonism of neurokinin-1 (NK-1) receptors.

The correct response is option **A.**

Murphy et al. (1991) proposed that drugs (e.g., metyrapone) that block an enzyme essential to the synthesis of cortisol would be a useful adjunct in treating patients who fail to respond to standard antidepressants. This proposal led to a number of studies using metyrapone or ketoconazole either alone or as adjuncts to antidepressants (Ghadirian et al. 1995; O'Dwyer et al. 1995; Thakore and Dinan 1995; Wolkowitz et al. 1993). **(p. 416)**

26.4   In two open-label studies, mifepristone, also known as RU-486 or C-1073, demonstrated efficacy in treating which of the following?

A. Manic symptoms.
B. Posttraumatic stress disorder symptoms.
C. Obsessive-compulsive symptoms.
D. Binge eating.
E. Psychotic symptoms.

The correct response is option **E.**

Several small studies with C-1073, a combined progesterone and glucocorticoid receptor antagonist, have been conducted. In two open-label studies (Belanoff et al. 2001, 2002), mifepristone (at high dosages) seemed to be very effective, resulting in significant reductions of psychotic symptoms in patients with psychotic depression. These preliminary findings warrant confirmation in larger studies. **(p. 417)**

26.5 Corticotropin-releasing hormone receptor 1 (CRHR1) is found in all of the following brain structures *except*

    A. Olfactory bulb.
    B. Amygdala.
    C. Cortex.
    D. Locus coeruleus.
    E. Anterior lobe of the pituitary gland.

The correct response is option **D**.

CRHR1 is expressed at high levels throughout the central nervous system, including the anterior pituitary, cortex, amygdala, brain stem, olfactory bulb, hippocampal formation, and basal ganglia. It is absent in the locus coeruleus. **(p. 408, see Table 26–1)**

References

Barden N, Daigle M, Picard V, et al: Perturbation of rat brain serotonergic systems results in an inverse relation between substance P and serotonin concentrations measured in discrete nuclei. J Neurochem 41:834–840, 1983

Belanoff JK, Flores BH, Kalezhan M, et al: Rapid reversal of psychotic depression using mifepristone. J Clin Psychopharmacol 21:516–521, 2001

Belanoff JK, Rothschild J, Cassidy F, et al: An open label trial of C-1073 (mifepristone) for psychotic major depression. Biol Psychiatry 52:386–392, 2002

Ghadirian A, Engelsmann F, Dhar V, et al: The psychotropic effects of inhibitors of steroid biosynthesis in depressed patients refractory to treatment. Biol Psychiatry 37:369–375, 1995

Keck ME, Wigger A, Welt T, et al: Vasopressin mediates the response of the combined dexamethasone/CRH test in hyper-anxious rats: implications for pathogenesis of affective disorders. Neuropsychopharmacology 26:94–105, 2002

Keck ME, Welt T, Müller MB, et al: Reduction of hypothalamic vasopressinergic hyperdrive contributes to clinically relevant behavioral and neuroendocrine effects of chronic paroxetine treatment in a psychopathological rat model. Neuropsychopharmacology 28:235–243, 2003

Kramer MS, Cutler N, Feighner J, et al: Distinct mechanism for antidepressant activity by blockade of central substance P receptors. Science 281:1640–1645, 1998

Modell S, Yassouridis A, Huber J, et al: Corticosteroid receptor function is decreased in depressed patients. Neuroendocrinology 65:216–222, 1997

Murphy BEP, Dhar V, Ghadirian AM, et al: Response to steroid suppression in major depression resistant to antidepressant therapy. J Clin Psychopharmacol 11:121–126, 1991

O'Dwyer AM, Lightman SL, Marks MN, et al: Treatment of major depression with metyrapone and hydrocortisone. J Affect Disord 33:123–128, 1995

Snider RM, Constantine JW, Lowe JA III, et al: A potent nonpeptide antagonist of the substance P (NK1) receptor. Science 251:435–437, 1991

Thakore JH, Dinan TG: Cortisol synthesis inhibition: a new treatment strategy for the clinical and endocrine manifestations of depression. Biol Psychiatry 37:364–368, 1995

Wolkowitz OM, Reus VI, Manfredi F, et al: Ketoconazole administration in hypercortisolemic depression. Am J Psychiatry 150:810–812, 1993

CHAPTER 27

Classic Antipsychotic Medications

Select the single best response for each question.

27.1 A 42-year-old woman with a diagnosis of schizophrenia is unwilling to take any of the atypical antipsychotics because she has heard that they cause weight gain. She has a seizure disorder that is being treated with gabapentin. Which of the following classic antipsychotics would be a logical choice for this patient?

A. Thioridazine.
B. Chlorpromazine.
C. Molindone.
D. Pimozide.
E. Perphenazine.

The correct response is option **C.**

Molindone is the only member of the dihydroindoles available in the United States. Sharing a similar structure with the indoleamines, such as serotonin, molindone has the distinction of being the only classic antipsychotic not associated with any weight gain or lowering of the seizure threshold. **(p. 429; see also Figure 27–1)**

27.2 A 28-year-old man with a diagnosis of Tourette's syndrome has failed to respond to trials with two different atypical antipsychotics. Which of the following classic antipsychotics would be a logical choice for this patient?

A. Thioridazine.
B. Chlorpromazine.
C. Molindone.
D. Pimozide.
E. Perphenazine.

The correct response is option **D.**

Pimozide, the only agent of the diphenylbutylpiperidine class available in the United States, is approved only for the treatment of Tourette's syndrome and has the distinction of possessing the highest selectivity and potency for dopamine$_2$ receptors among the conventional antipsychotics. **(p. 429)**

27.3 According to positron emission tomography (PET) data, a dopamine$_2$ (D$_2$) receptor occupancy of what percentage correlates with the appearance of extrapyramidal side effects (EPS)?

A. 20%.
B. 40%.
C. 60%.
D. 80%.
E. None of the above.

The correct response is option **D.**

EPS were considered a sign of therapeutic antipsychotic dosage by early clinicians, who failed to realize the serious consequences to patients of long-term EPS associated with excessive D$_2$ blockade. Decades later, PET data revealed that a D$_2$ receptor occupancy of 65%–70% correlates with maximal antipsychotic efficacy, with EPS appearing beyond 78% D$_2$ occupancy but no increase in benefits at higher rates of occupancy (Kapur and Seeman 2001). **(pp. 432, 433)**

27.4 Which traditional antipsychotic is effective for the treatment of nausea and intractable hiccups?

A. Haloperidol.
B. Chlorpromazine.
C. Molindone.
D. Pimozide.
E. Perphenazine.

The correct response is option **B.**

The lower-potency antipsychotics exert a potent antiemetic effect through histamine$_1$ receptor antagonism. This effect is closely related to their original role in reducing perioperative stress and emesis. Many well-known antiemetics, such as promethazine (Phenergan), are phenothiazines with a short-chain substitution. In addition, chlorpromazine is approved for oral, intramuscular, or intravenous therapy of intractable hiccups, depending on severity. **(p. 433)**

27.5 An 18-year-old cocaine user is given intramuscular haloperidol in the emergency room to manage serious aggression. Medical personnel should actively monitor this patient for which of the following potential adverse effects?

A. Antipsychotic-induced parkinsonism.
B. Tardive dyskinesia.
C. Tardive dystonia.
D. Tardive dysmentia.
E. Dystonia.

The correct response is option **E.**

Conventional antipsychotic agents can reverse the psychosis associated with acute and chronic amphetamine intoxication as well as that associated with cocaine use. However, the risk of acute dystonia must be considered in these populations, given that dopamine receptor downregulation is common, resulting in greater sensitivity to rapid dopamine$_2$ blockade. **(p. 432)**

27.6   A patient has received haloperidol for the acute treatment of aggression for 3 days in an inpatient unit in addition to his usual dose of olanzapine. He develops a fever, tachycardia, and extreme agitation. Which of the following laboratory studies should be ordered?

A. Creatinine.
B. Electrocardiogram.
C. Creatine phosphokinase.
D. Electroencephalogram.
E. None of the above.

The correct response is option **C.**

Neuroleptic malignant syndrome (NMS) is characterized by muscular rigidity, hyperpyrexia (101–107°F), autonomic instability (hypotension or hypertension, tachycardia, diaphoresis, pallor), and altered consciousness (Arana and Rosenbaum 2000). NMS has an estimated incidence of 0.02%–2% and carries a mortality rate of 20%–30%. Death often occurs secondary to dysrhythmias, renal failure secondary to rhabdomyolysis, aspiration pneumonia, or respiratory failure. Laboratory findings include elevated creatine phosphokinase, elevated white blood cell count, and elevated liver enzymes. **(p. 437)**

References

Arana G, Rosenbaum J: Handbook of Psychiatric Drug Therapy. Philadelphia, PA, Lippincott Williams & Wilkins, 2000

Kapur S, Seeman P: Does fast dissociation from the dopamine D_2 receptor explain the action of atypical antipsychotics? A new hypothesis. Am J Psychiatry 158:360–369, 2001

CHAPTER 28

Clozapine

Select the single best response for each question.

28.1 What is the primary reason that clozapine is a second-line rather than a first-line treatment for schizophrenia in the United States?

A. Side effects such as sedation, constipation, and sialorrhea are very common and difficult to manage.

B. Other chemically related medications, such as olanzapine and quetiapine, are equally efficacious with fewer side effects.

C. Clozapine is not a second-line treatment for schizophrenia in the United States; it is a first-line treatment.

D. Use of clozapine carries a risk of agranulocytosis.

E. Clozapine is associated with a higher risk of extrapyramidal side effects (EPS).

The correct response is option **D.**

Although clozapine has numerous troublesome side effects, it is the risk of agranulocytosis that led to clozapine's approval as a second-line agent in the treatment of schizophrenia in the United States. It is not clear that olanzapine and quetiapine are just as effective, and clozapine actually has a lower risk of EPS. **(pp. 443, 445)**

28.2 What serum level of clozapine is associated with greater toxicity with no apparent clinical benefit?

A. >600 ng/mL.

B. Serum levels have not been associated with efficacy or toxicity with clozapine.

C. >350 ng/mL.

D. >250 ng/mL.

E. >1,000 ng/mL.

The correct response is option **A.**

High clozapine serum levels, such as those greater than 600 ng/mL, are not associated with a greater likelihood of improvement than are moderate levels, and they may be associated with a higher incidence of side effects. **(pp. 444, 445)**

28.3 Which of the following statements best describes clozapine's unique receptor profile?

A. High affinity for dopamine$_2$ (D$_2$) receptors and low affinity for serotonin$_{2A}$ (5-hydroxytryptamine [5-HT]$_{2A}$) receptors.

B. Low affinity for both D$_2$ and 5-HT$_{2A}$ receptors.

C. Moderate affinity for D$_2$ receptors and a high affinity for 5-HT$_{2A}$ receptors.

D. Moderate affinity for both D$_2$ and D$_4$ receptors.

E. Low affinity for D$_2$ receptors and a moderate affinity for 5-HT$_{2A}$ receptors.

The correct response is option **C.**

Clozapine has a moderate affinity for D_2 receptors and a high affinity for several other receptors, including 5-HT$_{2A}$, 5-HT$_{1C}$, adrenergic, cholinergic, and D_4 receptors. **(p. 445)**

28.4 Clozapine has been shown to be effective in all of the following conditions *except*

A. Treatment-refractory schizophrenia.
B. Depression with psychotic features.
C. Mania.
D. Psychosis in Parkinson's disease.
E. Maintenance therapy in schizophrenia.

The correct response is option **B.**

The evidence for clozapine in the treatment of depression with psychosis is limited to case reports or reports of small numbers of cases (Ranjan and Meltzer 1996; Rothschild 1996). Controlled studies have demonstrated clozapine's efficacy in treatment-refractory schizophrenia (Kane et al. 1988), in mania (Barbini et al. 1997), in psychosis in Parkinson's disease (Parkinson Study Group 1999), and in maintenance therapy in schizophrenia (Rosenheck et al. 1997). **(pp. 446, 447, 448)**

28.5 Regarding the monitoring of hematological parameters during clozapine treatment, which of the following statements is *false*?

A. Agranulocytosis occurs in less than 1% of patients taking clozapine in the United States.
B. If leukopenia occurs with clozapine use, a patient can be rechallenged several months later without an increased risk of redevelopment of leukopenia or agranulocytosis.
C. Agranulocytosis is defined as an absolute neutrophil count of $<500/mm^3$.
D. If leukopenia is identified early, most patients recover within 2–3 weeks following cessation of clozapine.
E. With early identification and proper management, most patients with clozapine-associated agranulocytosis fully recover.

The correct response is option **B.**

When clozapine treatment is discontinued upon identification of marked leukopenia, patients usually recover within 14–24 days and without any long-term consequences (Honigfeld et al. 1998). However, rechallenging patients who have experienced agranulocytosis almost always leads to reoccurrence of the problem. The onset of the second episode is more aggressive than the first episode. In nine patients who were known to be rechallenged, the average time to onset was 10 weeks shorter (14 weeks) than the first episode (24 weeks) (Safferman et al. 1992). **(p. 448)**

28.6 Which of the following factors appears to be associated with a greater risk of clozapine-associated myocarditis and cardiomyopathy?

A. Male gender.
B. Female gender.
C. Older than 50 years of age.
D. Younger than 50 years of age.
E. No obvious risk factors have been associated with these rare side effects.

The correct response is option **C.**

Novartis (2002) reported 178 cases of clozapine-associated cardiomyopathy, 80% of which involved patients younger than age 50 years. Almost 20% of the incidents resulted in death—an alarming figure that may reflect delay in diagnosis and treatment. **(p. 449)**

28.7   Regarding the metabolic side effects of clozapine, all of the following statements are true *except*

    A. Serum triglyceride and cholesterol levels increase with clozapine treatment.

    B. The average 6-month weight gain with clozapine treatment is 6.9 kg.

    C. If diabetes occurs, it usually appears within the first 6 months of treatment.

    D. Prescribing guidelines recommend regular monitoring of weight and glucose levels.

    E. Weight gain can persist for several years after starting clozapine.

The correct response is option **A.**

Whereas clozapine has been shown in several studies to increase triglyceride levels (Gaulin et al. 1999; Ghaeli and Dufresne 1996), total cholesterol, low-density lipoprotein cholesterol, and high-density lipoprotein cholesterol levels have not been shown to change significantly with clozapine use (Dursun et al. 1999). **(pp. 449, 450, 451, 452)**

28.8   Clozapine is metabolized primarily by cytochrome P450 1A2. Which of the following drugs can substantially increase clozapine serum levels by inhibiting cytochrome P450 1A2?

    A. Fluoxetine.

    B. Sertraline.

    C. Paroxetine.

    D. Carbamazepine.

    E. Fluvoxamine.

The correct response is option **E.**

Fluvoxamine is a potent inhibitor of cytochrome P450 1A2, and concurrent use of this drug with clozapine can lead to substantial elevations in clozapine levels (Heeringa et al. 1999). Paroxetine and fluoxetine can raise clozapine levels by inhibiting cytochrome P450 2D6 (Joos et al. 1997; Spina et al. 1998). **(p. 453)**

References

Barbini B, Scherillo P, Benedetti F, et al: Response to clozapine in acute mania is more rapid than that of chlorpromazine. Int Clin Psychopharmacol 12:109–112, 1997

Dursun SM, Szemis A, Andrews H, et al: The effects of clozapine on levels of total cholesterol and related lipids in serum of patients with schizophrenia: a prospective study. J Psychiatry Neurosci 24:453–455, 1999

Gaulin BD, Markowitz JS, Caley CF, et al: Clozapine-associated elevation in serum triglycerides. Am J Psychiatry 156:1270–1272, 1999

Ghaeli P, Dufresne RL: Serum triglyceride levels in patients treated with clozapine. Am J Health Syst Pharm 53:2079–2081, 1996

Heeringa M, Beurskens R, Schouten W, et al: Elevated plasma levels of clozapine after concomitant use of fluvoxamine. Pharm World Sci 21:243–244, 1999

Honigfeld G, Arellano F, Sethi J, et al: Reducing clozapine-related morbidity and mortality: 5 years of experience with the Clozaril National Registry. J Clin Psychiatry 59 (suppl 3):3–7, 1998

Joos AA, Konig F, Frank UG, et al: Dose-dependent pharmacokinetic interaction of clozapine and paroxetine in an extensive metabolizer. Pharmacopsychiatry 30:266–270, 1997

Kane J, Honigfeld G, Singer J, et al: Clozapine for the treatment-resistant schizophrenic: a double-blind comparison with chlorpromazine. Arch Gen Psychiatry 45:789–796, 1988

Novartis: Association of Clozaril with cardiovascular toxicity (Dear Healthcare Professional letter). Dorval, QC, Canada, Novartis Pharmaceuticals, 2002

Parkinson Study Group: Low-dose clozapine for the treatment of drug-induced psychosis in Parkinson's disease. N Engl J Med 340:757–763, 1999

Ranjan R, Meltzer HY: Acute and long-term effectiveness of clozapine in treatment-resistant psychotic depression. Biol Psychiatry 40:253–258, 1996

Rosenheck R, Cramer J, Xu W, et al: A comparison of clozapine and haloperidol in hospitalized patients with refractory schizophrenia. Department of Veterans Affairs Cooperative Study Group on Clozapine in Refractory Schizophrenia. N Engl J Med 337:809–815, 1997

Rothschild AJ: Management of psychotic, treatment-resistant depression. Psychiatr Clin North Am 19:237–252, 1996

Safferman AZ, Lieberman JA, Alvir JM, et al: Rechallenge in clozapine-induced agranulocytosis (letter). Lancet 339:1296–1297, 1992

Spina E, Avenoso A, Facciola G, et al: Effect of fluoxetine on the plasma concentrations of clozapine and its major metabolites in patients with schizophrenia. Int Clin Psychopharmacol 13:141–145, 1998

CHAPTER 29

Olanzapine

Select the single best response for each question.

29.1 Olanzapine's chemical structure is closest to that of which of the following drugs?

A. Diazepam.
B. Clozapine.
C. Quetiapine.
D. Risperidone.
E. None of the above; olanzapine's chemical structure is unique and not related to other approved drugs.

The correct response is option **B.**

Olanzapine is a thienobenzodiazepine derivative and is chemically related to clozapine. Its similarity to clozapine is thought to confer high-affinity binding in vitro to a broad spectrum of neurotransmitter receptors. **(p. 458; see also Figure 29–1)**

29.2 Many of olanzapine's receptor-binding properties are similar to those of clozapine. Which of the following statements is *false*?

A. Olanzapine nonselectively binds to many different dopamine receptors, whereas clozapine is only partially selective for dopamine$_2$ (D$_2$) receptors.
B. Olanzapine and clozapine both inhibit the firing of A10 neurons without significant inhibition of A9 tracts of the nigrostriatal projections.
C. Olanzapine and clozapine both have a high affinity for serotonin$_{2A}$ (5-hydroxytryptamine [5-HT]$_{2A}$) receptors.
D. Olanzapine and clozapine both have a low affinity for 5-HT$_1$ receptors.
E. Olanzapine and clozapine have moderate binding affinities for 5-HT$_3$ receptors.

The correct response is option **A.**

Clozapine nonselectively binds to all five dopamine receptor subtypes, whereas olanzapine is only partially selective for the D$_2$-like group. **(pp. 458, 459)**

29.3 All of the following statements about olanzapine's pharmacokinetics and disposition are true *except*

A. Olanzapine's clearance is decreased in the elderly.
B. Olanzapine's pharmacokinetics in children and adolescents is similar to that in nonsmoking adults.
C. Smoking decreases the clearance of olanzapine.
D. Cytochrome P450 1A2 is the main enzyme responsible for the formation of 4′-*N*-desmethylolanzapine.
E. Food has little effect on olanzapine's bioavailability after oral intake.

The correct response is option **C.**

Smoking is known to induce cytochrome P450 1A2 and can increase the clearance of olanzapine. One study showed that clearance in nonsmokers was 37% lower in men and 48% lower in women compared with smokers (Patel et al. 1996). **(pp. 459, 460, 468)**

29.4   Olanzapine has been approved by the U.S. Food and Drug Administration for treatment of which of the following indications?

   A. Schizophrenia, bipolar disorder, and depression associated with psychosis.
   B. Schizophrenia, mania, and depression associated with psychosis.
   C. Psychosis, bipolar disorder, and agitation and psychosis in the elderly.
   D. Psychosis, schizophrenia, and bipolar mania.
   E. Schizophrenia and schizoaffective disorder only.

The correct response is option **D.**

Whereas olanzapine was originally approved for treatment of psychosis, its list of indications now includes schizophrenia and bipolar mania. **(p. 462)**

29.5   Olanzapine has been demonstrated in placebo-controlled studies to be efficacious in which of the following?

   A. Posttraumatic stress disorder (PTSD).
   B. Borderline personality disorder.
   C. Schizoaffective disorder.
   D. Anorexia nervosa.
   E. Panic disorder.

The correct response is option **C.**

In a study by Tran et al. (1999), schizoaffective disorder patients who received olanzapine had a superior outcome, compared with patients who received haloperidol, on many, but not all, measures. PTSD, borderline personality disorder, and anorexia nervosa have been studied in olanzapine only in small open-label studies or small case series. **(p. 464)**

29.6   The risk of tardive dyskinesia associated with olanzapine treatment has been reported as

   A. Negligible.
   B. An annual rate of 2%–3%.
   C. Similar to that associated with haloperidol.
   D. An annual rate of 5%.
   E. An annual rate of 0.5%.

The correct response is option **E.**

Olanzapine's adverse-effect profile is generally benign in regard to neurological effects. Extrapyramidal side effects, as manifested by dystonic reactions and parkinsonism, occur at a low rate with olanzapine treatment, and pooled data from long-term comparison trials of atypical antipsychotics (Beasley et al. 1999) showed that tardive dyskinesia is 10- to 15-fold less common in olanzapine-treated patients (annual rate: 0.52%) compared with haloperidol-treated patients (annual rate: 7.45%). **(p. 466)**

References

Beasley C, Deliva MA, Tamura RN, et al: Randomised double-blind comparison of the incidence of tardive dyskinesia in patients with schizophrenia during long-term treatment with olanzapine or haloperidol. Br J Psychiatry 174:23–30, 1999

Patel BR, Kurtz DL, Callaghan JT, et al: Effects of smoking and gender on population pharmacokinetics of olanzapine (OL) in a phase III clinical trial (abstract). Pharm Res 13 (9, suppl):S408, 1996

Tran PV, Tollefson GD, Sanger TM, et al: Olanzapine versus haloperidol in the treatment of schizoaffective disorder: acute and long-term therapy. Br J Psychiatry 174:15–22, 1999

CHAPTER 30

Quetiapine

Select the single best response for each question.

30.1   Given that quetiapine is metabolized primarily by cytochrome P450 3A4, which of the following statements is *false*?

   A.   Coadministration of lithium with quetiapine has little or no effect on quetiapine levels.
   B.   Quetiapine is not vulnerable to drug–drug interactions.
   C.   Quetiapine's levels can be lowered by 3A4-inducing agents such as carbamazepine.
   D.   Quetiapine has little effect on other drug levels.
   E.   Erythromycin can raise quetiapine levels.

The correct response is option **B.**

Although quetiapine is primarily metabolized via the cytochrome P450 enzyme 3A4, it does not appear to inhibit any of the cytochrome P450 enzymes, nor does it induce the 3A4 enzyme (Goldstein 1999). However, drugs that alter the activity of 3A4 have the potential for drug–drug interactions with quetiapine. Drugs that are potent inhibitors of 3A4, such as erythromycin, are likely to raise quetiapine levels; drugs that induce 3A4, such as carbamazepine and phenytoin, will decrease quetiapine levels (Nemeroff et al. 2002). Lithium levels are not changed by quetiapine (Potkin et al. 2002). **(pp. 474, 483)**

30.2   Which of the following statements regarding quetiapine and negative symptoms of schizophrenia is *true*?

   A.   Overall, studies indicate that quetiapine is much more effective than haloperidol in treating negative symptoms, as measured by the Scale for the Assessment of Negative Symptoms (SANS).
   B.   Negative symptoms do not improve with quetiapine.
   C.   Quetiapine's high affinity for serotonin$_{1A}$ (5-hydroxytryptamine [5-HT]$_{1A}$) receptors may increase dopamine levels in the hypoactive mesocortical dopaminergic pathway, thereby improving negative symptoms.
   D.   Both A and C are correct.
   E.   None of the above.

The correct response is option **C.**

Quetiapine's higher affinity for the 5-HT$_{1A}$ receptor relative to the dopamine$_2$ receptor indicates substantial occupancy of 5-HT$_{1A}$ sites at therapeutic doses. This partial agonist activity may increase dopamine levels in the hypoactive mesocortical dopaminergic pathway, thereby improving negative and cognitive symptoms of schizophrenia (Goldstein 2002). Studies appear to indicate that haloperidol and quetiapine are roughly equivalent in efficacy for negative symptoms, as measured by the SANS (Arvanitis and Miller 1997; Small et al. 1997). **(pp. 475, 479)**

30.3   In studies comparing quetiapine and haloperidol, for which cluster of symptoms did quetiapine show superior efficacy?

   A.   Aggression and cognitive symptoms.
   B.   Negative and cognitive symptoms.
   C.   Positive and negative symptoms.
   D.   Cognitive symptoms only.
   E.   Negative symptoms only.

The correct response is option **A**.

A prospective double-blind study indicated that quetiapine was superior to haloperidol for cognitive symptoms (Purdon and Hellewell 2001). In addition, in another study, the Brief Psychiatric Rating Scale hostility cluster score showed quetiapine to be superior to placebo and haloperidol (Chengappa et al. 2003). **(pp. 479, 480)**

30.4   Quetiapine's risk for extrapyramidal side effects (EPS)

   A.   Is similar to that of placebo.
   B.   Is slightly higher than that of placebo.
   C.   Is similar to that of risperidone.
   D.   Is similar to that of haloperidol.
   E.   Has not been established.

The correct response is option **A**.

In placebo-controlled trials, quetiapine produced EPS at a rate no different from that of placebo (Goldstein 1999; Nasrallah and Tandon 2002). **(p. 481)**

30.5   Regarding changes in prolactin levels with quetiapine use, which of the following statements is *true*?

   A.   Prolactin levels begin to increase as the daily dose of quetiapine exceeds 300 mg.
   B.   Prolactin levels begin to increase as the daily dose of quetiapine exceeds 500 mg.
   C.   Prolactin levels show no difference compared to placebo over a wide range of daily doses of quetiapine (75–750 mg/day).
   D.   Elevations in prolactin are common with quetiapine and are not necessarily dose related.
   E.   None of the above.

The correct response is option **C**.

In placebo-controlled trials, there was no difference between placebo- and quetiapine-treated patients in changes from baseline prolactin levels, and this was true across the dosage range of quetiapine (75–750 mg/day) and regardless of the length of therapy (Hamner and Goldstein 2001; Hamner et al. 1996). **(p. 481)**

30.6   Quetiapine, in common with other second-generation atypical antipsychotics, has been associated with weight gain. Which of the following orderings accurately represents these agents' relative propensity (from highest to lowest) to cause weight gain?

   A.   Clozapine ~ olanzapine > quetiapine > ziprasidone > risperidone.
   B.   Quetiapine > clozapine ~ olanzapine > risperidone > ziprasidone.
   C.   Clozapine ~ olanzapine > quetiapine > risperidone > ziprasidone.
   D.   Quetiapine > olanzapine > clozapine > risperidone > ziprasidone.
   E.   Clozapine ~ olanzapine > risperidone > quetiapine > ziprasidone.

The correct response is option **E.**

Weight gain is a common adverse effect of many antipsychotic drugs; however, the propensity to produce weight gain differs among the various antipsychotics (Allison et al. 1999; Sussman 2001). During long-term treatment (1 year), the order of the atypical antipsychotics in terms of their relative amounts of weight gain has been reported to be clozapine ~ olanzapine > risperidone > quetiapine > ziprasidone (Nasrallah and Mulvihill 2001). Aripiprazole would likely follow ziprasidone (i.e., be associated with the least weight gain of the atypical antipsychotics). **(p. 481)**

References

Allison DB, Mentore JL, Heo M, et al: Antipsychotic-induced weight gain: a comprehensive research synthesis. Am J Psychiatry 156:1686–1696, 1999

Arvanitis LA, Miller BG. Multiple fixed doses of "Seroquel" (quetiapine) in patients with acute exacerbation of schizophrenia: a comparison with haloperidol and placebo. The Seroquel Trial 13 Study Group. Biol Psychiatry 42:233–246, 1997

Chengappa KN, Goldstein JM, Greenwood M, et al: A post hoc analysis of the impact on hostility and agitation of quetiapine and haloperidol among patients with schizophrenia. Clin Ther 25:530–541, 2003

Goldstein J: Quetiapine fumarate (Seroquel): a new atypical antipsychotic. Drugs Today (Barc) 35:193–210, 1999

Goldstein JM: Mechanism of action of quetiapine, a modulator of dopamine at the D_2 receptor. Presentation at the Society for Neuroscience, Orlando, FL, November 2–7, 2002

Hamner MB, Goldstein J: Acute and long-term effects of quetiapine on plasma prolactin levels. Presentation at the Society of Biological Psychiatry, New Orleans, LA, May 3–5, 2001

Hamner MB, Arvanitis LA, Miller BG, et al: Plasma prolactin in schizophrenia subjects treated with Seroquel (ICI 204, 636). Psychopharmacol Bull 32:107–110, 1996

Nasrallah HA, Mulvihill T: Iatrogenic disorders associated with conventional vs atypical antipsychotics. Ann Clin Psychiatry 13:215–227, 2001

Nasrallah H, Tandon R: Efficacy, safety and tolerability of quetiapine in patients with schizophrenia. J Clin Psychiatry 63 (suppl 13):12–20, 2002

Nemeroff CB, Kinkead B, Goldstein J: Quetiapine: preclinical studies, pharmacokinetics, drug interactions, and dosing. J Clin Psychiatry 63 (suppl 13):5–11, 2002

Potkin SG, Thyrum PT, Bera R, et al: Open-label study of the effect of combination quetiapine/lithium therapy on lithium pharmacokinetics and tolerability. Clin Ther 24:1809–1823, 2002

Purdon SE, Hellewell JSE: The effect of quetiapine in improving cognitive impairment in schizophrenia. Presentation at the International Congress on Schizophrenia Research, Whistler, BC, Canada, April 28–May 2, 2001

Small JG, Hirsch SR, Arvanitis LA, et al: Quetiapine in patients with schizophrenia: a high- and low-dose double-blind comparison with placebo. Seroquel Study Group. Arch Gen Psychiatry 54:549–557, 1997

Sussman N: Review of atypical antipsychotics and weight gain. J Clin Psychiatry 62 (suppl 23):5–12, 2001

CHAPTER 31

Aripiprazole

Select the single best response for each question.

31.1   Which of the following statements best describes the receptor profile of aripiprazole?

A. Dopamine$_2$ (D$_2$) partial antagonist, serotonin$_{1A}$ (5-hydroxytryptamine [5-HT]$_{1A}$) partial agonist, 5-HT$_{2A}$ agonist.

B. D$_2$ and 5-HT$_{1A}$ partial agonist, 5-HT$_{2A}$ agonist.

C. D$_2$ and 5-HT$_{1A}$ partial agonist, 5-HT$_{2A}$ antagonist.

D. D$_2$ partial antagonist, 5-HT$_{1A}$ partial agonist, 5-HT$_{2A}$ antagonist.

E. D$_2$ partial antagonist, 5-HT$_{1A}$ partial antagonist, 5-HT$_{2A}$ agonist.

The correct response is option **C**.

Aripiprazole exhibits potent partial-agonist activity at the D$_2$ (Burris et al. 2002) and 5-HT$_{1A}$ (Jordan et al. 2002) receptors, together with potent antagonist activity at the 5-HT$_{2A}$ receptor. **(p. 489)**

31.2   Which of the following describes the likely outcome if carbamazepine is coadministered with aripiprazole?

A. Carbamazepine will increase the blood levels of aripiprazole, and adverse effects from aripiprazole will ensue.

B. Aripiprazole will increase the blood levels of carbamazepine, and adverse effects from carbamazepine will ensue.

C. Aripiprazole will decrease the blood levels of carbamazepine.

D. Carbamazepine will decrease the blood levels of aripiprazole.

E. No drug–drug interaction will arise between aripiprazole and carbamazepine.

The correct response is option **D**.

In vivo studies show decreased levels of aripiprazole and dehydro-aripiprazole in the plasma when aripiprazole is coadministered with carbamazepine, a cytochrome P450 3A4 inducer. The aripiprazole dose should therefore be increased when the drug is administered concomitantly with carbamazepine. **(p. 492)**

31.3   Aripiprazole is associated with which of the following potential adverse effects?

A. Extreme weight gain.

B. Increases in triglycerides.

C. Increases in fasting blood glucose.

D. Increases in prolactin levels.

E. None of the above.

The correct response is option **E**.

Minimal changes in mean body weight were observed with aripiprazole treatment in short-term studies (Marder et al. 2003) and long-term studies (Carson et al. 2002; Kujawa et al. 2002). Aripiprazole treatment was not associated with increases in prolactin levels, or with adverse changes in glucose or lipid levels, during short- or long-term studies. Overall, aripiprazole treatment is associated with a very low incidence of extrapyramidal symptoms and with minimal or no effects on weight gain, QTc interval, or circulating levels of cholesterol, glucose, and prolactin. A pooled analysis of safety and tolerability data from the five short-term studies (Marder et al. 2003; Stock et al. 2002) showed that aripiprazole treatment was well tolerated. **(p. 492)**

31.4 A 62-year-old woman with schizophrenia is about to begin a trial of aripiprazole. Which of the following dosing adjustments may be necessary?

A. The initial dose must be lowered to 5 mg because of gender-related decreases in kidney function.
B. The initial dose must be increased to 20 mg because of gender-related increases in cytochrome P450 1A2 activity.
C. The initial dose must be increased to 20 mg if the patient smokes cigarettes.
D. No specific changes in dosing requirements are necessary.
E. Because she is older than 60 years, the initial dose must be increased because of the increased glomerular filtration rate.

The correct response is option **D**.

Patient demographic characteristics have not been shown to have any clinically significant impact on the pharmacokinetics of aripiprazole. In general, dosing does not need to be adjusted in regard to a patient's age, gender, race, smoking status, or hepatic or renal function. **(p. 489)**

References

Burris KD, Molski TF, Xu C, et al: Aripiprazole, a novel antipsychotic, is a high-affinity partial agonist at human dopamine D_2 receptors. J Pharmacol Exp Ther 302:381–389, 2002

Carson WH, Pigott TA, Saha AR, et al: Aripiprazole vs placebo in the treatment of chronic schizophrenia (abstract). Int J Neuropsychopharmacol 5 (suppl 1):S187, 2002

Jordan S, Koprivica V, Chen R, et al: The antipsychotic aripiprazole is a potent, partial agonist at the human 5-HT$_{1A}$ receptor. Eur J Pharmacol 441:137–140, 2002

Kujawa M, Saha AR, Ingenito GG, et al: Aripiprazole for long-term maintenance treatment of schizophrenia (abstract). Int J Neuropsychopharmacol 5 (suppl 1):S186, 2002

Marder SR, McQuade RD, Stock E, et al: Aripiprazole in the treatment of schizophrenia: safety and tolerability in short-term placebo-controlled trials. Schizophr Res 61:123–136, 2003

Stock E, Marder SR, Saha AR, et al: Safety and tolerability meta-analysis of aripiprazole in schizophrenia (abstract). Int J Neuropsychopharmacol 5 (suppl 1):S185, 2002

CHAPTER 32

Risperidone

Select the single best response for each question.

32.1   Which of the following statements best describes the receptor profile of risperidone?

   A.   Serotonin$_{2A}$ (5-hydroxytryptamine [5-HT]$_{2A}$) and dopamine$_2$ (D$_2$) agonism.
   B.   5-HT$_{2A}$ antagonism and D$_2$ agonism, modest histamine$_1$ (H$_1$) activity, and no affinity for α_1-adrenergic receptors.
   C.   5-HT$_{2A}$ and D$_2$ agonism and no affinity for histamine or α_1-adrenergic receptors.
   D.   5-HT$_{2A}$ and D$_2$ antagonism.
   E.   None of the above.

The correct response is option **D.**

Risperidone is a benzisoxazole derivative characterized by very high affinity for the 5-HT$_{2A}$ receptor and a moderately high affinity for the D$_2$, H$_1$, and α_1- and α_2-adrenergic receptors. In vitro, the affinity of risperidone for the 5-HT$_{2A}$ receptor is roughly 10- to 20-fold greater than that for the D$_2$ receptor (Leysen et al. 1994; Schotte et al. 1996). **(p. 495)**

32.2   A patient with bipolar mania is about to begin a trial with risperidone. Which of the following describes the likely time course of risperidone's absorption following oral administration?

   A.   Peak plasma level of risperidone will be reached only after 8 hours.
   B.   Because of its active metabolite, peak plasma levels will be reached in 12 hours.
   C.   Peak plasma levels of risperidone will be reached only after 16 hours.
   D.   Peak plasma levels of risperidone will be reached within 1 hour.
   E.   Peak plasma levels of risperidone will be reached in 6 hours.

The correct response is option **D.**

Risperidone is rapidly absorbed after oral administration, with peak plasma levels achieved within 1 hour (Heykants et al. 1994). **(p. 496)**

32.3   A 27-year-old man with schizophrenia is receiving risperidone 16 mg/day. Which of the following statements regarding likely side effects or interactions is *true*?

   A.   Because of his low dose of risperidone, he is likely to experience few adverse events.
   B.   If paroxetine is added, he is likely to have a decrease in his blood levels of risperidone.
   C.   He is unlikely to experience sexual adverse effects.
   D.   He is unlikely to experience parkinsonian symptoms.
   E.   He is at risk for parkinsonian symptoms.

The correct response is option **E.**

Risperidone generally has been very well tolerated in clinical trials. In a U.S. multicenter trial reported by Marder and Meibach (1994), only headache and dizziness were significantly more frequent with risperidone 6 mg/day, compared with placebo, whereas the group receiving higher-dose (16 mg/day) risperidone treatment also reported more extrapyramidal side effects and dyspepsia than did the group receiving placebo. Fatigue, sedation, accommodation disturbances, orthostatic dizziness, palpitations or tachycardia, weight gain, diminished sexual desire, and erectile dysfunction displayed a statistically significant relationship to risperidone dose. In the North American trials (Chouinard et al. 1993; Marder and Meibach 1994), risperidone produced significantly fewer parkinsonian side effects than did haloperidol (20 mg/day). Patients receiving risperidone (2 and 6 mg/day) did not differ from the group receiving placebo in mean ratings of parkinsonism and in the use of anticholinergic medication. Parkinsonism change scores were significantly correlated with the risperidone dosage ($r = 0.94$); however, risperidone (16 mg/day) was associated with fewer parkinsonian side effects than was haloperidol. Drug–drug interactions have not been convincingly demonstrated with risperidone (Byerly and DeVane 1996) **(pp. 500, 501, 502, 503)**

32.4 In clinical studies, risperidone's efficacy has been demonstrated for which of the following conditions?

   A. Schizophrenia, bipolar mania, and attention-deficit/hyperactivity disorder.
   B. Generalized anxiety disorder, and attention-deficit/hyperactivity disorder.
   C. Schizophrenia, bipolar mania, and autistic disorder.
   D. Oppositional defiant disorder, trichotillomania, and schizophrenia.
   E. None of the above.

The correct response is option **C**.

Risperidone has been found to be well tolerated and effective in subgroups of patients with schizophrenia, including first-episode patients and elderly patients. There is convincing evidence of the clinical utility of risperidone in other disorders. Sachs et al. (2002) compared flexible-dose risperidone with haloperidol added to mood stabilizers in a 3-week placebo-controlled trial in 156 patients with acute mania. Risperidone was also studied in a large placebo-controlled, 8-week trial in 101 children with autism accompanied by severe tantrums, aggression, or self-injurious behavior (McCracken et al. 2002). In this study, there was a reduction of 57% in irritability, compared with a decrease of 14% in the placebo group, and the response rate was 69% with risperidone, compared with 12% with placebo. **(p. 500)**

32.5 Risperidone is metabolized by which cytochrome P540 enzyme?

   A. 2C19.
   B. 2D6.
   C. 2E1.
   D. 3A4.
   E. None of the above.

The correct response is option **B**.

Hydroxylation of risperidone is catalyzed by cytochrome P450 2D6, and the half-life of the parent compound varies according to the relative activity of this enzyme. **(p. 497)**

References

Byerly M, DeVane L: Pharmacokinetics of clozapine and risperidone: a review of the literature. J Clin Psychopharmacol 16:177–187, 1996

Chouinard G, Jones B, Remington G, et al: A Canadian multicenter placebo-controlled study of fixed doses of risperidone and haloperidol in the treatment of chronic schizophrenic patients. J Clin Psychopharmacol 13:25–40, 1993

Heykants J, Huang ML, Mannens G, et al: The pharmacokinetics of risperidone in humans: a summary. J Clin Psychiatry 55 (suppl):13–17, 1994

Leysen JE, Janssen PMF, Megens AAHP, et al: Risperidone: a novel antipsychotic with balanced serotonin-dopamine antagonism, receptor occupancy profile, and pharmacologic activity. J Clin Psychiatry 55 (suppl 5):5–12, 1994

Marder SR, Meibach RC: Risperidone in the treatment of schizophrenia. Am J Psychiatry 151:825–835, 1994

McCracken JT, McGough J, Shah B, et al: Risperidone in children with autism and serious behavioral problems. N Engl J Med 347:314–321, 2002

Sachs GS, Grossman F, Ghaemi SN, et al: Combination of a mood stabilizer with risperidone or haloperidol for treatment of acute mania: a double-blind, placebo-controlled comparison of efficacy and safety. Am J Psychiatry 159:1146–1154, 2002

Schotte A, Janssen PF, Gommeren W, et al: Risperidone compared with new and reference antipsychotic drugs: in vitro and in vivo receptor binding. Psychopharmacology (Berl) 124:57–73, 1996

CHAPTER 33

Ziprasidone

Select the single best response for each question.

33.1 Which of the following uniquely characterizes ziprasidone's receptor profile in comparison with other atypical antipsychotics?

A. Blockade of serotonin reuptake.
B. Blockade of norepinephrine reuptake.
C. Blockade of dopamine reuptake.
D. Blockade of serotonin and norepinephrine reuptake.
E. Blockade of serotonin, norepinephrine, and dopamine reuptake.

The correct response is option **D.**

Ziprasidone exhibits moderate reuptake blockade at serotonin and norepinephrine reuptake proteins, which may partially mediate its efficacy in the treatment of affective or negative symptoms associated with schizophrenia and schizoaffective disorder. **(p. 507)**

33.2 A 22-year-old man with schizophrenia is about to begin a trial of ziprasidone. Which of the following dosing considerations are important?

A. Monitoring of aldehyde oxidase levels will be needed.
B. Expect that doubling the ziprasidone dosage will produce a doubling of the drug's blood levels.
C. If the patient is taking warfarin, expect increases in the international normalized ratio (INR).
D. If the patient is a cigarette smoker, expect to decrease the dosage of ziprasidone.
E. If the patient is also taking a cytochrome P450 2D6 inhibitor, expect ziprasidone blood levels to be extremely elevated.

The correct response is option **B.**

Ziprasidone is extensively metabolized after oral administration. Approximately two-thirds of ziprasidone metabolism is via reduction by aldehyde oxidase; less than one-third of its metabolism is mediated by cytochrome P450 3A4- and 1A2-catalyzed oxidation ("Ziprasidone" 2002). There are currently no known clinically relevant inhibitors or inducers of aldehyde oxidase that provide potential drug interaction liability ("Ziprasidone" 2002). Multiple-dose pharmacokinetics of ziprasidone is dose proportionate, and accumulation is predictable within the recommended dosage range. Ziprasidone is more than 99% bound to plasma proteins (primarily albumin and α_1-acid glycoprotein). In vitro binding of ziprasidone in human plasma was not affected by warfarin or propranolol; thus, ziprasidone is unlikely to interfere with the metabolism of other drugs metabolized by cytochrome P450 enzymes ("Ziprasidone" 2002). **(pp. 509, 510)**

33.3 In which of the following patients would ziprasidone be a reasonable first-choice medication for treatment of schizophrenia?

A. A patient currently taking quinidine who is extremely thin.
B. A patient currently taking amiodarone who is extremely obese.
C. A patient currently taking warfarin who is extremely obese.
D. A patient who is a smoker and is extremely thin.
E. A patient currently taking carbamazepine who is extremely obese.

The correct response is option **C**.

There are currently no known clinically relevant inhibitors or inducers of aldehyde oxidase that provide potential drug interaction liability. In vitro binding of ziprasidone in human plasma was not affected by warfarin or propranolol; thus, ziprasidone is unlikely to interfere with the metabolism of other drugs metabolized by cytochrome P450 enzymes ("Ziprasidone" 2002). Ziprasidone produced only modest weight gain in short-term (4- to 6-week) trials (Pfizer 2000). Compounds that induce cytochrome P450 3A4 activity could potentially increase ziprasidone metabolic clearance (administration with carbamazepine [200 mg twice a day] showed a 36% and 27% mean decrease in steady-state area under the curve $[AUC]_{0-12}$ and C_{max}, respectively) ("Ziprasidone" 2002). It should be noted that an amendment to the current labeling notes that pharmacokinetic/pharmacodynamic studies between ziprasidone and other drugs that prolong the QTc interval have not been performed and that an additive effect cannot be ruled out. **(pp. 509, 510, 513, 515)**

33.4 A 28-year-old man with schizophrenia has failed to respond to olanzapine, and a switch to ziprasidone is planned. Assuming that no contraindications exist, which of the following statements describes the best protocol?

A. Stop olanzapine and start ziprasidone the same day to avoid the sedating effects of ziprasidone.
B. Stop olanzapine and start ziprasidone the same day to avoid the hypotensive effects of ziprasidone.
C. Gradually cross-taper the two drugs to avoid the hypotensive effects of ziprasidone.
D. Gradually cross-taper the two drugs to avoid the activating effects of ziprasidone.
E. Gradually cross-taper the two drugs to avoid the parkinsonian effects of ziprasidone.

The correct response is option **D**.

Anecdotally, clinicians frequently report that after a switch to ziprasidone, patients often experience a subjective enhanced sense of alertness, awareness of feelings, and clarity of thinking. However, clinicians also occasionally report a less desirable "activation." **(p. 515)**

33.5 After successful use of parenteral ziprasidone (20 mg im) for acute agitation with psychosis in the emergency department, how is the transition to oral ziprasidone accomplished?

A. Cross-taper intramuscular preparation and oral preparation for 3–7 days as tolerated.
B. Initiate oral therapy the day after intramuscular therapy ceases, at 40 mg po twice a day.
C. Allow 36–48 hours after intramuscular therapy ceases before administering 40 mg po twice a day.
D. Initiate oral therapy the day after intramuscular therapy ceases, at 200 mg po twice a day.
E. None of the above.

The correct response is option **B**.

In clinical trials, the transition to oral ziprasidone therapy was accomplished smoothly the day after intramuscular therapy ceased by initiating oral ziprasidone (40 mg po twice a day with meals) (Daniel et al. 2002). Given the relatively rapid elimination of the intramuscular formulation, it may also be reasonable to begin oral treatment later in the day following an earlier intramuscular dose. **(p. 512)**

References

Daniel D, Brook S, Benattia I: Transition from IM to oral ziprasidone: clinical, efficacy, and safety data (abstract). Int J Psychopharmacol 5 (suppl 1):S124, 2002 (Abstracts from the XXIII CINP Congress, Montreal, QC, Canada, June 23–27, 2002)

Pfizer: Briefing document for Zeldox capsules (ziprasidone HCl). U.S. Food and Drug Administration Web site. July 19, 2000. Available at http://www.fda.gov/OHRMS/. Accessed April 22, 2002.

Ziprasidone (package insert). New York, Pfizer, 2002

CHAPTER 34

Drugs to Treat
Extrapyramidal Side Effects

Select the single best response for each question.

34.1   The form of extrapyramidal side effects (EPS) most likely to appear within days of initiating an antipsychotic agent is

   A. Akathisia.
   B. Rabbit syndrome.
   C. Acute dystonic reaction.
   D. Tardive dyskinesia.
   E. Pseudoparkinsonism.

The correct response is option **C**.

Acute dystonic reactions are generally the first EPS to appear and are often the most dramatic (Angus and Simpson 1970). Dystonias are involuntary sustained or spasmodic muscle contractions that cause abnormal twisting or rhythmic movements and/or postures. **(p. 520)**

34.2   Benztropine and trihexyphenidyl are able to prevent and treat antipsychotic-induced parkinsonism and acute dystonic reactions through blockade of which receptor?

   A. Dopamine$_2$ (D$_2$).
   B. Serotonin$_{2C}$ (5-hydroxytryptamine [5-HT]$_{2C}$).
   C. Histamine$_1$ (H$_1$).
   D. Muscarinic.
   E. Nicotinic.

The correct response is option **D**.

Trihexyphenidyl, a tertiary-amine analogue of atropine, is a competitive antagonist of acetylcholine and other muscarinic agonists that compete for a common binding site on muscarinic receptors (Yamamura and Snyder 1974). It exerts little blockade at nicotinic receptors (Timberlake et al. 1961). Trihexyphenidyl and all drugs in this class are referred to as anticholinergic, antimuscarinic, or atropine-like drugs. As a tertiary amine, trihexyphenidyl readily crosses the blood-brain barrier (Brown and Taylor 1996). **(pp. 523, 525)**

34.3   Benztropine, trihexyphenidyl, and other anticholinergic drugs can produce all of the following side effects *except*

A. Miosis.
B. Tachycardia.
C. Urinary retention.
D. Constipation.
E. Dry mouth.

The correct response is option **A.**

In the eye, anticholinergic drugs block both the sphincter muscle of the iris, causing the pupil to dilate (mydriasis), and the ciliary muscle of the lens, preventing accommodation and causing cycloplegia. In the heart, anticholinergic drugs usually produce a mild tachycardia through vagal blockade at the sinoatrial node pacemaker, although a mild slowing can occur. In the gastrointestinal tract, anticholinergic drugs reduce salivary and gastric secretions. Salivary secretion is particularly sensitive and can be completely abolished. In the respiratory system, anticholinergic agents reduce secretions and can produce mild bronchodilatation. Anticholinergics inhibit the activity of sweat glands and mildly inhibit urinary bladder function and bowel motility, which can produce urinary retention, constipation, and obstipation (Brown and Taylor 1996). **(pp. 523, 524, 525)**

34.4   Amantadine has demonstrated effectiveness in the treatment of which of the following?

A. Acute dystonic reactions.
B. Influenza A.
C. Akathisia.
D. Tardive dyskinesia.
E. Tardive dystonia.

The correct response is option **B.**

Amantadine is effective in preventing and treating illness from influenza A virus (Hay 1992). It also reduces the symptoms of parkinsonism, including akinesia (generalized slowing of movement), masked facies, cogwheeling, rigidity, resting tremor, and hypersalivation. **(pp. 527, 528)**

34.5   Of the following drugs, the agent most effective in the treatment of akathisia is

A. Benztropine.
B. Lorazepam.
C. Vitamin E.
D. Atenolol.
E. Propranolol.

The correct response is option **E.**

β-Blockers, including propranolol, have been studied primarily for the treatment of akathisia. Both nonselective and selective β-blockers have been reported to be efficacious (Fleischhacker et al. 1990). **(p. 529)**

34.6   Which of the following antipsychotic agents is *least* likely to produce extrapyramidal side effects?

    A. Risperidone.

    B. Chlorpromazine.

    C. Perphenazine.

    D. Clozapine.

    E. Olanzapine.

The correct response is option **D**.

Patients treated with clozapine were found to have significantly less parkinsonism than patients treated with the combination of chlorpromazine and an antiparkinsonian agent (Kane et al. 1988). The prevalence and incidence of akathisia have also been shown to be lower in patients treated with clozapine than in patients treated with typical antipsychotics (Chengappa et al. 1994; Kurz et al. 1995; Stanilla et al. 1995). At lower doses, risperidone usually does not produce significant parkinsonism, but unlike clozapine, it can produce significant parkinsonism at higher doses (Chouinard et al. 1993). **(pp. 533, 534)**

References

Angus JWS, Simpson GM: Hysteria and drug-induced dystonia. Acta Psychiatr Scand Suppl 21:52–58, 1970

Brown JH, Taylor P: Muscarinic receptor agonists and antagonists, in Goodman and Gilman's The Pharmacological Basis of Therapeutics, 9th Edition. Edited by Hardman JG, Limbird LE, Molinoff PB, et al. New York, McGraw-Hill, 1996, pp 141–160

Chengappa KN, Shelton MD, Baker RW, et al: The prevalence of akathisia in patients receiving stable doses of clozapine. J Clin Psychiatry 55:142–145, 1994

Chouinard G, Jones B, Remington G, et al: A Canadian multicenter placebo-controlled study of fixed doses of risperidone and haloperidol in the treatment of chronic schizophrenic patients. J Clin Psychopharmacol 13:25–40, 1993 (Erratum appears in J Clin Psychopharmacol 13:149, 1993)

Fleischhacker WW, Roth SD, Kane JM: The pharmacologic treatment of neuroleptic-induced akathisia. J Clin Psychopharmacol 10:12–21, 1990

Hay AJ: The action of amantadine against influenza A viruses: inhibition of the M2 ion channel protein. Seminars in Virology 3:21–30, 1992

Kane J, Honigfeld G, Singer J, et al: Clozapine for the treatment-resistant schizophrenic. A double-blind comparison with chlorpromazine. Arch Gen Psychiatry 45:789–796, 1988

Kurz M, Hummer M, Oberbauer H, et al: Extrapyramidal side effects of clozapine and haloperidol. Psychopharmacology (Berl) 118:52–56, 1995

Stanilla JK, Nair C, de Leon J, et al: Clozapine does not produce akathisia or parkinsonism. Poster presented at the 34th annual meeting of the American College of Neuropsychopharmacology, San Juan, PR, December 11–15, 1995

Timberlake WH, Schwab RS, England AC Jr: Biperiden (Akineton) in parkinsonism. Arch Neurol 5:560–564, 1961

Yamamura HI, Snyder SH: Muscarinic cholinergic receptor binding in the longitudinal muscle of the guinea pig ileum with [^{3}H]quinuclidinyl benzilate. Mol Pharmacol 10:861–867, 1974

C H A P T E R 3 5

Lithium

Select the single best response for each question.

35.1   Which of the following is a predictor of poor antimanic response to lithium?

A. Late age at first manic episode.
B. Grandiosity.
C. Euphoria.
D. Rapid cycling.
E. Pregnancy.

The correct response is option **D.**

Predictors of a poor antimanic response to lithium include rapid cycling and substance abuse (Dunner and Fieve 1974; Goodwin and Jamison 1990; Himmelhoch et al. 1976). Mixed mania, the co-occurrence of mania with depression, may also predict poor response to lithium (Swann et al. 1997). **(p. 550)**

35.2   Lithium has demonstrated efficacy for which of the following?

A. Treatment of obsessive-compulsive disorder.
B. Treatment of hyperthyroidism.
C. Antidepressant augmentation in unipolar depression.
D. Treatment of anorexia nervosa.
E. Correction of syndrome of inappropriate antidiuretic hormone secretion (SIADH).

The correct response is option **C.**

Analysis of five controlled trials of lithium augmentation for unipolar depression found significant improvement in 56%–96% of patients (Austin et al. 1991; Heit and Nemeroff 1998; Heninger et al. 1983; Kantor et al. 1986; Schopf et al. 1989; Stein and Bernadt 1993; Zusky et al. 1988). **(p. 552)**

35.3   Lithium levels may be increased by all of the following *except*

A. Osmotic diuretics.
B. Thiazide diuretics.
C. Nonsteroidal anti-inflammatory drugs (NSAIDs).
D. Angiotensin-converting enzyme inhibitors.
E. Sodium restriction.

The correct response is option **A.**

Volume depletion, use of NSAIDs, and use of thiazide diuretics can increase lithium levels (Stoudemire et al. 1990). When lithium is used concurrently with NSAIDs, signs and symptoms of toxicity and lithium levels must be monitored more carefully because NSAIDs increase the risk of toxicity (Johnson et al. 1993). Because lithium excretion relies on renal clearance, diuretic medications may affect lithium levels, depending on their site of action. Thiazide diuretics trigger a compensatory increase in reabsorption in the proximal tubule and lead to elevations in lithium levels, whereas loop diuretics do not promote lithium reabsorption and do not greatly affect lithium levels (Finley et al. 1995). Osmotic diuretics enhance lithium excretion and may serve to counteract lithium toxicity, and either no change or a slight increase in lithium levels has been reported with potassium-sparing diuretics. Angiotensin-converting enzyme inhibitors may raise lithium levels (DasGupta et al. 1992; Finley et al. 1996). Lithium serum levels may increase in the context of sodium restriction (Bennett 1997). **(pp. 553, 558)**

35.4   The cardiac malformation most associated with the use of lithium during pregnancy is

A. Patent ductus arteriosus.
B. Dextrocardia.
C. Ventricular septal defect.
D. Atrial septal defect.
E. Dysplastic tricuspid valve.

The correct response is option **E.**

Ebstein's anomaly, a cardiac malformation, was in the past thought to be a relatively high risk of lithium use in the first trimester of pregnancy (Weinstein and Goldfield 1975). In Ebstein's anomaly, a dysplastic tricuspid valve may yield tricuspid regurgitation, and clinical manifestations include cyanosis and atrial tachyarrhythmias. First-trimester exposure to lithium results in 0.05%–0.1% prevalence of Ebstein's anomaly, and relative risk is 10–20 compared with the general population (Cohen and Rosenbaum 1998). **(p. 554)**

35.5   Lithium is associated with all of the following side effects *except*

A. Cognitive dulling.
B. Weight loss.
C. Tremor.
D. Hypothyroidism.
E. Diabetes insipidus.

The correct response is option **B.**

Cognitive side effects and weight *gain* have been reported to be the most disturbing side effects for patients receiving lithium maintenance treatment. A fine postural tremor affects 4%–5% of the patients who receive lithium (Gelenberg and Jefferson 1995). In a study of patients receiving lithium, Kirov (1998) found that 14.9% of the females and 3.4% of the males developed hypothyroidism. Diabetes insipidus, caused by unresponsiveness of the kidneys to antidiuretic hormone, occurs in approximately 10% of the patients who receive long-term lithium therapy (Bendz and Aurell 1999). **(pp. 555, 556)**

35.6   Which of the following is relatively contraindicated in combination with lithium?

   A. Olanzapine.
   B. Valproate.
   C. Electroconvulsive therapy (ECT).
   D. Nortriptyline.
   E. Gabapentin.

The correct response is option **C.**

Patients who concurrently receive ECT and lithium treatment may experience neurotoxic reactions, including delirium and memory deficits (Ayd 1981; DePaulo et al. 1982; El-Mallakh 1988; Jefferson et al. 1987; Mielke et al. 1984). Preliminary data suggest that the combination of lithium and olanzapine is efficacious and well tolerated in acute mania (Madhusoodanan et al. 2000; Sanger et al. 2001). Gabapentin is also used adjunctively in the treatment of bipolar disorder, and because gabapentin has no known drug interactions, it is likely safe with lithium use (Frye et al. 1998; Vollmer et al. 1986). The combination of lithium and valproate is a strategy in the treatment of mania refractory to monotherapy with either lithium or valproate (Frances et al. 1996). Interactions may include additive side effects, such as sedation, tremor, or weight gain, but the pharmacokinetics of lithium is not altered by the addition of valproate (Granneman et al. 1996). **(pp. 557, 558)**

References

Austin MPV, Souza FGM, Goodwin GM: Lithium augmentation in antidepressant-resistant patients: a quantitative analysis. Br J Psychiatry 159:510–514, 1991

Ayd FJ: Lithium-ECT induced cerebral toxicity. Int Drug Ther Newsl 16:21–23, 1981

Bendz H, Aurell M: Drug-induced diabetes insipidus: incidence, prevention and management. Drug Saf 21:449–456, 1999

Bennett WM: Drug interactions and consequences of sodium restriction. Am J Clin Nutr 65:678–681, 1997

Cohen LS, Rosenbaum JF: Psychotropic drug use during pregnancy: weighing the risks. J Clin Psychiatry 59 (suppl 2):18–28, 1998

DasGupta K, Jefferson JW, Kobak KA, et al: The effect of enalapril on serum lithium levels in healthy men. J Clin Psychiatry 53:398–400, 1992

DePaulo JR, Folstein MF, Correa EI: The course of delirium due to lithium intoxication. J Clin Psychiatry 43:447–449, 1982

Dunner DL, Fieve RR: Clinical factors in lithium prophylaxis failure. Arch Gen Psychiatry 30:229–233, 1974

El-Mallakh RS: Complications of concurrent lithium and electroconvulsive therapy: a review of clinical material and theoretical considerations. Biol Psychiatry 23:595–601, 1988

Finley P, Warner M, Peabody C: Clinical relevance of drug interactions with lithium. Clin Pharmacokinet 29:172–191, 1995

Finley PR, O'Brien JG, Coleman RW: Lithium and angiotensin-converting enzyme inhibitors: evaluation of a potential interaction. J Clin Psychopharmacol 16:68–71, 1996

Frances A, Docherty JP, Kahn DA: Treatment of bipolar disorder. J Clin Psychiatry 57 (suppl 12A):5–58, 1996

Frye MA, Kimbrell TA, Dunn RT, et al: Gabapentin does not alter single-dose lithium pharmacokinetics. J Clin Psychopharmacol 18:461–464, 1998

Gelenberg AJ, Jefferson JW: Lithium tremor. J Clin Psychiatry 56:283–287, 1995

Goodwin FK, Jamison KR: Manic Depressive Illness. New York, Oxford University Press, 1990

Granneman GR, Schneck DW, Cavanaugh JH, et al: Pharmacokinetic interactions and side effects resulting from concomitant administration of lithium and divalproex sodium. J Clin Psychiatry 57:204–206, 1996

Heit S, Nemeroff CB: Lithium augmentation of antidepressants in treatment-refractory depression. J Clin Psychiatry 59 (suppl 6):28–33, 1998

Heninger GR, Charney DS, Sternberg DE: Lithium carbonate augmentation of antidepressant treatment. Arch Gen Psychiatry 40:1335–1342, 1983

Himmelhoch JM, Mulla D, Neil JF, et al: Incidence and significance of mixed affective states in a bipolar population. Arch Gen Psychiatry 33:1062–1066, 1976

Jefferson JW, Greist JH, Ackerman DL, et al: Lithium Encyclopedia for Clinical Practice, 2nd Edition. Washington, DC, American Psychiatric Press, 1987

Johnson AG, Seideman P, Day RO: Adverse drug interactions with nonsteroidal anti-inflammatory drugs (NSAIDs): recognition, management and avoidance. Drug Saf 8:99–127, 1993

Kantor D, McNevin S, Leichner P, et al: The benefit of lithium carbonate adjunct in refractory depression. Am J Psychiatry 31:416–418, 1986

Kirov G: Thyroid disorders in lithium-treated patients. J Affect Disord 50:33–40, 1998

Madhusoodanan S, Brenner R, Suresh P, et al: Efficacy and tolerability of olanzapine in elderly patients with psychotic disorders: a prospective study. Ann Clin Psychiatry 12:11–18, 2000

Mielke DH, Winstead DK, Goethe JW: Multiple-monitored electroconvulsive therapy: safety and efficacy in elderly depressed patients. J Am Geriatr Soc 32:180–182, 1984

Sanger TM, Grundy SL, Gibson PJ, et al: Long-term olanzapine therapy in the treatment of bipolar I disorder: an open-label continuation phase study. J Clin Psychiatry 62:273–281, 2001

Schopf J, Baumann P, Lemarchand T, et al: Treatment of endogenous depressions resistant to tricyclic antidepressants or related drugs by lithium addition: results of a placebo-controlled double-blind study. Pharmacopsychiatry 22:183–187, 1989

Stein G, Bernadt B: Lithium augmentation therapy in tricyclic-resistant depression. Br J Psychiatry 162:634–640, 1993

Stoudemire A, Moran MG, Fogel BS: Psychotropic drug use in the medically ill. Psychosomatics 21:377–391, 1990

Swann AC, Bowden CL, Morris D, et al: Depression during mania. Treatment response to lithium or divalproex. Arch Gen Psychiatry 54:37–42, 1997

Vollmer KO, Von Hodenberg A, Kolle EU: Pharmacokinetics and metabolism of gabapentin in rat, dog, and man. Arzneimittelforschung 36:830–839, 1986

Weinstein MR, Goldfield MD: Cardiovascular malformations with lithium use during pregnancy. Am J Psychiatry 132:529–531, 1975

Zusky PM, Biederman J, Rosenbaum JF, et al: Adjunct low dose lithium carbonate in lithium-resistant depression: a placebo-controlled study. J Clin Psychopharmacol 8:120–124, 1988

CHAPTER 36

Valproate

Select the single best response for each question.

36.1 U.S. Food and Drug Administration (FDA)–approved indications for the use of valproate include all of the following *except*

A. Bipolar mania.
B. Bipolar maintenance.
C. Migraine prophylaxis.
D. Monotherapy for absence seizures.
E. Adjunctive therapy for other seizure types.

The correct response is option **B**.

The indications for valproate that are currently recognized by the FDA are for the treatment of the manic episodes associated with bipolar disorder, for sole and adjunctive therapy in the treatment of simple and complex absence seizures, for adjunctive therapy in multiple seizure types that include absence seizures, and for prophylaxis of migraine. **(p. 570)**

36.2 Valproate-induced hair loss may be minimized by taking a multivitamin containing which of the following?

A. Magnesium.
B. Calcium.
C. Inositol.
D. Danshen (*Salvia miltiorrhiza*).
E. Zinc and selenium.

The correct response is option **E**.

Hair loss may occur early in valproate treatment and is usually transient. Frequency of hair loss may be greater in women than in men (Lajee and Parsonage 1980). Hair loss may be minimized by cotreatment with a multivitamin containing zinc and selenium (Hurd et al. 1984). **(p. 574)**

36.3 The greatest teratogenic risk posed by valproate is for which of the following?

A. Tricuspid atresia.
B. Cleft palate.
C. Neural tube defects.
D. Bone marrow suppression.
E. Floppy baby syndrome.

The correct response is option **C**.

Serious side effects of valproate include teratogenicity (particularly neural tube defects with first-trimester exposure). Offspring of mothers taking valproate have been reported to have an incidence of neural tube defects of 1%–1.5%. **(p. 575)**

36.4   The free concentration of valproate is most likely to be increased by which of the following?

A. Aspirin.
B. Fluvoxamine.
C. Phenytoin.
D. Risperidone.
E. Lithium.

The correct response is option **A.**

Because valproate is highly protein-bound and extensively metabolized by the liver, a number of potential drug–drug interactions may occur with other protein-bound or metabolized drugs. Free-fraction concentrations of valproate in serum can be increased by coadministration of other highly protein-bound drugs (e.g., aspirin) that can displace valproate from its protein binding sites. **(p. 575)**

36.5   The ability of valproate to inhibit phase II glucuronidation can lead to increased levels of coadministered drugs. Which of the following drugs, if taken concomitantly with valproate, is susceptible to this effect?

A. Glyburide.
B. Warfarin.
C. Alprazolam.
D. Lamotrigine.
E. Zonisamide.

The correct response is option **D.**

Valproate's competitive inhibition of excretion of lamotrigine via glucuronidation requires that lamotrigine be started at a lower dose, usually 25 mg every other day, and increased more cautiously. **(p. 576)**

36.6   A 25-year-old medically healthy man who has been receiving valproate monotherapy for migraine prophylaxis for about 1 month experiences sudden, sharp midepigastric pain. Which of the following laboratory studies is most likely to reveal the cause of this pain?

A. Alkaline phosphatase.
B. Mean corpuscular volume.
C. Serum amylase.
D. Valproate blood level.
E. Creatine phosphokinase.

The correct response is option **C.**

Pancreatitis occurs on an idiosyncratic basis early in treatment in a small proportion of young patients (Asconape et al. 1993). The low rate does not justify routine monitoring of serum amylase, but psychiatrists should be alert to the symptoms of pancreatitis. **(p. 575)**

References

Asconape JJ, Penry JK, Dreifuss FE, et al: Valproate-associated pancreatitis. Epilepsia 34:177–183, 1993

Hurd RW, Van Rinsvelt HA, Wilder BJ, et al: Selenium, zinc, and copper changes with valproic acid: possible relation to drug side effects. Neurology 34:1393–1395, 1984

Lajee HCK, Parsonage MJ: Unwanted effects of sodium valproate in the treatment of adult patients with epilepsy, in The Place of Sodium Valproate in the Treatment of Epilepsy. Edited by Parsonage MJ, Caldwell ADS. London, Royal Society of Medicine, 1980, pp 141–158

CHAPTER 37

Carbamazepine and Oxcarbazepine

Select the single best response for each question.

37.1   In the treatment of mood disorders, the oxcarbazepine dosage is gradually raised

A. To a usual dose of 3,600 mg/day.
B. To clinically desired effect.
C. To a serum level of 50–150 µg/mL.
D. Until the patient develops diplopia, at which point the dosage is gradually tapered until diplopia resolves.
E. None of the above.

The correct response is option **B**.

Oxcarbazepine can be tolerated at dosages up to about 2,400 mg/day. For bipolar disorder, oxcarbazepine is titrated to clinical desired effect as tolerated. **(p. 585)**

37.2   Which of the following is *not* considered a clinical action of carbamazepine?

A. Decreasing sodium influx and glutamate release.
B. Acting on peripheral benzodiazepine receptors.
C. Acting on α_2-adrenergic receptors.
D. Inhibiting monoamine reuptake.
E. All of the above.

The correct response is option **D**.

Carbamazepine's cellular actions include decreasing sodium influx and glutamate release, increasing potassium conductance, and acting on peripheral benzodiazepine and α_2-adrenergic receptors. Carbamazepine lacks major effects on monoamine reuptake or high affinity for histaminergic or cholinergic receptors and, unlike many antidepressants, fails to downregulate β-adrenergic receptors. Also, carbamazepine, unlike antipsychotics, does not block dopamine receptors. **(pp. 585, 586)**

37.3   Which of the following statements concerning carbamazepine is *true*?

A. Carbamazepine is ineffective in treating acute mania.
B. Carbamazepine does not autoinduce its own metabolism.
C. Carbamazepine has equal acute antimanic and antidepressant effects.
D. Carbamazepine has equal prophylactic antimanic and antidepressant effects.
E. None of the above.

The correct response is option **D**.

Carbamazepine appears to have equal *prophylactic* antidepressant and antimanic efficacy, in contrast to its lesser potent *acute* antidepressant compared with antimanic effects. Carbamazepine is a robust inducer of catabolic enzymes (including cytochrome P450 3A3/4) and decreases the serum concentrations not only of itself (*autoinduction*) but also of many other medications (*heteroinduction*). Across studies of acute mania that used diverse paradigms, overall response rates with carbamazepine were generally comparable to those seen with lithium or antipsychotics or in other studies with valproate. **(p. 588)**

37.4 Which of the following adverse events is *not* associated with the rapid titration of carbamazepine?

A. Extrapyramidal side effects (EPS).
B. Diplopia and nystagmus.
C. Ataxia.
D. Sedation.
E. All of the above are associated with rapid carbamazepine titration.

The correct response is option **A.**

Carbamazepine has several common dose-related adverse effects that generally can be minimized by gradual titration of dosage or reversed by decreasing dosage. At high doses, patients can develop neurotoxicity, with sedation, ataxia, diplopia, and nystagmus. However, in contrast to treatment with neuroleptics, carbamazepine therapy is not associated with EPS. **(pp. 590–591)**

37.5 During gradual titration of carbamazepine dosage, the emergence of dizziness, ataxia, and diplopia 1–2 hours after an individual dose may indicate that

A. The patient has misunderstood the dosing schedule.
B. The adverse-effect threshold has been exceeded, requiring dosage redistribution.
C. A drug–drug interaction has occurred.
D. The patient needs reassurance that the symptoms will subside.
E. None of the above.

The correct response is option **B.**

Dizziness, ataxia, or diplopia emerging 1–2 hours after an individual dose is often a sign that the adverse-effect threshold has been exceeded and that dosage redistribution (spreading out the total dose or giving more of the total dose at bedtime) or dosage reduction may be required. **(p. 591)**

37.6 Patients taking carbamazepine should be alerted to seek immediate medical attention if they experience which of the following symptoms?

A. Oral ulcers.
B. Petechiae.
C. Easy bruising and bleeding.
D. Rash.
E. All of the above.

The correct response is option **E.**

In view of the risk of rare but serious decreases in blood counts, which resulted in a "black box" warning in the carbamazepine product information, it is important to alert patients to seek immediate medical evaluation if they develop signs and symptoms of possible hematological reactions, such as fever, sore throat, oral ulcers, petechiae, and easy bruising or bleeding. **(p. 591)**

37.7 Laboratory monitoring during carbamazepine therapy is performed after 2, 4, 6, and 8 weeks postinitiation and every 3 months thereafter. This laboratory testing includes which of the following?

A. Thyroid panel.
B. Clean-catch urinalysis.
C. Complete blood count (CBC) and liver-associated enzymes.
D. Electrocardiogram.
E. Urine metabolites.

The correct response is option **C**.

Conservative laboratory monitoring during carbamazepine therapy includes baseline studies and reevaluation of CBC, differential, platelets, and hepatic indices initially at 2, 4, 6, and 8 weeks and then every 3 months (American Psychiatric Association 1994, 2002). Serum carbamazepine concentrations can be assessed at steady state and then as clinically indicated. **(p. 591)**

37.8 Inhibition of which metabolic cytochrome P450 enzyme causes carbamazepine toxicity?

A. 1A2.
B. 2D6.
C. 3A3/4.
D. 2C19.
E. 2E1.

The correct response is option **C**.

Carbamazepine metabolism (which is primarily by cytochrome P450 3A3/4) can be inhibited by certain enzyme inhibitors, yielding increases in serum carbamazepine concentrations and causing carbamazepine intoxication. Autoinduction makes carbamazepine particularly vulnerable to the effects of enzyme inhibitors. Thus, a variety of agents that inhibit 3A3/4 can yield increased serum carbamazepine concentrations and intoxication. **(pp. 594, 596 [Table 37–5]; see also Figure 37–1)**

37.9 Which cytochrome P450 metabolic enzyme is induced by both carbamazepine and oxcarbazepine?

A. 1A2.
B. 2D6.
C. 3A3/4.
D. 2C19.
E. 2E1.

The correct response is option **C**.

Carbamazepine is a robust inducer of cytochrome P450 3A3/4 and decreases the serum concentrations of many medications, including carbamazepine itself. By contrast, oxcarbazepine is only a modest to moderate inducer of 3A3/4. **(pp. 594, 595 [Table 37–4], 598)**

References

American Psychiatric Association: Practice guideline for the treatment of patients with bipolar disorder. Am J Psychiatry 151:1–36, 1994

American Psychiatric Association: Practice guideline for the treatment of patients with bipolar disorder (revision). Am J Psychiatry 159:1–50, 2002

CHAPTER 38

Gabapentin

Select the single best response for each question.

38.1 Gabapentin is thought to exert its effects through which of the following mechanisms?

  A. Directly regulating the benzodiazepine receptor.
  B. Acting as a monoamine reuptake inhibitor.
  C. Blocking dopamine release primarily in limbic structures.
  D. Increasing brain intracellular γ-aminobutyric acid (GABA) via blood-brain barrier amino acid transporter and other enzymatic regulatory mechanisms.
  E. None of the above.

The correct response is option **D**.

The mechanism of gabapentin's anticonvulsant and psychotropic action is not fully understood. Gabapentin was originally developed as an analogue of GABA, the major inhibitory neurotransmitter in the cerebral cortex. Gabapentin does not act as a GABA precursor, agonist, or antagonist. Preclinical studies have suggested that gabapentin increases brain and intracellular GABA by an amino acid active transporter at the blood-brain barrier and multiple enzymatic regulatory mechanisms, respectively. **(p. 607)**

38.2 Gabapentin has a benign drug-interaction profile because

  A. It has no active metabolites.
  B. It has no protein binding.
  C. It has no cytochrome P450 interactions.
  D. All of the above.
  E. None of the above.

The correct response is option **D**.

Gabapentin has a benign drug interaction profile because there is no active metabolite, and it has nonlinear bioavailability most likely related to an active, saturable amino acid transport carrier present in gut and blood-brain barrier (McLean 1999). There is no evidence of plasma protein binding, hepatic metabolism, or cytochrome P450 autoinduction. **(p. 608)**

38.3 Controlled studies have shown that gabapentin is clearly beneficial in the treatment of which of the following?

  A. Migraine headaches.
  B. Diabetic neuropathy.
  C. Postherpetic neuralgia.
  D. All of the above.
  E. None of the above.

The correct response is option **D.**

Gabapentin has been systematically evaluated for the treatment of diabetic neuropathy and postherpetic neuralgia (Backonja et al. 1998; Rowbotham et al. 1998). A more recent study also suggests that gabapentin is an effective agent for migraine prophylaxis (Mathew et al. 2001). **(pp. 608, 609)**

38.4   Gabapentin shows promise in the treatment of

   A. Bipolar disorder.
   B. Social phobia.
   C. Major depression.
   D. Schizophrenia.
   E. None of the above.

The correct response is option **B.**

Pande et al. (1999) investigated gabapentin in a two-site, 14-week, randomized, double-blind, placebo-controlled study of 69 outpatients with DSM-IV–confirmed social phobia. Gabapentin was more effective than placebo in the reduction of social phobia symptoms. **(p. 609)**

38.5   Although gabapentin has a benign side-effect profile, which serious adverse effect has been associated with use of gabapentin in pediatric epilepsy and adult mania?

   A. Torsades de pointes.
   B. Serotonin syndrome.
   C. Aggression.
   D. Tics.
   E. Sleepwalking.

The correct response is option **C.**

Adverse events caused by gabapentin have been few but have important psychiatric implications. In addition to reports of gabapentin-induced hypomania and mania (Leweke et al. 1999; Short and Cooke 1995), gabapentin has been associated with aggression both in pediatric epilepsy (Wolf et al. 1996) and in adult mania (Pinninti and Mahajan 2001). **(p. 611)**

References

Backonja M, Beydoun A, Edwards KR, et al: Gabapentin for the symptomatic treatment of painful neuropathy in patients with diabetes mellitus. JAMA 280:1831–1836, 1998

Leweke FM, Bauer J, Elger CE: Manic episode due to gabapentin treatment (letter). Br J Psychiatry 175:291, 1999

Mathew NT, Rapoport A, Saper J, et al: Efficacy of gabapentin in migraine prophylaxis. Headache 41:119–128, 2001

McLean MJ: Gabapentin in the management of convulsive disorders. Epilepsia 40 (suppl 6):S39–S50, 1999

Pande AC, Davidson JRT, Jefferson JW, et al: Treatment of social phobia with gabapentin: a placebo-controlled study. J Clin Psychopharmacol 19:341–348, 1999

Pinninti NR, Mahajan DS: Gabapentin-associated aggression. J Neuropsychiatry Clin Neurosci 13:424–429, 2001

Rowbotham M, Harden N, Stacey B, et al: Gabapentin for the treatment of postherpetic neuralgia. JAMA 280:1837–1842, 1998

Short C, Cooke L: Hypomania induced by gabapentin (letter). Br J Psychiatry 166:679–680, 1995

Wolf SM, Shinnar S, Kang H, et al: Gabapentin toxicity in children manifesting as behavioral changes. Epilepsia 36:1203–1205, 1996

CHAPTER 39

Lamotrigine

Select the single best response for each question.

39.1 Lamotrigine's mechanism of action is not fully understood but is presumed to be associated with

    A. Its effects on dopamine$_1$ (D$_1$) or dopamine$_2$ (D$_2$) receptors.
    B. Its effects on γ-aminobutyric acid B (GABA$_B$) receptors.
    C. Inhibition of glutamine-induced burst firing and decreased release of glutamate.
    D. Its effects on histamine$_1$ (H$_1$) receptors.
    E. All of the above.

The correct response is option **C**.

Lamotrigine at concentrations of up to 10^{-4} M shows no effect on D$_1$ or D$_2$, GABA$_B$, α$_1$-, α$_2$-, or β-adrenergic, muscarinic M$_1$ or M$_2$, histamine$_1$, adenosine$_2$, opioid κ or σ, or serotonin (5-hydroxytryptamine)$_2$ (5-HT$_2$) receptors. A weak inhibitory effect is reported on the 5-HT$_3$ receptor. Lamotrigine's psychotropic mechanism of action is not clear but is presumed to be associated with its antiepileptic activity. Lamotrigine-associated inhibition of glutamine-induced repetitive burst firing has been detected (Cheung et al. 1992; Miller et al. 1986). Initial, but not subsequent, stimuli of burst-firing wave trains are comparatively unimpeded by lamotrigine at high concentrations. This effect is attenuated by hyperpolarization. The presynaptic inhibitory effects of lamotrigine on use-dependent and voltage-sensitive sodium, calcium, and potassium channels result in decreased release of the excitatory amino acid glutamate that may account in part for observations of lamotrigine's mood stabilization (Calabrese et al. 2000; Frye et al. 2000) and neuroprotective properties (Graham et al. 1993; Leach et al. 1993; McGeer and Zhu 1990). **(pp. 616, 617)**

39.2 The side effects most commonly associated with lamotrigine include

    A. Tremor, headache, and rash.
    B. Dizziness, headache, diplopia, nausea, and ataxia.
    C. Extrapyramidal symptoms, nausea, diarrhea, and rash.
    D. All of the above.
    E. None of the above.

The correct response is option **B**.

The spectrum of side effects reported with lamotrigine have included dizziness, headache, diplopia, nausea, and ataxia (Messenheimer et al. 1998; Schachter et al. 1995). Although the prevalence of rash with lamotrigine in randomized mood disorder trials did not exceed the prevalence seen with placebo, rash is generally recognized as the side effect that is most likely to significantly complicate the drug's clinical use. **(p. 619)**

39.3 Which of the following dosing strategies would best minimize the risk of lamotrigine-associated rash?

A. Rapid escalation of dosage.
B. 25 mg daily for 2 weeks if coadministered with valproic acid.
C. Starting at dosages above 25 mg/day.
D. 25 mg every other day for 2 weeks if coadministered with valproic acid.
E. 50 mg daily for 14 days if coadministered with valproic acid.

The correct response is option **D.**

In open-label and placebo-controlled clinical trials, the risk of rash was increased when valproic acid was coadministered with lamotrigine or when the recommended initial dosage or rate of dosage escalation of lamotrigine was exceeded. The recommended titration schedule for lamotrigine added to valproate in patients older than 12 years begins at 25 mg every other day for 14 days, advances to 25 mg daily for 14 days, and then increases by 25–50 mg/day every 1–2 weeks. **(p. 623; see also Table 39–1)**

39.4 Which of the following best describes the currently recommended clinical management strategy for lamotrigine-associated rash?

A. Hold the next dose and seek immediate medical attention.
B. Revert to the previous lower dose and monitor via telephone daily.
C. Double the dose to "shoot through" the rash-inducing dosage.
D. Hold the current dosage for 2 weeks before resuming dosage escalation.
E. None of the above.

The correct response is option **A.**

The most common lamotrigine-associated eruption is maculopapular or morbilliform and is benign; however, a clinically similar eruption may accompany rare but more serious systemic hypersensitivity reactions (Guberman et al. 1999). All patients who develop rash during the first few months of lamotrigine therapy should be instructed to hold the next dose and immediately seek medical consultation. **(p. 621)**

39.5 Drug interaction warnings for lamotrigine include which of the following?

A. Reduced plasma concentration of lamotrigine when coadministered with carbamazepine.
B. Reduced plasma concentration of lamotrigine when coadministered with oral contraceptives.
C. Increased plasma concentration of lamotrigine when coadministered with valproic acid.
D. All of the above.
E. None of the above.

The correct response is option **D.**

Addition of adjunctive lamotrigine to enzyme inducers such as carbamazepine, phenytoin, and phenobarbital decreases the lamotrigine plasma concentration by approximately 40%–50%. Introduction of adjunctive valproate (an enzyme inhibitor) results in immediate and successful competition for metabolism, with resultant increases in half-life; the steady-state half-life for lamotrigine in the presence of valproate is 69.6 hours (Yau et al. 1992). Sabers et al. (2001) reported decreased plasma lamotrigine levels (mean 49%, range 41%–64%) in seven patients taking oral contraceptives containing ethinylestradiol. **(p. 624)**

References

Calabrese J, Suppes T, Bowden C, et al. for the Lamictal 614 Study Group: A double-blind, placebo-controlled, prophylaxis study of lamotrigine in rapid-cycling bipolar disorder. J Clin Psychiatry 61:841–850, 2000

Cheung H, Kamp D, Harris E: An in vitro investigation of the action of lamotrigine on neuronal voltage-activated sodium channels. Epilepsy Res 13:107–112, 1992

Frye M, Ketter T, Kimbrell T, et al: A placebo-controlled study of lamotrigine and gabapentin monotherapy in refractory mood disorders. J Clin Psychopharmacol 20:607–614, 2000

Graham S, Chen J, Leach M, et al: BW619C89 decreases glutamate release and infarction volume after MCA occlusion in the rat (abstract). Can J Neurol Sci 20 (suppl 4):S138, 1993

Guberman A, Besag F, Brodie M, et al: Lamotrigine-associated rash: risk/benefit considerations in adults and children. Epilepsia 40:985–991, 1999

Leach M, Swan J, Eisenthal D, et al: BW619C89, a glutamate release inhibitor, protects against focal cerebral ischemic damage. Stroke 24:1063–1067, 1993

McGeer E, Zhu S: Lamotrigine protects against kainate but not ibotenate lesions in rat striatum. Neurosci Lett 112:348–351, 1990

Messenheimer JA, Mullens EL, Giorgi L, et al: Safety review of adult clinical trial experience with lamotrigine. Drug Saf 18:281–296, 1998

Miller AA, Wheatley P, Sawyer DA, et al: Pharmacological studies on lamotrigine, a novel antiepileptic drug: anticonvulsant profile in mice and rats. Epilepsia 27:483–489, 1986

Sabers A, Buchholt J, Uldall P, et al: Lamotrigine plasma levels reduced by oral contraceptives. Epilepsy Res 47:151–154, 2001

Schachter S, Leppik E, Matsuo F, et al: Lamotrigine: a 6-month, placebo-controlled, safety and tolerance study. J Epilepsy 8:201–209, 1995

Yau M, Wargin W, Wolf K, et al: Effect of valproate on the pharmacokinetics of lamotrigine at steady state (abstract). Epilepsia 33 (suppl 3):82, 1992

CHAPTER 40

Topiramate

Select the single best response for each question.

40.1 Topiramate has been approved by the U.S. Food and Drug Administration (FDA) for use in which of the following psychiatric disorders?

A. Bipolar disorder in adolescents only.
B. Bipolar disorder in adults only.
C. Bipolar disorder in adolescents and adults.
D. Rapid-cycling bipolar disorder.
E. None of the above.

The correct response is option **E.**

Topiramate is not currently approved by the FDA for use in the treatment of any psychiatric disorder. However, the drug is becoming increasingly used off-label in the acute and maintenance treatment of bipolar disorder with manic and depressive symptoms; for episodes that are resistant to lithium, valproate, carbamazepine, and antipsychotics; or in cases in which the patient is unable to tolerate these agents (Chengappa et al. 2001a). **(p. 629)**

40.2 In a placebo-controlled study of topiramate in acute bipolar mania, the drug's efficacy was demonstrated in adolescent patients taking topiramate who completed the study. This study was prematurely discontinued for which of the following reasons?

A. Patients lost too much weight.
B. A high proportion of patients developed acidosis.
C. Topiramate demonstrated no benefit in the adult cohort of this study.
D. Common side effects, such as dizziness, were too difficult to manage, causing most patients to drop out of the study.
E. There were ethical concerns about research on adolescents.

The correct response is option **C.**

Johnson & Johnson Pharmaceutical Research and Development, the discoverer and manufacturer of topiramate, conducted a large clinical study program of topiramate in the treatment of bipolar disorder. Controlled trials of the drug in adults with acute bipolar mania failed to demonstrate significant separation between the topiramate and placebo groups. In contrast, a double-blind, placebo-controlled study of topiramate in adolescents with acute bipolar mania, which was prematurely discontinued when the adult mania studies were found to be negative, demonstrated significant improvement in Young Mania Rating Scale scores for patients taking topiramate who completed the study (Johnson & Johnson Pharmaceutical Research and Development, data on file). **(pp. 627, 629)**

40.3   In an 8-week comparison of topiramate and sustained-release bupropion in 36 patients with bipolar depression (McIntyre et al. 2002), mean weight loss with bupropion was 1.2 kg. What was the mean weight loss for topiramate-treated patients?

A. 7.6 kg.
B. 6.6 kg.
C. 8.6 kg.
D. 5.6 kg.
E. 3.6 kg.

The correct response is option **D.**

The 8-week comparison showed patients treated with topiramate had an average weight loss of 5.6 kg (McIntyre et al. 2002). Other reports (Chengappa et al. 2001b; McElroy et al. 2000) suggest that this weight loss can persist for up to 2 years. **(p. 632)**

40.4   Regarding findings from the first controlled study of topiramate monotherapy in acute bipolar disorder, which of the following statements about side effects is *true*?

A. Significant dropout due to side effects was found in the topiramate-treated group compared with the placebo-treated group.
B. Discontinuation due to side effects was no different with topiramate than it was with placebo.
C. Discontinuation was higher in the placebo-treated group than the topiramate-treated group.
D. Dyspepsia was the most common side effect in topiramate-treated patients.
E. None of the above.

The correct response is option **B.**

In the first controlled study of topiramate monotherapy in acute bipolar mania, relatively fast titration of topiramate (256 or 512 mg/day in 10 days) was well tolerated, and discontinuations because of side effects were not significantly different between topiramate and placebo (Johnson & Johnson Pharmaceutical Research and Development, data on file). **(p. 633)**

40.5   Two uncommon but potentially serious side effects of topiramate are

A. Reversible metabolic acidosis and weight loss.
B. Nephrolithiasis and secondary angle-closure glaucoma.
C. Nephrolithiasis and weight loss.
D. Myopia and breakthrough bleeding in females on birth control pills.
E. Secondary angle-closure glaucoma and reversible metabolic acidosis.

The correct response is option **B.**

All of the side effects listed may occur with the use of topiramate. However, the most serious, and uncommon, side effects—which would require immediate medical attention—are nephrolithiasis and myopia with secondary angle-closure glaucoma. Although one could argue that metabolic acidosis is serious, it is usually mild and easily treated, with few or no long-term consequences compared with angle-closure glaucoma or the pain associated with angle-closure glaucoma or nephrolithiasis. **(p. 633)**

References

Chengappa K, Gershon S, Levine J: The evolving role of topiramate among other mood stabilizers in the management of bipolar disorder. Bipolar Disord 3:215–232, 2001a

Chengappa K, Levine J, Rathore D, et al: Long-term effects of topiramate on bipolar mood instability, weight change and glycemic control: a case-series. Eur Psychiatry 16:186–190, 2001b

McElroy SL, Suppes T, Keck PE Jr, et al: Open-label adjunctive topiramate in the treatment of bipolar disorders. Biol Psychiatry 47:1025–1033, 2000

McIntyre RS, Mancini DA, McCann S, et al: Topiramate versus bupropion SR when added to mood stabilizer therapy for the depressive phase of bipolar disorder: a preliminary single-blind study. Bipolar Disord 4:207–213, 2002

CHAPTER 41

Cognitive Enhancers

Select the single best response for each question.

41.1   Evidence of cholinergic system involvement in the pathophysiology of Alzheimer's disease (AD) includes all of the following *except*

A.   Greater reactivity to cholinergic blockade demonstrated by patients with AD compared with age-matched control subjects.
B.   Reduced ChAT cell bodies in the basal forebrain at autopsy in patients with AD.
C.   Deficits in attention and learning in animals with cholinergic system lesions.
D.   Precipitation of age-dependent learning impairments in humans through blockade of the central cholinergic system with anticholinergic drugs such as scopolamine.
E.   Increased choline acetyltransferase (ChAT) activity in the hippocampus and cerebral cortex in patients with AD.

The correct response is option **E.**

The involvement of the cholinergic system in the pathophysiology of AD has been known and carefully investigated for more than two decades. Among the earliest biochemical changes recognized in AD was the loss of ChAT activity in the hippocampus and cerebral cortex (Davies and Maloney 1976). Cell bodies responsible for ChAT production are primarily located in the basal forebrain (Mesulam and Geula 1988), and a major early pathological finding was that these cell bodies were reduced in number in AD subjects at autopsy (Whitehouse et al. 1982). Furthermore, an important role for the cholinergic system in memory formation was supported by the findings that lesion studies of the cholinergic system in animals show deficits in attention (Robbins et al. 1989) and learning (Ridley et al. 1986). From a pharmacological perspective, blockade of the central cholinergic system with the anticholinergic drug scopolamine causes age-dependent learning impairments in human control subjects without AD (Molchan et al. 1992; Tariot et al. 1996). In addition, AD subjects themselves are much more reactive to cholinergic blockade than are age-matched control subjects, suggesting increased sensitivity (Sunderland et al. 1988). Together, this large body of supportive data placed the cholinergic system in the forefront as a therapeutic target for AD. **(p. 639)**

41.2   Regarding shared characteristics of the acetylcholinesterase inhibitors (AChEIs) donepezil, rivastigmine, and galantamine, all of the following statements are correct *except*

A.   They are all approved by the U.S. Food and Drug Administration for use in Alzheimer's disease.
B.   They are all reversible AChEIs.
C.   They are all naturally occurring substances derived from herbs or plants.
D.   They have not been demonstrated to differ from one another in efficacy.
E.   All of the above are correct.

The correct response is option **C.**

Of these AChEIs, only galantamine is naturally occurring; it is an alkaloid extracted from the bulb of the daffodil (Fulton and Benfield 1996; Giacobini 2000; Harvey 1995). All other statements are correct. **(pp. 640–641)**

41.3   All of the following cholinergic-active substances have been shown to improve cognitive functioning in Alzheimer's disease *except*

   A. Nicotine.
   B. Huperzine-α.
   C. Tacrine.
   D. Rivastigmine.
   E. Physostigmine.

The correct response is option **E.**

Evidence for physostigmine's effectiveness in symptomatic treatment of Alzheimer's disease is limited. Even in a controlled-release formulation, physostigmine showed no convincing benefits (Coelho and Birks 2001). Nicotine, huperzine-α, tacrine, and rivastigmine, through direct or indirect influences on the cholinergic system, have all been shown to improve cognitive symptoms in Alzheimer's disease. **(pp. 640–641)**

41.4   Which of the following statements regarding studies using nonsteroidal anti-inflammatory drugs (NSAIDs) in Alzheimer's disease (AD) is *true?*

   A. Retrospective studies have indicated that NSAIDs could delay the onset of AD, but prospective studies did not find such an effect.
   B. Meta-analysis of studies in patients taking NSAIDs for rheumatoid arthritis indicated a substantially decreased risk of developing AD.
   C. In one prospective study, AD patients treated with indomethacin showed no differences compared with placebo-treated patients after 6 months.
   D. There is only indirect evidence for inflammatory and immunological abnormalities in the AD brain.
   E. All of the above.

The correct response is option **B.**

In a small trial of NSAIDs in Alzheimer's disease, patients taking indomethacin had no progression of cognitive impairment after 6 months, whereas placebo-treated patients had a 10%–12% decline in cognitive function scores (Rogers et al. 1993). Direct evidence of inflammatory and immunological abnormalities in the AD brain has been extensively documented (Aisen and Davis 1994). More than 20 epidemiological studies have suggested that NSAIDs can slow the progression of AD and may delay its onset. In a longitudinal study of aging, the risk of developing AD decreased with increasing duration of NSAID use (Stewart et al. 1997). Meta-analysis of 17 retrospective studies indicated that chronic NSAID use by rheumatoid arthritis patients may have decreased their risk of developing AD by as much as 50% and may have delayed the onset of AD by 5–7 years (McGeer et al. 1996). **(p. 642)**

41.5   *Ginkgo biloba*'s mechanism of action in preserving cognitive function is due to

   A. Its acetylcholinesterase activity.
   B. Its antioxidant activity.
   C. It ability to reduce cholesterol.
   D. Its activity with *N*-methyl-D-aspartate (NMDA) receptors.
   E. Its effects on estrogen hormone.

The correct response is option **B.**

Ginkgo biloba is a flavonoid that has anti-inflammatory, anti-ischemic and antioxidant properties. The antioxidant properties are likely a result of the presence of several flavonoids found in ginkgo. **(p. 643)**

41.6   Memantine has been shown to improve cognition and/or reduce deterioration in which of the following?

   A. Alzheimer's disease only.
   B. Vascular dementia only.
   C. Both Alzheimer's disease and vascular dementia.
   D. Alzheimer's disease only, when used in combination with acetylcholinesterase inhibitors.
   E. None of the above.

The correct response is option **C**.

A randomized, placebo-controlled trial showed that memantine improved cognitive function in mild to moderate vascular dementia (Orgogozo et al. 2002; Wilcock et al. 2002). A multicenter study showed that memantine reduced clinical deterioration in moderate to severe Alzheimer's disease (Rossouw et al. 2002). **(pp. 644, 645)**

References

Aisen PS, Davis KL: Inflammatory mechanisms in Alzheimer's disease: implications for therapy. Am J Psychiatry 151:1105–1113, 1994

Coelho F, Birks J: Physostigmine for Alzheimer's disease. Cochrane Database Syst Rev 2:CD001499, 2001

Davies P, Maloney AFJ: Selective loss of central cholinergic neurons in Alzheimer's disease (letter). Lancet 2:1403, 1976

Fulton B, Benfield P: Galanthamine. Drugs Aging 9:60–65; discussion 66–67, 1996

Giacobini E: Cholinesterase inhibitors: from the Calabar bean to Alzheimer therapy, in Cholinesterase and Cholinesterase Inhibitors. Edited by Giacobini E. London, Martin Dunitz, 2000, pp 181–226

Harvey AL: The pharmacology of galanthamine and its analogues. Pharmacol Ther 68:113–128, 1995

McGeer PL, Schulzer M, McGeer EG: Arthritis and anti-inflammatory agents as possible protective factors for Alzheimer's disease: a review of 17 epidemiologic studies. Neurology 47:425–432, 1996

Mesulam MM, Geula C: Nucleus basalis (Ch4) and cortical cholinergic innervation in the human brain: observations based on the distribution of acetylcholinesterase and choline acetyltransferase. J Comp Neurol 275:216–240, 1988

Molchan SE, Martinez RA, Hill JL, et al: Increased cognitive sensitivity to scopolamine with age and a perspective on the scopolamine model. Brain Res Brain Res Rev 17:215–226, 1992

Orgogozo JM, Rigaud AS, Stoffler A, et al: Efficacy and safety of memantine in patients with mild to moderate vascular dementia: a randomized, placebo-controlled trial (MMM 300). Stroke 33:1834–1839, 2002

Ridley RM, Murray TK, Johnson JA, et al: Learning impairment following lesion of the basal nucleus of Meynert in the marmoset: modification by cholinergic drugs. Brain Res 376:108–116, 1986

Robbins TW, Everitt BJ, Marston HM, et al: Comparative effects of ibotenic acid- and quisqualic acid-induced lesions of the substantia innominata on attentional function in the rat: further implications for the role of the cholinergic neurons of the nucleus basalis in cognitive processes. Behav Brain Res 35:221–240, 1989

Rogers J, Kirby LC, Hempelman SR, et al: Clinical trial of indomethacin in Alzheimer's disease. Neurology 43:1609–1611, 1993

Rossouw JE, Anderson GL, Prentice RL, et al: Risks and benefits of estrogen plus progestin in healthy postmenopausal women: principal results from the Women's Health Initiative randomized controlled trial. JAMA 288:321–333, 2002

Stewart WF, Kawas C, Corrada M, et al: Risk of Alzheimer's disease and duration of NSAID use. Neurology 48:626–632, 1997

Sunderland T, Tariot PN, Newhouse PA: Differential responsivity of mood, behavior, and cognition to cholinergic agents in elderly neuropsychiatric populations. Brain Res 472:371–389, 1988

Tariot PN, Patel SV, Cox C, et al: Age-related decline in central cholinergic function demonstrated with scopolamine. Psychopharmacology (Berl) 125:50–56, 1996

Whitehouse PJ, Price DL, Struble RG, et al: Alzheimer's disease and senile dementia: loss of neurons in the basal forebrain. Science 215:1237–1239, 1982

Wilcock G, Mobius HJ, Stoffler A: A double-blind, placebo-controlled multicentre study of memantine in mild to moderate vascular dementia (MMM500). Int Clin Psychopharmacol 17:297–305, 2002

CHAPTER 42

Sedative-Hypnotics

Select the single best response for each question.

42.1   Regarding the pharmacological profile of benzodiazepines, which of the following statements is *true?*

A. They alter GABAergic (γ-aminobutyric acid [GABA]) receptors directly.
B. They chemically bind to and permanently alter GABA receptors.
C. They influence the influx of chloride ions into the cell.
D. They do not have specific receptors in the central nervous system.
E. None of the above.

The correct response is option **C.**

The GABA$_A$ receptor is a ligand-gated ion channel that mediates fast synaptic neurotransmission in the central nervous system. When the GABA$_A$ receptor is occupied by GABA or GABA agonists, the chloride channels open and chloride ions diffuse into the cell. Schmidt et al. in 1967 first reported that diazepam could potentiate the inhibitory effects of GABA on the spinal cord in cats. Later, it was shown that the effect of diazepam could be abolished if the endogenous content of GABA was depleted. These findings established that diazepam (and related benzodiazepines) did not act directly through GABA but modulated inhibitory transmission through the GABA$_A$ receptor in some other way. It was subsequently reported that benzodiazepines bind specifically to neural elements in the mammalian brain with high affinity and that an excellent correlation exists between drug affinities for these specific binding sites and in vivo pharmacological potencies (Möhler and Okada 1977; Squires and Braestrup 1977). **(p. 656)**

42.2   All of the following statements regarding the GABA$_A$ receptor are true *except*

A. It consists of five subunits, which form a rosette surrounding an ion channel pore for chloride ions.
B. When activated by conformational changes due to the presence of a benzodiazepine, chloride ions exit the cell.
C. Activation causes neuronal inhibition.
D. The GABAergic system is widespread throughout the central nervous system.
E. All of the above statements are true.

The correct response is option **B.**

It is postulated that the binding of GABA to *N*-terminal extracellular domains of α and β subunits causes conformational changes within the subunits. Ion channel pores subsequently open, and chloride ions flow across the neuronal membrane, resulting in neuronal inhibition (Amin and Weiss 1993; Boileau et al. 1999; Sigel et al. 1992; Smith and Olsen 1994). **(pp. 656, 657; see also Figure 42–3)**

42.3 Which of the following statements about desmethyldiazepam is *true?*

A. As a metabolite, it has a short half-life, and it is quickly excreted from the body.
B. It is a metabolite only of diazepam.
C. It has a long half-life and is ultimately oxidated to other compounds that are then conjugated and excreted.
D. It has a long half-life, but it is directly conjugated and excreted.
E. It undergoes oxidation to clorazepate and is then excreted.

The correct response is option **C.**

Desmethyldiazepam is a direct metabolite of diazepam and an indirect metabolite of chlordiazepoxide and clorazepate, among others. It is a critically important metabolite for biological activity because of its long half-life of more than 72 hours. Desmethyldiazepam undergoes oxidation to oxazepam, which is rapidly conjugated with glucuronic acid and excreted. **(p. 660)**

42.4 Which of the following statements concerning the effects of most benzodiazepines on sleep architecture is *true?*

A. Decrease sleep latency, increase the time in stage 2 sleep, and increase rapid eye movement (REM) latency.
B. Decrease sleep latency, decrease the time in stage 2 sleep, and decrease REM latency.
C. Suppress stage 3 and 4 sleep and decrease REM latency.
D. Increase stage 3 and 4 sleep and increase REM latency.
E. Lengthen slow-wave sleep and decrease REM latency.

The correct response is option **A.**

Most benzodiazepines decrease sleep latency, increase time spent in stage 2 sleep, suppress stage 3 and 4 sleep, and increase REM latency. **(p. 661; see also Table 42–1)**

42.5 Which of the following represents a contraindication to the use of a benzodiazepine for insomnia?

A. Multiple sclerosis.
B. Asthma.
C. Anxiety disorders.
D. Jet lag.
E. Myasthenia gravis.

The correct response is option **E.**

Benzodiazepines can increase the frequency of apnea and exacerbate oxygen desaturation in healthy subjects and in subjects with chronic bronchitis (Geddes et al. 1976). Although many reports suggest that benzodiazepines are safe in patients with obstructive sleep apnea, other authors disagree, and it seems wise to avoid hypnotics in patients with severe sleep apnea. One of the only other contraindications is myasthenia gravis, a condition in which muscle relaxation with benzodiazepines can exacerbate muscle atonia. **(p. 662)**

42.6   Which of the following statements concerning benzodiazepines is *false*?

A. Overdose of benzodiazepines is usually not fatal.
B. Benzodiazepines are safe for use during early pregnancy.
C. Mental/cognitive impairment is clearly shown when using benzodiazepines.
D. Benzodiazepine use can improve mental/cognitive function in very anxious patients.
E. None of the above.

The correct response is option **B.**

Because the safety of benzodiazepines in early pregnancy is not established, they should be avoided unless absolutely necessary. Diazepam is secreted in breast milk and may make the infant sleepy, unresponsive, and slow to feed. Overdoses of benzodiazepines reportedly are not fatal unless alcohol or other psychotropic drugs are taken simultaneously. Otherwise asymptomatic subjects clearly show mental impairment with benzodiazepines; however, because anxiety itself interferes with mental performance, alleviation of anxiety may result in improved functioning, which more than compensates for the direct drug-related decrement. **(p. 663)**

42.7   Reasons that benzodiazepines are preferred to barbiturates include all of the following *except*

A. Barbiturates can depress respiration.
B. Barbiturates cause patients to feel more "drugged" the next day.
C. Barbiturates do not decrease sleep latency.
D. Barbiturates are less safe in overdose compared with benzodiazepines.
E. All of the above reasons are correct.

The correct response is option **C.**

Barbiturates and benzodiazepines both decrease sleep latency. However, barbiturates generally compare poorly with benzodiazepines. The patient feels "drugged" the next day, and there is always the risk of fatal overdose because of the depressant effect on respiration. Barbiturates suppress respiration, and the therapeutic dose of barbiturates may cause fatal respiratory depression in patients with sleep apnea. Patients with sleep apnea should therefore avoid taking barbiturates. Because of these risks, many clinicians have stopped using barbiturates as hypnotics and sedatives and prescribe them only as anticonvulsants. **(p. 653)**

42.8   The most common reason/presentation for insomnia is

A. Insomnia associated with psychiatric disorders.
B. Insomnia associated with psychological factors and/or physiological tension/arousal.
C. Insomnia associated with sleep-induced respiratory impairment.
D. Insomnia perceived by a patient but not demonstrated by objective polysomnography.
E. Insomnia associated with alcohol and/or drug use.

The correct response is option **A.**

Data from the Association of Sleep Disorders Centers National Case Series (Coleman 1983), which involved approximately 2,000 patients with a diagnosed disorder related to initiating and maintaining sleep, showed that insomnia associated with psychiatric disorders accounted for the greatest proportion (35%) of insomnia diagnoses. Insomnia associated with psychological factors and/or physiological tension/arousal accounted for 15% of insomnia diagnoses, and insomnia associated with sleep-induced respiratory impairment and insomnia associated with sleep-state misperception (a subjective insomnia complaint not substantiated by polysomnography) each accounted for 5%–10% of insomnia diagnoses. **(p. 666; see Table 42–3)**

References

Amin J, Weiss DS: GABAA receptor needs two homologous domains of the beta-subunit for activation by GABA but not by pentobarbital. Nature 366:565–569, 1993

Boileau AJ, Evers AR, Davis AF, et al: Mapping the agonist binding site of the GABAA receptor: evidence for a beta-strand. J Neurosci 19:4847–4854, 1999

Coleman RM: Diagnosis, treatment, and follow-up of about 8,000 sleep/wake disorder patients, in Sleep/Wake Disorders: Natural History, Epidemiology, and Long-Term Evolution. Edited by Guilleminault C, Lugarese E. New York, Raven, 1983, pp 29–35

Geddes DM, Rudorf M, Saunders KB: Effect of nitrazepam and flurazepam on the ventilatory response to carbon dioxide. Thorax 31:548–551, 1976

Möhler H, Okada T: Benzodiazepine receptor: demonstration in the central nervous system. Science 198:849–851, 1977

Schmidt RF, Vogel ME, Zimmermann M: Effect of diazepam on presynaptic inhibition and other spinal reflexes. Naunyn Schmiedebergs Arch Pharmacol 258:69–82, 1967

Sigel E, Baur R, Kellenberger S, et al: Point mutations affecting antagonist affinity and agonist dependent gating of GABA$_A$ receptor channels. EMBO J 11:2017–2023, 1992

Smith GB, Olsen RW: Identification of a [^{3}H]muscimol photoaffinity substrate in the bovine gamma-aminobutyric acid$_A$ receptor alpha subunit. J Biol Chem 269:20380–20387, 1994

Squires RF, Braestrup C: Benzodiazepine receptors in rat brain. Nature 266:732–734, 1977

CHAPTER 43

Psychostimulants in Psychiatry: Amphetamine, Methylphenidate, and Modafinil

Select the single best response for each question.

43.1 The action of which molecular structure provides the rate-limiting step in the clinical effects of amphetamines?

A. *N*-Methyl-D-aspartate (NMDA) receptors.
B. Dopamine transporter (DAT).
C. G-protein complex.
D. γ-Aminobutyric acid B ($GABA_B$) receptors.
E. Norepinephrine transporter (NET).

The correct response is option **B.**

The classic mechanism of action of amphetamines involves rapid diffusion directly into neuron terminals; through dopamine (DA) and norepinephrine (NE) transporters, amphetamine enters vesicles, causing release of DA and NE. The release of these neurotransmitters into the synapse mediates some of the psychological and motoric effects of amphetamine, including euphoria, increased energy, and locomotor activation. However, the actual mechanism of action of amphetamine appears to be more complex than simply promoting DA or NE efflux. This is most notably observed with respect to DA. Release of DA is a two-step process: 1) release from the vesicles into the *presynaptic* terminal and then 2) release from the presynaptic terminal into the synaptic cleft. Although amphetamines rapidly cause the release of DA from the vesicles into the presynaptic terminal, in knockout mice lacking an intact DAT, DA was not released into the synaptic cleft, thus showing that the action of the DAT constitutes the rate-limiting step in the effects of amphetamine (Jones et al. 1998). **(p. 674)**

43.2 What is a known neurotoxic effect of methamphetamine and its potential consequences?

A. The drug destroys acetylcholine neurons and increases the risk of cortical dementia.
B. The drug destroys γ-aminobutyric acid B ($GABA_B$) receptors and increases the risk of panic disorder.
C. The drug destroys dopaminergic neurons and may increase the risk of Parkinson's disease.
D. All of the above.
E. None of the above.

The correct response is option **C.**

Methamphetamine is more neurotoxic than amphetamine; it can cause destruction of dopaminergic neurons in the basal ganglia and, thus, is widely suspected to increase the likelihood of future parkinsonism (Guilarte 2001). **(p. 675)**

43.3 Amphetamine is partially metabolized by which of the following cytochrome P450 enzymes?

A. 1A2.
B. 2C9 and 2C19.
C. 2D6.
D. 2E1.
E. 3A4/5.

The correct response is option **C.**

A comprehensive review found that drug interactions with amphetamine were mostly pharmacodynamic in nature (Markowitz and Patrick 2001); however, because a small portion of amphetamine's metabolism occurs via cytochrome P450 2D6, those drugs that inhibit 2D6 metabolism can, theoretically, have the effect of increasing the plasma level of amphetamines. **(p. 674; see also p. 676)**

43.4 Potential adverse effects associated with methylphenidate use include which of the following?

A. Nervousness and insomnia.
B. Growth impairment.
C. Worsened tics.
D. All of the above.
E. None of the above.

The correct response is option **A.**

The common side effects of methylphenidate are similar to those of amphetamine and include nervousness, insomnia, and anorexia, as well as dose-related systemic effects such as increased heart rate and blood pressure. Although worry over the possibility that methylphenidate worsens tics is common, controlled trials indicate that this concern may be unfounded (Castellanos et al. 1997; Law and Schachar 1999). At least one such controlled study found that in children with comorbid tic disorder, tic severity was no worse with methylphenidate than with placebo until approximately 12 weeks, at which point the tic severity actually improved with methylphenidate (The Tourette's Syndrome Study Group 2002). There are case reports of growth impairment in children, possibly due to an effect on growth hormone secretion (Holtkamp et al. 2002), although numerous studies have not found such an effect on growth (Kramer et al. 2000; Lahat et al. 2000; Toren et al. 1997). **(pp. 676, 677)**

43.5 Which of the following statements best describes modafinil's cytochrome P450 metabolism?

A. Modafinil's metabolism occurs primarily via cytochrome P450 3A4/5.
B. Modafinil induces metabolism at cytochrome P450 3A4/5, which can reduce the effectiveness of medications such as triazolam.
C. Modafinil increases levels of medications metabolized at cytochrome P450 2C19, such as tricyclic antidepressants, phenytoin, and propranolol.
D. All of the above.
E. None of the above.

The correct response is **D.**

Modafinil induces cytochrome P450 3A4/5 and thus conceivably could lower the plasma concentrations of medications with substantial 3A4/5 metabolism. However, it is not clear whether this induction substantially affects only the gastrointestinal cytochrome and is thus relevant only for other drugs undergoing significant first-pass metabolism. Modafinil inhibits cytochrome P450 2C19 in vitro (Robertson et al. 2000). **(pp. 677–678)**

References

Castellanos X, Giedd J, Elia J, et al: Controlled stimulant treatment of ADHD and comorbid Tourette's syndrome: effects of stimulant and dose. J Am Acad Child Adolesc Psychiatry 36:589–596, 1997

Guilarte TR: Is methamphetamine abuse a risk factor in parkinsonism? Neurotoxicology 22:725–731, 2001

Holtkamp K, Peters-Wallraf B, Wüller S, et al: Methylphenidate-related growth impairment. J Child Adolesc Psychopharmacol 12:55–61, 2002

Jones SR, Gainetdinov RR, Wightman RM, et al: Mechanisms of amphetamine action revealed in mice lacking the dopamine transporter. J Neurosci 18:1979–1986, 1998

Kramer JR, Loney J, Ponto LB, et al: Predictors of adult height and weight in boys treated with methylphenidate for childhood behavior problems. J Am Acad Child Adolesc Psychiatry 39:517–524, 2000

Lahat E, Weiss M, Ben-Shlomo A, et al: Bone mineral density and turnover in children with attention-deficit/hyperactivity disorder receiving methylphenidate. J Child Neurol 15:436–439, 2000

Law SF, Schachar RJ: Do typical clinical doses of methylphenidate cause tics in children treated for attention-deficit/hyperactivity disorder? J Am Acad Child Adolesc Psychiatry 38:944–951, 1999

Markowitz JS, Patrick KS: Pharmacokinetic and pharmacodynamic drug interactions in the treatment of attention-deficit/hyperactivity disorder. Clin Pharmacokinet 40:753–772, 2001

Robertson P, DeCory HH, Madan A, et al: In vitro inhibition and induction of human hepatic cytochrome P450 enzymes by modafinil. Drug Metab Dispos 28:664–671, 2000

Toren P, Silbergeld A, Eldar S, et al: Lack of effect of methylphenidate on serum growth hormone (GH), GH-binding protein, and insulin-like growth factor I. Clin Neuropharmacol 20:264–269, 1997

The Tourette's Syndrome Study Group: Treatment of ADHD in children with tics: a randomized controlled trial. Neurology 58:527–536, 2002

CHAPTER 44

Electroconvulsive Therapy

Select the single best response for each question.

44.1 Electroconvulsive therapy (ECT) has been found to be effective in which of the following conditions?

A. Atypical depression, hypomania, and schizoaffective disorder.
B. Depression, mania, and drug-related psychosis.
C. Depression, mania, and schizotypal personality disorder.
D. Depression, mania, and schizoid personality disorder.
E. Depression, mania, and schizophrenia.

The correct response is option **E.**

Since ECT was first developed, almost 70 years ago, it has been found to be consistently effective in the treatment of depression, mania, and schizophrenia (Abrams 1992). **(p. 685)**

44.2 Electroconvulsive therapy (ECT) has been found to be effective in treating what percentage of individuals with treatment-resistant unipolar or bipolar depression?

A. 20%.
B. 40%.
C. 60%.
D. 80%.
E. 100%.

The correct response is option **D.**

ECT is an effective treatment in more than 80% of patients with treatment-resistant unipolar or bipolar major depression (Abrams 1992; Fink 1979; O'Connor et al. 2001; Petrides et al. 2001). **(p. 689)**

44.3 Electroconvulsive therapy (ECT) is effective in treating which of the following?

A. Acute psychotic break.
B. Catatonic schizophrenia.
C. Neuroleptic malignant syndrome.
D. All of the above.
E. None of the above.

The correct response is option **D.**

ECT continues to have an important role in the treatment of an acute psychotic break, catatonic schizophrenia, and neuroleptic malignant syndrome. **(p. 690)**

44.4   Which of the following medical conditions increases the risk of complications from electroconvulsive therapy (ECT)?

A. Increased intracranial pressure.
B. Recent myocardial infarction.
C. Severe chronic obstructive pulmonary disease.
D. Recent cerebral infarction.
E. All of the above.

The correct response is option **E**.

Several clinical conditions may increase the risk of complications from ECT: recent myocardial infarction or unstable cardiac conditions; any illness that increases intracranial pressure; recent cerebral infarction, particularly hemorrhagic infarction; aneurysm or vascular malformation; an American Society of Anesthesiology (ASA) physical-status classification of level 4 or 5; and severe pulmonary disease. **(p. 694)**

44.5   Which of the following statements best characterizes the memory loss attributed to ECT?

A. Anterograde memory loss can be temporary and retrograde memory loss can be permanent.
B. Anterograde memory loss can be permanent and retrograde memory loss can be temporary.
C. Both anterograde and retrograde memory loss can be temporary.
D. Both anterograde and retrograde memory loss can be permanent.
E. Anterograde memory loss can be permanent.

The correct response is option **A**.

The memory loss attributed to ECT is typically anterograde and retrograde and has a temporal gradient, being more profound around the time of the treatments and extending back months before the treatment and several weeks after the ECT course (American Psychiatric Association Task Force on Electroconvulsive Therapy 2001; Sackeim 2000). In most patients, the anterograde memory loss clears quickly after ECT, but in some patients, the retrograde memory loss can be permanent and may extend back years before ECT. **(p. 700)**

References

Abrams R: Electroconvulsive Therapy, 2nd Edition. New York, Oxford University Press, 1992

American Psychiatric Association Task Force on Electroconvulsive Therapy: The Practice of Electroconvulsive Therapy: Recommendations for Treatment, Training and Privileging. Task Force Report on ECT. Washington, DC, American Psychiatric Association, 2001

Fink M: Convulsive Therapy: Theory and Practice. New York, Raven, 1979

O'Connor MK, Knapp R, Husain M, et al: The influence of age on response of major depression to electroconvulsive therapy: a C.O.R.E. Report. Am J Geriatr Psychiatry 9:382–390, 2001

Petrides G, Fink M, Husain MM, et al: ECT remission rates in psychotic versus nonpsychotic depressed patients: a report from CORE. J ECT 17:244–253, 2001

Sackeim HA: Memory and ECT: from polarization to reconciliation (editorial; comment). J ECT 16:87–96, 2000

CHAPTER 45

Biology of Mood Disorders

Select the single best response for each question.

45.1   Which of the following statements best describes the state of current knowledge about genetic markers for bipolar disorder?

    A. Chromosome 21 has definitely been implicated.

    B. Chromosome 21 and the Y chromosome have definitely been implicated.

    C. After studies implicating chromosome 11 and the X chromosome were published, further studies have not supported these findings.

    D. After studies implicating chromosome 11 and the Y chromosome were published, further studies have not supported these findings.

    E. Chromosome 21 and the X chromosome have definitely been implicated.

The correct response is option **C.**

Two teams of investigators have reported two different genes associated with manic-depressive disorder. In a Pennsylvania Amish community, the gene reported to produce manic-depressive disorder was found to be positioned on chromosome 11 and inherited by autosomal dominant transmission (Egeland et al. 1987). Unfortunately, subsequent analysis did not confirm this finding in an expanded data set of the same population (Kelsoe et al. 1989). In an Israeli population, Baron et al. (1987) localized another gene responsible for bipolar disorder on the long arm of the X chromosome; this finding was later retracted (Baron et al. 1993). **(p. 723)**

45.2   Which of the following clinical findings has been demonstrated in patients with bipolar disorder?

    A. Decreased plasma cortisol concentration.

    B. Decreased cortisol in cerebrospinal fluid.

    C. Suppression of plasma glucocorticoid concentration after dexamethasone administration.

    D. Nonsuppression of plasma glucocorticoid concentration after dexamethasone administration.

    E. Increased diurnal variation of plasma cortisol concentrations.

The correct response is option **D.**

Alterations in the activity of the hypothalamic-pituitary-adrenal (HPA) axis in bipolar disorder include increased plasma cortisol concentrations, blunted diurnal variation of plasma cortisol concentrations, increased cortisol in cerebrospinal fluid, and nonsuppression of plasma glucocorticoid concentrations after dexamethasone administration. **(p. 725; see Table 45–2)**

45.3   Clinical response of depressed patients to antidepressant treatment has been associated with which of the following physiological measures?

   A. Increased metabolic activity in the rostral cingulate cortex.
   B. Decreased metabolic activity in the rostral cingulate cortex.
   C. Increased ventral prefrontal cortical activity.
   D. Increased metabolic activity in the left posterior cingulate cortex.
   E. None of the above.

The correct response is option **A.**

Among patients with major depression, antidepressant treatment response and symptom remission appear to be correlated with increased metabolic activity in the rostral cingulate cortex (Mayberg 2002). Ventral prefrontal cortical activity has been found to decrease among antidepressant treatment responders and found to be positively correlated with improvement in Hamilton Rating Scale for Depression scores (Brody et al. 1999). Lower metabolic activity in the left anterior cingulate gyrus at pretreatment seems to be associated with a greater degree of antidepressant treatment response (Brody et al. 1999). **(pp. 746–747; see also Table 45–18)**

45.4   Which of the following changes in the serotonergic system has been associated with depression?

   A. Decreased postsynaptic serotonin$_2$ (5-hydroxytryptamine [5-HT]$_2$) receptors.
   B. Increased plasma tryptophan concentrations.
   C. Increased prolactin response to fenfluramine.
   D. Increased postsynaptic 5-HT$_2$ receptors.
   E. Increased serotonin transporter (5-HTT) binding in midbrain.

The correct response is option **D.**

Alterations in the serotonergic system in depression include decreased plasma tryptophan concentrations (Deakin et al. 1990; Maes et al. 1990), increased postsynaptic 5-HT$_2$ receptors (Mann et al. 1986), blunted prolactin response to fenfluramine (Cowen and Charig 1987; Siever et al. 1984), and decreased 5-HTT binding in the midbrain (Malison et al. 1997). **(pp. 737–739; see also Table 45–8)**

45.5   Which of the following statements best describes the dexamethasone suppression test (DST)?

   A. The rate of cortisol nonsuppression correlates best with a diagnosis of atypical depression.
   B. The rate of cortisol nonsuppression correlates best with a diagnosis of nonpsychotic depression.
   C. The rate of cortisol nonsuppression correlates best with a diagnosis of psychotic depression.
   D. The rate of cortisol nonsuppression correlates best with a diagnosis of depression not otherwise specified (NOS).
   E. The rate of cortisol nonsuppression correlates best with a diagnosis of seasonal affective disorder.

The correct response is option **C.**

Another indication of hypothalamic-pituitary-adrenal (HPA) axis hyperactivity in depression is cortisol hypersecretion, which is reflected in elevated plasma corticosteroid concentrations (Carpenter and Bunney 1971; Gibbons and McHugh 1962), increased levels of cortisol metabolites (Sachar et al. 1970), elevated 24-hour urinary free cortisol concentrations, and nonsuppression of plasma hydroxycorticosteroid levels after the administration of dexamethasone (the DST). Since Carroll's (1968) initial report and subsequent claims for diagnostic utility (Carroll 1982), the DST has generated considerable controversy (Arana and Mossman 1988). The rate of cortisol nonsuppression after dexamethasone administration generally has been found to be correlated with the severity of the subtype of depression (i.e., nearly all patients with major depression with psychotic features show DST nonsuppression) (Arana et al. 1985; Evans and Nemeroff 1983; Krishnan et al. 1985; Schatzberg et al. 1984). For instance, a meta-analysis of 19 studies examining DST nonsuppression in patients with depression found that 64% of the subjects with psychotic depression showed nonsuppression of cortisol on the DST as compared with 41% of the nonpsychotic patients (Nelson and Davis 1997). (p. 726)

References

Arana GW, Mossman D: The DST and depression: approaches to the use of a laboratory test in psychiatry. Neurol Clin 6:21–39, 1988

Arana GW, Baldessarini RJ, Ornsteen M: The dexamethasone suppression test for diagnosis and prognosis in psychiatry. Arch Gen Psychiatry 42:1193–1204, 1985

Baron M, Risch N, Hamburger R, et al: Genetic linkage between X-chromosome markers and bipolar affective illness. Nature 326:289–292, 1987

Baron M, Freimer NF, Risch N: Diminished support for linkage between manic depressive illness and X-chromosome markers in three Israeli pedigrees. Nat Genet 3:49–55, 1993

Brody AL, Saxena S, Silverman DHS, et al: Brain metabolic changes in major depressive disorder from pre- to post-treatment with paroxetine. Psychiatry Res 91:127–139, 1999

Carpenter W, Bunney W: Adrenal cortical activity in depressive illness. Am J Psychiatry 128:31–40, 1971

Carroll BJ: Pituitary-adrenal function in depression. Lancet 1(7556):1373–1374, 1968

Carroll BJ: Use of the dexamethasone suppression test in depression. J Clin Psychiatry 43:44–50, 1982

Cowen PJ, Charig EM: Neuroendocrine responses to tryptophan in major depression. Arch Gen Psychiatry 44:958–966, 1987

Deakin JFW, Pennell I, Upadhyaya AJ, et al: A neuroendocrine study of 5-HT function in depression: evidence for biological mechanisms of endogenous and psychosocial causation. Psychopharmacology (Berl) 101:85–92, 1990

Egeland JA, Gerhard DS, Pauls DL, et al: Bipolar affective disorders linked to DNA markers on chromosome 11. Nature 325:783–787, 1987

Evans DL, Nemeroff CB: Use of the dexamethasone suppression test using DSM-III criteria on an inpatient psychiatric unit. Biol Psychiatry 18:505–511, 1983

Gibbons JL, McHugh PR: Plasma cortisol in depressive illness. J Psychiatr Res 1:162–171, 1962

Kelsoe JR, Ginns EI, Egeland JA, et al: Re-evaluation of the linkage relationship between chromosome 11p loci and the gene for bipolar affective disorder in the Old Order Amish. Nature 342:238–243, 1989

Krishnan KRR, France RD, Pelton S, et al: What does the dexamethasone suppression test identify? Biol Psychiatry 20:957–964, 1985

Maes M, Jacobs M-P, Suy E, et al: Suppressant effects of dexamethasone on the availability of plasma L-tryptophan and tyrosine in healthy controls and in depressed patients. Acta Psychiatr Scand 81:19–23, 1990

Malison RT, Pelton G, Carpenter L, et al: Reduced midbrain serotonin transporter binding in depressed vs. healthy subjects as measured by [^{123}I]beta-CIT SPECT. Society for Neuroscience Abstracts 23:1220, 1997

Mann JJ, Stanley M, McBride PA, et al: Increased serotonin 2 and beta-adrenergic receptor binding in the frontal cortices of suicide victims. Arch Gen Psychiatry 43:954–959, 1986

Mayberg HS: Depression, II: localization of pathophysiology. Am J Psychiatry 159:1979, 2002

Nelson JC, Davis JM: DST studies in psychotic depression: a meta-analysis. Am J Psychiatry 154:1497–1503, 1997

Sachar E, Hellman L, Fukushima D, et al: Cortisol production in depressive illness. Arch Gen Psychiatry 23:289–298, 1970

Schatzberg AF, Rothschild AJ, Bond TC, et al: The DST in psychotic depression: diagnostic and pathophysiologic implications. Psychopharmacol Bull 20:362–364, 1984

Siever LJ, Murphy DL, Slater S, et al: Plasma prolactin change following fenfluramine in depressed patients compared to controls: an evaluation of central serotonergic responsivity in depression. Life Sci 34:1029–1039, 1984

CHAPTER 46

Neurobiology of Schizophrenia

Select the single best response for each question.

46.1 Which of the following sensory modalities is consistently impaired in individuals with schizophrenia?

A. Sight.
B. Hearing.
C. Touch.
D. Taste.
E. Smell.

The correct response is option **E**.

Olfactory deficits have been noted in schizophrenia: patients with schizophrenia are impaired in their ability to detect and identify odors. Olfactory deficits are present at the onset of illness, do not relate to disease severity or treatment, and are possibly progressive (Kopala et al. 1993). It is unclear whether the deficits are part of the generalized neurocognitive impairment. The neuroanatomic differences noted in patients (Turetsky et al. 2000) suggest that olfactory bulb changes and medial temporal lobe abnormalities could mediate the observed behavioral aberrations. **(p. 766)**

46.2 Reduced volume of anterior, posterior, and (less consistently) total superior temporal gyrus has been correlated with which of the following clinical measures?

A. Persistence of negative symptoms.
B. Severity of auditory hallucinations and thought disorder.
C. Deficits in working memory.
D. Impaired processing of auditory evoked potentials.
E. Magnitude of comorbid mood dysregulation.

The correct response is option **B**.

Cortical temporal regions, especially the superior temporal gyrus, have been examined in patients with schizophrenia. Reduced volume has been observed in anterior (Barta et al. 1990; Pearlson et al. 1997), posterior (Shenton et al. 1992), and total superior temporal gyrus (Flaum et al. 1995; Marsh et al. 1999) and has been related to severity of auditory hallucinations (Barta et al. 1990) and thought disorder (Shenton et al. 1992). However, superior temporal gyrus volume reductions have not been noted in other studies (DeLisi et al. 1994; Kulynych et al. 1996). **(p. 767)**

46.3   In 1991, McCarley et al. found the greatest P300 amplitude separation between persons with schizophrenia and controls for which of the following electrode sites?

   A. Nondominant parietal lobe.
   B. Left occipital lobe.
   C. Left temporal lobe.
   D. Dominant frontal lobe.
   E. Nondominant frontal lobe.

The correct response is option **C**.

The greatest P300 amplitude separation between schizophrenia patients and healthy participants was reported for the left temporal electrode sites (McCarley et al. 1991). **(p. 768)**

46.4   The developmental histories of individuals with schizophrenia reveal higher rates of all of the following *except*

   A. Heavy maternal alcohol use during the first trimester.
   B. Maternal starvation during the first trimester.
   C. Maternal influenza infection during the second trimester.
   D. Rhesus and ABO blood-type incompatibility.
   E. Perinatal anoxic birth injuries.

The correct response is option **A**.

Higher frequencies of gestational and perinatal events and obstetrical complications have been noted in prospective studies of people who later manifest schizophrenia. Thus, for example, maternal starvation during the first trimester of pregnancy (Susser et al. 1996), maternal influenza infection during the second trimester (Mednick et al. 1988), rhesus and ABO blood-type incompatibility (Hollister et al. 1996), and perinatal anoxic birth injuries (Cannon et al. 2002) have been observed to occur at higher rates in the early development of persons who subsequently develop schizophrenia. **(p. 770)**

46.5   One of the most consistent neuroanatomic findings in schizophrenia has been

   A. Enlarged hippocampal volumes.
   B. Underdevelopment of the corpus callosum.
   C. Enlarged amygdala.
   D. Enlarged lateral ventricles.
   E. Pituitary hyperplasia.

The correct response is option **D**.

One of the most consistent neuroanatomic findings in schizophrenia has been an increase in size of the lateral ventricles, evident in early computed tomography studies as well as in magnetic resonance imaging studies (Liddle 1995). The degree of ventricular enlargement correlates with poor premorbid adjustment, and the enlargement has been found at the initial presentation. **(p. 770)**

46.6 The genetic contributions to schizophrenia may be best described as

A. Sex-linked.
B. Multifactorial.
C. Mendelian.
D. Mutations.
E. Iatrogenic.

The correct response is option **B**.

Schizophrenia is a heritable brain disorder with evidence of complex neural aberrations affecting frontotemporal brain networks. Current views are that genetic liability and environmental factors combine to produce the symptomatic manifestations. Advances in genetics have fueled intensified efforts to apply molecular methodologies in family study designs that include affected sibling pairs and other multiplex family paradigms, with symptoms providing the phenotypic characterization. A complementary approach is to study the genetics of schizophrenia from the neurobiological perspective as a culmination of genetic and environmental processes that lead to disruption in neurodevelopment (Freedman et al. 1999; Kendler 1999). This approach is advantageous considering the need, once candidate allelic involvement is established, to elucidate the pathophysiology leading to clinical manifestations (Goldman 1999). To date, no single gene has been associated with schizophrenia, although positive linkage results have been found for several chromosomal loci. A problem in linkage studies is that "schizophrenia" encompasses a broad range of complex behaviors, with variability even within families. **(pp. 768, 769)**

References

Barta PE, Pearlson GD, Powers RE, et al: Auditory hallucinations and smaller superior temporal gyral volume in schizophrenia. Am J Psychiatry 147:1457–1462, 1990

Cannon TD, van Erp TG, Rosso IM, et al: Fetal hypoxia and structural brain abnormalities in schizophrenic patients, their siblings, and controls. Arch Gen Psychiatry 59:35–41, 2002

DeLisi LE, Hoff AL, Chance N, et al: Asymmetries in the superior temporal lobe in male and female first-episode schizophrenic patients: measures of the planum temporale and superior temporal gyrus by MRI. Schizophr Res 12:19–28, 1994

Flaum M, Swayze VW II, O'Leary DS, et al: Effects of diagnosis, laterality, and gender on brain morphology in schizophrenia. Am J Psychiatry 152:704–714, 1995

Freedman R, Adler LE, Leonard S: Alternative phenotypes for the complex genetics of schizophrenia. Biol Psychiatry 45:551–558, 1999

Goldman D: Big mountain (editorial). Arch Gen Psychiatry 56:553, 1999

Hollister JM, Laing P, Mednick SA: Rhesus incompatibility as a risk factor for schizophrenia in male adults. Arch Gen Psychiatry 53:19–24, 1996

Kendler KS: Preparing for gene discovery. Arch Gen Psychiatry 56:554–555, 1999

Kopala LC, Clark C, Hurwitz T: Olfactory deficits in neuroleptic naive patients with schizophrenia. Schizophr Res 8:245–250, 1993

Kulynych JJ, Vladar K, Jones DW, et al: Superior temporal gyrus volume in schizophrenia: a study using MRI morphometry assisted by surface rendering. Am J Psychiatry 153:50–56, 1996

Liddle PF: Brain imaging, in Schizophrenia. Edited by Hirsch SR, Weinberger DR. London, Blackwood, 1995, pp 295–323

Marsh L, Lim KO, Hoff AL, et al: Severity of schizophrenia and magnetic resonance imaging abnormalities: a comparison of state and veterans hospital patients. Biol Psychiatry 45:49–61, 1999

McCarley RW, Faux SF, Shenton ME, et al: Event-related potentials in schizophrenia: their biological and clinical correlates and a new model of schizophrenic pathophysiology. Schizophr Res 4:209–231, 1991

Mednick SA, Machon RA, Huttunen M, et al: Adult schizophrenia following prenatal exposure to an influenza epidemic. Arch Gen Psychiatry 45:189–192, 1988

Pearlson GD, Barta PE, Powers RE, et al: Medial and superior temporal gyral volumes and cerebral asymmetry in schizophrenia versus bipolar disorder. Biol Psychiatry 41:1–14, 1997

Shenton ME, Kikinis R, Jolesz RA, et al: Left-lateralized temporal lobe abnormalities in schizophrenia and their relationship to thought disorder: a computerized, quantitative MRI study. N Engl J Med 327:604–612, 1992

Susser E, Neugebauer R, Hoek HW, et al: Schizophrenia after prenatal famine. Arch Gen Psychiatry 53:25–31, 1996

Turetsky BI, Moberg PJ, Yousem DM, et al: Reduced olfactory bulb volume in patients with schizophrenia. Am J Psychiatry 157:828–830, 2000

CHAPTER 47

Neurobiology of Anxiety Disorders

Select the single best response for each question.

47.1 The involvement of noradrenergic systems in enhanced memory consolidation of emotional material is evidenced by the blocking of this effect by

A. Clonidine.
B. Guanfacine.
C. Propranolol.
D. Yohimbine.
E. Bupropion.

The correct response is option **C**.

Animal data have shown that administration of cortisol, epinephrine, and norepinephrine at the times of training and testing enhances consolidation and retrieval of memory, respectively (Roozendaal 2000; Southwick et al. 1999). Propranolol, administered pre- or posttraining (Cahill et al. 2000), abolishes these effects. In humans, memory for an emotional story is superior to memory for a nonemotional story (Cahill et al. 1994). Propranolol blocks the superior mnemonic encoding of the emotional story but does not alter memory for the emotionally neutral story (Cahill et al. 1994). Pitman et al. (2002) administered propranolol to trauma survivors in an emergency department within 6 hours of exposure to trauma. Propranolol was more effective than placebo in preventing the development of posttraumatic stress disorder at 1 and 3 months, although the difference did not reach statistical significance. A recent human study reported that the magnitude of increase in noradrenergic activity after viewing an emotional story is related to the extent of recall of this story (Southwick et al. 2002). Corticotropin-releasing hormone (CRH) infusions in the hippocampus enhance memory consolidation. This enhancement is blocked by propranolol. These results support the concept that CRH, glucocorticoids, and the noradrenergic system interact to consolidate traumatic memories, enhancing fear conditioning in vulnerable subjects (see McGaugh 2002). Administration of CRH antagonists, glucocorticoids, and adrenergic receptor antagonists may prevent these effects. **(p. 776)**

47.2 Fear- or anxiety-inducing stimuli in which sensory modality are transmitted to the amygdala rather than to the dorsal thalamus?

A. Sight.
B. Hearing.
C. Touch.
D. Smell.
E. Taste.

The correct response is option **D**.

The sensory information contained in a fear- or anxiety-inducing stimulus is transmitted from peripheral receptor cells to the dorsal thalamus (LeDoux 2000). An exception is the olfactory system, which does not relay information through the thalamus and whose principal targets in the brain are the amygdala and entorhinal cortex. **(p. 777)**

47.3 Each of the following agents has been used to provoke panic attacks in experimental protocols *except*

A. Disulfiram.
B. Carbon dioxide (CO_2).
C. Cholecystokinin-4 (CCK-4).
D. Yohimbine.
E. Lactate.

The correct response is option **A.**

Decreased bilateral resting perfusion was reported in lactate-sensitive subjects with panic disorder compared with control subjects. Anxiety attacks induced in healthy humans with CCK-4 also were associated with regional cerebral blood flow (CBF) increases in similar regions and the anterior cingulate cortex. Yohimbine administration increased medial frontal CBF in healthy control subjects but decreased relative prefrontal cortical perfusion in patients with panic disorder relative to control subjects. Patients with panic disorder, but not healthy control subjects, had reductions in absolute measures of global CBF under CO_2 provocation (Ponto et al. 2002). **(pp. 778, 779)**

47.4 Fear and anxiety states activate noradrenergic neurons in which of the following brain structures?

A. Amygdala.
B. Ventromedial hypothalamus.
C. Thalamus.
D. Hippocampus.
E. Locus coeruleus.

The correct response is option **E.**

The locus coeruleus is the major noradrenergic cell body aggregate in the brain. Neurons in the locus coeruleus are activated during fear and anxiety states (see Charney and Drevets 2002 for review). Limbic and cortical regions innervated by the locus coeruleus are involved in the elaboration of adaptive responses to stress. **(p. 781)**

47.5 Early and chronic exposures to stressors may be associated with hippocampal damage, mediated through elevated levels of

A. Testosterone.
B. Corticotropin-releasing hormone (CRH).
C. Growth hormone.
D. Prolactin.
E. Substance P.

The correct response is option **B.**

Exposure to stress in early life can produce long-term elevation of CRH (i.e., exaggerated CRH release) and sensitization of CRH neurons to subsequent stress. The long-term response to heightened CRH is individual and may depend on social environment, trauma history, and behavioral dominance (Strome et al. 2002). Early exposure of the hippocampus to elevated levels of CRH may be associated with hippocampal damage later in life (Brunson et al. 2001). **(p. 783)**

47.6   Dysregulation of dopaminergic release in which of the following brain structures is associated with helplessness behaviors and delayed extinction of conditioned fear responses?

   A. Amygdala.
   B. Nucleus accumbens.
   C. Medial prefrontal cortex.
   D. Tuberoinfundibular tract.
   E. Cingulate gyrus.

The correct response is option **C**.

Dopamine innervation of the medial prefrontal cortex appears to be particularly susceptible to stress. Increasing intensity and/or duration of stress can enhance dopamine release and metabolism in other areas receiving dopamine innervation (i.e., the mesolimbic and nigrostriatal systems). Uncontrollable stress activates dopamine release in the medial prefrontal cortex (Ventura et al. 2002) and inhibits it in the nucleus accumbens (Cabib and Puglisi-Allegra 1996). Lesions of medial prefrontal cortex dopamine neurons or reduced medial prefrontal cortex dopamine release delays extinction of the conditioned fear stress response, a situation hypothesized to occur in posttraumatic stress disorder (Morrow et al. 1999). Increased medial prefrontal cortex dopamine release thus enhances extinction while contributing to helplessness behavior. There may be an optimal range of medial prefrontal cortex dopamine release that facilitates adaptive behavioral responses, extinction of conditioned emotional memories without features of learned helplessness. Too much dopamine release (as in uncontrollable stress) could produce learned helplessness behavior, whereas insufficient medial prefrontal cortex dopamine release could prolong conditioned fear responses. **(p. 785)**

47.7   Stimulation of which of the following neurotransmitter receptors is anxiolytic?

   A. Corticotropin-releasing hormone receptor 1 (CRHR1).
   B. Serotonin (5-hydroxytryptamine)$_{1A}$ (5-HT$_{1A}$).
   C. 5-HT$_{2A}$.
   D. Dopamine$_2$ (D$_2$).
   E. α_1-Adrenergic.

The correct response is option **B**.

5-HT release has both anxiogenic and anxiolytic effects, depending on the region involved and the receptor subtype activated. Most anxiogenic effects are mediated via the 5-HT$_{2A}$ receptor, whereas stimulation of 5-HT$_{1A}$ receptors is anxiolytic and may even relate to adaptive responses to aversive events. **(p. 786)**

References

Brunson KL, Eghbal-Ahmadi M, Bender R, et al: Long-term, progressive hippocampal cell loss and dysfunction induced by early life administration of corticotropin-releasing hormone reproduce the effects of early life stress. Proc Natl Acad Sci U S A 98:8856–8861, 2001

Cabib S, Puglisi-Allegra S: Different effects of repeated stressful experiences on mesocortical and mesolimbic dopamine metabolism. Neuroscience 73:375–380, 1996

Cahill L, Prins B, Weber M, et al: Beta-adrenergic activation and memory for emotional events. Nature 371:702–704, 1994

Cahill L, Pham CA, Setlow B: Impaired memory consolidation in rats produced with beta-adrenergic blockade. Neurobiol Learn Mem 74:259–266, 2000

Charney DS, Drevets WD: Neurobiological basis of anxiety disorders, in Neuropsychopharmacology: The Fifth Generation of Progress. Edited by Davis KL, Charney D, Coyle JT, et al. Baltimore, MD, Lippincott Williams & Wilkins, 2002, pp 901–930

LeDoux JE: Emotion circuits in the brain. Annu Rev Neurosci 23:155–184, 2000

McGaugh JL: Memory consolidation and the amygdala. Trends Neurosci 25:456–461, 2002

Morrow BA, Elsworth JD, Rasmusson AM, et al: The role of mesoprefrontal dopamine neurons in the acquisition and expression of conditioned fear in the rat. Neuroscience 92:553–564, 1999

Pitman RK, Sanders KM, Zusman RM, et al: Pilot study of secondary prevention of posttraumatic stress disorder with propranolol. Biol Psychiatry 51:189–192, 2002

Ponto LL, Kathol RG, Kettelkamp R, et al: Global cerebral blood flow after CO_2 inhalation in normal subjects and patients with panic disorder determined with [^{15}O]water and PET. J Anxiety Disord 16:247–258, 2002

Roozendaal B: 1999 Curt P. Richter award: glucocorticoids and the regulation of memory consolidation. Psychoneuroendocrinology 25:213–238, 2000

Southwick SM, Paige S, Morgan CA 3rd, et al: Neurotransmitter alterations in PTSD: catecholamines and serotonin. Semin Clin Neuropsychiatry 4:242–248, 1999

Southwick SM, Davis M, Horner B, et al: Relationship of enhanced norepinephrine activity during memory consolidation to enhanced long-term memory in humans. Am J Psychiatry 159:1420–1422, 2002

Strome EM, Wheler GH, Higley JD, et al: Intracerebroventricular corticotropin-releasing factor increases limbic glucose metabolism and has social context-dependent behavioral effects in nonhuman primates. Proc Natl Acad Sci U S A 99:15749–15754, 2002

Ventura R, Cabib S, Puglisi-Allegra S: Genetic susceptibility of mesocortical dopamine to stress determines liability to inhibition of mesoaccumbens dopamine and to behavioral 'despair' in a mouse model of depression. Neuroscience 115:999–1007, 2002

CHAPTER 48

Biology of Alzheimer's Disease

Select the single best response for each question.

48.1 Of all the pathological alterations seen in Alzheimer's disease (AD), which of the following best correlates with cognitive deficits?

   A. Number of neurofibrillary tangles.
   B. Number of neuritic plaques.
   C. Location of amyloid deposition.
   D. Amount of cortical cellular loss.
   E. Loss of cortical synapses.

The correct response is option **E.**

A–D are all important in understanding the pathophysiology of AD, but of all pathological alterations, synapse loss best correlates with cognitive deficits. **(p. 794)**

48.2 All of the following point to failed neurotransmission at cholinergic synapses in the neocortex and hippocampus in Alzheimer's disease (AD) *except*

   A. Acetylcholinesterase (AChE) inhibitors achieve a high degree (over 80%) of AChE inhibition, which explains their efficacy in AD.
   B. Presynaptic cholinergic markers are decreased in AD.
   C. Basal forebrain neurons degenerate in AD.
   D. Pharmacological blockage of basal forebrain muscarinic acetylcholine receptors impairs learning and memory.
   E. AChE inhibitors improve cognitive and behavioral problems associated with AD.

The correct response is option **A.**

The typical degree of AChE inhibition achievable with available drugs is only about 30% (Kuhl et al. 2000), which provides one explanation for their modest efficacy. Abundant evidence suggests that AD involves failed neurotransmission at cholinergic synapses in neocortex and hippocampus (Coyle et al. 1983). This concept is based on several observations. First, presynaptic cholinergic markers are decreased in neocortex and hippocampus in AD, and they have been found to correlate with dementia severity (Bowen and Francis 1990). Second, basal forebrain neurons, which provide the majority of cholinergic innervation of neocortex and hippocampus, degenerate in AD (Whitehouse et al. 1982). Third, basal forebrain lesions or pharmacological blockade of muscarinic acetylcholine receptors impairs learning, memory, and attention (Damasio et al. 1985). Finally, clinical trials of AChE inhibitors show improved cognition and quality of life, reduced behavioral problems, and delayed institutionalization (see Cummings and Cole 2002). **(p. 795)**

48.3   Which of the following statements regarding muscarinic and nicotinic receptors is *true*?

A. Muscarinic$_4$ (M$_4$) receptors are decreased in Alzheimer's disease (AD).
B . A muscarinic$_1$ (M$_1$) agonist has been shown to reduce hallucinations and agitation in AD.
C. M$_4$ is the most abundant receptor in the cortex and hippocampus.
D. M$_1$ is primarily an autoreceptor on cholinergic terminals.
E. Nicotinic receptors have a very well-defined role in cholinergic transmission in AD.

The correct response is option **B.**

One of the first selective M$_1$ agonists, xanomeline, showed significant clinical efficacy in a double-blind, multicenter study (Bodick et al. 1997), with some of the benefits being reduced agitation, delusions, and hallucinations. M$_4$ is actually increased in Alzheimer's disease. M$_1$ is the most abundant receptor in the cortex and hippocampus. M$_2$ is primarily an autoreceptor on cholinergic terminals. Nicotinic receptors also play a role, albeit a poorly defined one, in cholinergic transmission. **(pp. 796–797)**

48.4   The biggest risk factor for Alzheimer's disease (AD) is

A. Presence of the apolipoprotein-E (APOE) ε4 allele.
B. Poor linguistic abilities in early life.
C. Age.
D. Mutations in the amyloid precursor protein (*APP*) gene on chromosome 21, the presenilin 1 (*PS1*) gene on chromosome 4, and the presenilin 2 (*PS2*) gene on chromosome 1.
E. None of the above.

The correct response is option **C.**

Aging is the biggest risk factor for AD. Inheritance of the APOE ε4 allele; poor linguistic abilities in early life; and mutations in *APP*, *PS1*, and *PS2* do confer possible risks for Alzheimer's disease, but not to the degree that age does. **(pp. 797, 798)**

48.5   Regarding prospective clinical trials of nonsteroidal anti-inflammatory drugs (NSAIDs) in Alzheimer's disease (AD), which of the following statements is *true*?

A. NSAIDs have been found to reduce the risk of developing AD by 30%–80%.
B. NSAIDs have shown no benefit in patients with AD.
C. No prospective studies have been conducted, only retrospective studies.
D. NSAID use has proven too risky, because of these agents' side effects.
E. Studies have yielded mixed results, with some showing benefit for NSAIDs in AD and others not.

The correct response is option **B.**

Prospective clinical trials of NSAIDs have thus far been negative. However, several epidemiological investigations, including a large prospective population-based study, found that the relative risk of AD was lower with long-term use of NSAIDs (in t' Veld et al. 2001; Stewart et al. 1997). The magnitude of the reduced risk associated with NSAIDs ranged from 30% to 80%. Nonetheless, it is posited that anti-inflammatory agents may have a protective role in earlier preclinical stages of AD, and prospective studies examining this possibility are currently under way. **(pp. 798, 803)**

48.6   Which of the following is the primary focus of the leading theory of Alzheimer's disease (AD) pathogenesis?

A. Inflammation.
B. Oxidative injury.
C. Mitochondrial dysfunction.
D. Amyloid cascade.
E. None of the above.

The correct response is option **D.**

The amyloid cascade hypothesis has gained increasing support in recent years and is the theory currently favored by many investigators of AD (Hardy and Selkoe 2002). Other theories with particular relevance for current clinical practice have focused on the roles of cholinergic systems, inflammation, and oxidative injury in the pathogenesis of AD. **(pp. 799, 800, 802, 803)**

References

Bodick NC, Offen WW, Levey AI, et al: Effects of xanomeline, a selective muscarinic receptor agonist, on cognitive function and behavioral symptoms in Alzheimer disease. Arch Neurol 54:465–473, 1997

Bowen D, Francis P: Neurochemistry, neuropharmacology, and aetiological factors in Alzheimer's disease. Semin Neurosci 2:101–108, 1990

Coyle J, Price D, DeLong M: Alzheimer's disease: disorder of cortical cholinergic innervation. Science 219:1184–1190, 1983

Cummings JL, Cole G: Alzheimer disease. JAMA 287:2335–2338, 2002

Damasio AR, Graff-Radford N, Eslinger PJ, et al: Amnesia following basal forebrain lesions. Arch Neurol 42:263–271, 1985

Hardy J, Selkoe DJ: The amyloid hypothesis of Alzheimer's disease: progress and problems on the road to therapeutics. Science 297:353–356, 2002

in t' Veld BA, Ruitenberg A, Hofman A, et al: Nonsteroidal antiinflammatory drugs and the risk of Alzheimer's disease. N Engl J Med 345:1515–1521, 2001

Kuhl DE, Minoshima S, Frey KA, et al: Limited donepezil inhibition of acetylcholinesterase measured with positron emission tomography in living Alzheimer cerebral cortex. Ann Neurol 48:391–395, 2000

Stewart WF, Kawas C, Corrada M, et al: Risk of Alzheimer's disease and duration of NSAID use. Neurology 48:626–632, 1997

Whitehouse PJ, Price DL, Struble RG, et al: Alzheimer's disease and senile dementia: loss of neurons in the basal forebrain. Science 215:1237–1239, 1982

CHAPTER 49

Neurobiology of Substance Abuse Disorders

Select the single best response for each question.

49.1   The neural substrates of drug reward and reinforcement include which of the following?

    A. Extrapyramidal system.
    B. Dorsal raphe nuclei.
    C. Tegmental fields.
    D. Mesolimbic projections to the nucleus accumbens.
    E. All of the above.

The correct response is option **D.**

Animal models have implicated brain dopamine systems, specifically the mesolimbic projection to the nucleus accumbens (a component of the ventral striatum), as the neural substrate of drug reward and reinforcement (Di Chiara and Imperato 1988). **(p. 810)**

49.2   The primary receptor site of action of cocaine is

    A. Dopamine transporter (DAT).
    B. Vesicular monoamine transporter (VMAT).
    C. Nicotinic acetylcholine (ACh) receptors.
    D. γ-Aminobutyric acid (GABA) receptors.
    E. *N*-Methyl-D-aspartate (NMDA) receptors.

The correct response is option **A.**

Cocaine's three known molecular targets are the DAT, the serotonin transporter (5-HTT), and the norepinephrine transporter (NET). **(p. 811; see Table 49–1)**

49.3   The primary receptor site of action of ethanol is

    A. Dopamine transporter (DAT).
    B. Vesicular monoamine transporter (VMAT).
    C. Nicotinic acetylcholine (ACh) receptors.
    D. γ-Aminobutyric acid (GABA) and *N*-methyl-D-aspartate (NMDA) receptors.
    E. G proteins.

The correct response is option **D.**

Ethanol's primary molecular targets are the GABA and NMDA receptors. **(p. 811; see Table 49–1)**

49.4 Functional neuroimaging studies have implicated which of the following mechanisms in opiate and nicotine dependence?

A. Lack of reward-related striatal activation and lack of reinforcement-related activation of brain areas involved in reward processes.

B. Significant reward-related striatal activation and lack of reinforcement-related activation of brain areas involved in reward processes.

C. Significant reward-related striatal activation and significant reinforcement-related activation of brain areas involved in reward processing.

D. Lack of reward-related striatal activation and significant reinforcement-related activation of brain areas involved in reward processing.

E. None of the above.

The correct response is option **A**.

Recent functional neuroimaging findings suggest that drug addiction is associated with neurobiological evidence for deficits in processing rewards. Martin-Soelch et al. (2001a, 2001b) reported that opiate- and nicotine-dependent subjects had distinct patterns, relative to non-drug-dependent subjects, of distributed neural activity related to processing monetary rewards and nonmonetary behavioral reinforcers. Drug dependence was associated with a lack of reward-related striatal activation and a lack of reinforcement-related activation of brain areas involved in reward processing. **(p. 812)**

49.5 Positron emission tomography (PET) imaging has been used to assess the effects of cocaine craving in cocaine-dependent subjects. Conditioned cocaine cues were found to be associated with activation of which of the following brain structures?

A. Amygdala.

B. Prefrontal cortex.

C. Anterior cingulate cortex.

D. All of the above.

E. None of the above.

The correct response is option **D**.

Both PET and functional magnetic resonance imaging (fMRI) have been used to localize the hemodynamic correlates of alterations in brain activity in response to drug use reminders in drug-dependent subjects. Videotapes of simulated drug use and the handling of drug paraphernalia, script-guided mental imagery of drug use, and olfactory associations have been used as conditioned drug cues in abstinent cocaine, ethanol, and nicotine abusers. Grant et al. (1996) used PET imaging to assess the effects of cocaine craving induced by discriminative stimuli that predicted availability of cocaine on metabolic correlates of brain activity in cocaine-dependent men and women. Relative to a drug-free videotape and object-handling control condition, cocaine-related stimuli were associated with activation of the amygdala and dorsolateral prefrontal cortex. Subsequent PET (Childress et al. 1999) and fMRI (Maas et al. 1998) studies of similar conditioned cocaine cues in cocaine-dependent subjects further implicated the amygdala and prefrontal cortex, as well as the anterior cingulate cortex, in the craving response. The anterior cingulate response to conditioned cocaine cues was subsequently shown to precede the experience of cocaine craving (Wexler et al. 2001). **(p. 813)**

References

Childress AR, Mozley PD, McElgin W, et al: Limbic activation during cue-induced cocaine craving. Am J Psychiatry 156:11–18, 1999

Di Chiara G, Imperato A: Drugs abused by humans preferentially increase synaptic dopamine concentrations in the mesolimbic system of freely moving rats. Proc Natl Acad Sci U S A 85:5274–5278, 1988

Grant S, London ED, Newlin DB, et al: Activation of memory circuits during cue-induced cocaine craving. Proc Natl Acad Sci U S A 93:12040–12045, 1996

Maas LC, Lukas SE, Kaufman MJ, et al: Functional magnetic resonance imaging of human brain activation during cue-induced cocaine craving. Am J Psychiatry 155:124–126, 1998

Martin-Soelch C, Leenders KL, Chevalley AF, et al: Reward mechanisms in the brain and their role in dependence: evidence from neurophysiological and neuroimaging studies. Brain Res Brain Res Rev 36:139–149, 2001a

Martin-Soelch C, Magyar S, Künig G, et al: Changes in brain activation associated with reward processing in smokers and nonsmokers. Exp Brain Res 139:278–286, 2001b

Wexler BE, Gottschalk CH, Fulbright RK, et al: Functional magnetic resonance imaging of cocaine craving. Am J Psychiatry 158:86–95, 2001

CHAPTER 50

Biology of Eating Disorders

Select the single best response for each question.

50.1   Individuals with the binge-eating/purging subtype of anorexia nervosa are more likely than those with the restricting subtype to have a history of which of the following?

A. Behavioral dyscontrol.
B. Substance abuse.
C. Overt family conflict.
D. All of the above.
E. None of the above.

The correct response is option **D.**

Individuals with the binge-eating/purging subtype of anorexia nervosa are more likely to have histories of behavioral dyscontrol, substance abuse, and overt family conflict in comparison with those with the restricting subtype. **(p. 820)**

50.2   Which of the following statements concerning anorexia nervosa is *true*?

A. When at normal weight, patients with anorexia nervosa have increased plasma cortisol secretion.
B. Once increased, plasma and cerebrospinal fluid (CSF) levels of corticotropin-releasing hormone (CRH) never return to normal.
C. Intracerebroventricular CRH administration in experimental animals fails to produce physiological and behavioral changes similar to anorexia nervosa in humans.
D. The hypothalamic-pituitary-thyroid axis is activated by weight gain.
E. When underweight, patients with anorexia nervosa have increased plasma cortisol secretion.

The correct response is option **E.**

When underweight, patients with anorexia nervosa have increased plasma cortisol secretion that is thought to be at least in part a consequence of hypersecretion of endogenous CRH (Gold et al. 1986; Kaye et al. 1987; Licinio et al. 1996; Walsh et al. 1987). In that the plasma and CSF measures return toward normal, it appears likely that activation of the hypothalamic-pituitary-thyroid axis is precipitated by weight loss. The observation of increased CRH activity is of great theoretical interest in anorexia nervosa, because intracerebroventricular CRH administration in experimental animals produces many of the physiological and behavioral changes that are associated with anorexia nervosa, including markedly decreased eating behavior (Glowa and Gold 1991). **(p. 824)**

50.3 Which of the following statements about patients with bulimia nervosa is *true*?

    A. In comparison with control subjects, patients with bulimia nervosa have diminished release of cholecystokinin (CCK) following ingestion of a standardized test meal.

    B. In comparison with control subjects, patients with bulimia nervosa have excessive release of CCK following ingestion of a standardized test meal.

    C. In comparison with control subjects, patients with bulimia nervosa have no release of CCK following ingestion of a standardized test meal.

    D. Standardized test meals have no effect on CCK levels in patients with bulimia nervosa.

    E. None of the above.

The correct response is option **A.**

CCK is a peptide secreted by the gastrointestinal system in response to food intake. Release of CCK is thought to be one means of transmitting satiety signals to the brain by way of vagal afferents (Gibbs et al. 1973). In parallel to its role in satiety in rodents, exogenously administered CCK reduces food intake in humans. The preponderance of data suggests that patients with bulimia nervosa, in comparison with control subjects, have diminished release of CCK following ingestion of a standardized test meal (Devlin et al. 1997; Geracioti and Liddle 1988; Phillipp et al. 1991; Pirke et al. 1994). **(p. 824)**

50.4 In patients who achieve sustained recovery from bulimia nervosa, serum levels of leptin

    A. Gradually increase over time.

    B. Remain decreased.

    C. Are associated with increased metabolic rate.

    D. Are associated with reduced metabolic rate.

    E. None of the above.

The correct response is option **B.**

Leptin is secreted predominantly by adipose tissue cells and acts in the central nervous system to decrease food intake, thus regulating body fat stores. Initial findings in individuals who achieved sustained recovery from bulimia nervosa, when compared with control subjects with closely matched percentage body fat, suggest that serum leptin levels remain decreased (Baranowska et al. 2001; Brewerton et al. 2000). This finding may be related to evidence for a persistent decrease in activity in the hypothalamic-pituitary-thyroid axis in individuals in long-term recovery from bulimia nervosa. These alterations could be associated with decreased metabolic rate and a tendency toward weight gain, contributing to the preoccupation with body weight characteristic of bulimia nervosa. **(p. 825)**

50.5 Which of the following statements regarding serotonin metabolism in anorexia nervosa is *true*?

    A. Cerebrospinal fluid (CSF) concentrations of 5-hydroxyindoleacetic acid (5-HIAA) are decreased in individuals with long-term weight recovery.

    B. When underweight, women with anorexia nervosa show significant elevations in basal CSF concentrations of 5-HIAA.

    C. Resumption of normal eating may unmask intrinsic abnormalities in serotonergic systems that mediate certain core behavioral or temperamental underpinnings of risk and vulnerability.

    D. All of the above.

    E. None of the above.

The correct response is option **C**.

Serotonergic pathways play an important role in postprandial satiety, and there has been considerable interest in the role that serotonin may play in anorexia nervosa and bulimia nervosa (Brewerton 1995; Jimerson et al. 1990; Kaye and Weltzin 1991; Kaye et al. 1998; Treasure and Campbell 1994). In part, this is related to the fact that studies have found that patients with anorexia nervosa and bulimia nervosa have alterations in serotonin metabolism. When underweight, women with anorexia nervosa show significant reductions in basal CSF concentrations of the serotonin metabolite 5-HIAA compared with healthy control subjects, as well as blunted plasma prolactin response to drugs with serotonergic activity and reduced [^{3}H]imipramine binding. Together, these findings suggest reduced serotonergic activity, although this may arise secondarily from reductions in dietary supplies of the serotonin precursor amino acid tryptophan. By contrast, CSF concentrations of 5-HIAA are reported to be elevated in individuals with long-term weight recovery from anorexia nervosa. These contrasting findings of reduced and heightened serotonergic activity in individuals who are acutely ill and have been in long-term recovery from anorexia nervosa, respectively, may seem counterintuitive; however, because dieting lowers plasma tryptophan levels in otherwise healthy women (Anderson et al. 1990), resumption of normal eating in individuals with anorexia nervosa may unmask intrinsic abnormalities in serotonergic systems that mediate certain core behavioral or temperamental underpinnings of risk and vulnerability. **(p. 826)**

References

Anderson IM, Parry-Billings M, Newsholme EA, et al: Dieting reduces plasma tryptophan and alters brain 5-HT function in women. Psychol Med 20:785–791, 1990

Baranowska B, Wolinska-Witort E, Wasilewska-Dziubinska E, et al: Plasma leptin, neuropeptide Y (NPY) and galanin concentrations in bulimia nervosa and in anorexia nervosa. Neuro Endocrinol Lett 22:356–358, 2001

Brewerton TD: Toward a unified theory of serotonin dysregulation in eating and related disorders. Psychoneuroendocrinology 20:561–590, 1995

Brewerton TD, Lesem MD, Kennedy A, et al: Reduced plasma leptin concentration in bulimia nervosa. Psychoneuroendocrinology 25:649–658, 2000

Devlin MJ, Walsh BT, Guss JL, et al: Postprandial cholecystokinin release and gastric emptying in patients with bulimia nervosa. Am J Clin Nutr 65:114–120, 1997

Geracioti TD Jr, Liddle RA: Impaired cholecystokinin secretion in bulimia nervosa. N Engl J Med 319:683–688, 1988

Gibbs J, Young RC, Smith GP: Cholecystokinin decreases food intake in rats. J Comp Physiol Psychol 84:488–495, 1973

Glowa JR, Gold PW: Corticotropin releasing hormone produces profound anorexigenic effects in the rhesus monkey. Neuropeptides 18:55–61, 1991

Gold PW, Gwirtsman H, Avgerinos PC, et al: Abnormal hypothalamic-pituitary-adrenal function in anorexia nervosa: pathophysiologic mechanisms in underweight and weight-corrected patients. N Engl J Med 314:1335–1342, 1986

Jimerson DC, Lesem MD, Kaye WH, et al: Eating disorders and depression: is there a serotonin connection? Biol Psychiatry 28:443–454, 1990

Kaye WH, Weltzin TE: Serotonin activity in anorexia and bulimia nervosa: relationship to the modulation of feeding and mood. J Clin Psychiatry 52(suppl):41–48, 1991

Kaye WH, Gwirtsman HE, George DT, et al: Elevated cerebrospinal fluid levels of immunoreactive corticotropin-releasing hormone in anorexia nervosa: relation to state of nutrition, adrenal function, and intensity of depression. J Clin Endocrinol Metab 64:203–208, 1987

Kaye WH, Greeno CG, Moss H, et al: Alterations in serotonin activity and psychiatric symptomatology after recovery from bulimia nervosa. Arch Gen Psychiatry 55:927–935, 1998

Licinio J, Wong ML, Gold PW: The hypothalamic-pituitary-adrenal axis in anorexia nervosa. Psychiatry Res 62:75–83, 1996

Phillipp E, Pirke KM, Kellner MB, et al: Disturbed cholecystokinin secretion in patients with eating disorders. Life Sci 48:2443–2450, 1991

Pirke KM, Kellner MB, Friess E, et al: Satiety and cholecystokinin. Int J Eat Disord 15:63–69, 1994

Treasure J, Campbell I: The case for biology in the aetiology of anorexia nervosa. Psychol Med 24:3–8, 1994

Walsh BT, Roose SP, Katz JL, et al: Hypothalamic-pituitary-adrenal-cortical activity in anorexia nervosa and bulimia. Psychoneuroendocrinology 12:131–140, 1987

CHAPTER 51

Biology of Personality Disorders

Select the single best response for each question.

51.1   Which of the following diagnoses is found at increased prevalence among the first-degree relatives of patients with schizophrenia?

A. Antisocial personality disorder.
B. Generalized anxiety disorder.
C. Borderline personality disorder.
D. Schizotypal personality disorder.
E. Attention-deficit/hyperactivity disorder.

The correct response is option **D**.

Schizotypal personality disorder is more prevalent among first-degree relatives of persons with schizophrenia. This also may be true, although to a lesser extent, of paranoid, schizoid, and avoidant personality disorders but not borderline personality disorder (Kendler et al. 1993). Given the strong familial relationship between schizophrenia and schizotypal personality disorder, it follows that investigations of abnormalities found in schizophrenia might be applied to schizotypal personality disorder. Such an investigation would help to define a dimension of schizotypy or of its components (e.g., psychosis proneness, negative symptoms). **(p. 837)**

51.2   In response to amphetamine challenge, individuals with which of the following diagnoses are more likely than control subjects to become psychotic?

A. Antisocial personality disorder.
B. Generalized anxiety disorder.
C. Borderline personality disorder.
D. Avoidant personality disorder.
E. Attention-deficit/hyperactivity disorder.

The correct response is option **C**.

Individuals with borderline personality disorder are more likely than control subjects without borderline personality disorder to develop psychotic symptoms in response to amphetamine challenge (Schulz et al. 1985, 1988). **(p. 838)**

51.3   There is substantial comorbidity between which of the following diagnoses?

   A. Generalized social phobia and avoidant personality disorder.
   B. Panic disorder and avoidant personality disorder.
   C. Generalized social phobia and schizotypal personality disorder.
   D. Generalized social phobia and borderline personality disorder.
   E. Generalized anxiety disorder and avoidant personality disorder.

The correct response is option **A.**

Given the substantial comorbidity between generalized social phobia and avoidant personality disorder (Liebowitz et al. 1985; Widiger 1992), investigations into the neurobiology of social phobia may provide some clues about avoidant personality disorder. **(p. 840)**

51.4   Structural magnetic resonance imaging (MRI) studies of subjects with schizotypal personality disorder have shown which of the following?

   A. Larger left and right caudate nucleus volumes compared with non–schizotypal personality disorder subjects.
   B. Larger relative size of putamen compared with schizophrenic or control subjects.
   C. Higher regional glucose metabolic rate in caudate compared with control subjects.
   D. Ventricular enlargement intermediate between that in control subjects and schizophrenic subjects.
   E. Smaller hippocampal volumes compared with control subjects.

The correct response is option **D.**

Structural MRI studies have found evidence of ventricular enlargement in subjects with schizotypal personality disorder compared with control subjects (Siever et al. 1995). **(p. 838)**

51.5   Borderline personality disorder is associated with which of the following cognitive and perceptual disturbances?

   A. Odd thinking and speech.
   B. Ideas of reference.
   C. Odd beliefs.
   D. Transient, stress-related paranoid ideation.
   E. Superstitiousness.

The correct response is option **D.**

Borderline personality disorder is associated with transient, stress-related paranoid ideation or severe dissociative symptoms (American Psychiatric Association 2000). **(p. 837)**

References

American Psychiatric Association: Diagnostic and Statistical Manual of Mental Disorders, 4th Edition, Text Revision. Washington, DC, American Psychiatric Association, 2000

Kendler KS, McGuire M, Gruenberg AM, et al: The Roscommon Family study, III: schizophrenia-related personality disorders in relatives. Arch Gen Psychiatry 50:781–788, 1993

Liebowitz MR, Gorman JM, Feyuer AJ, et al: Social phobia: review of a neglected anxiety disorder. Arch Gen Psychiatry 42:729–736, 1985

Schulz SC, Schulz P, Dommisse C, et al: Amphetamine response in borderline patients. Psychiatry Res 15:97–108, 1985

Schulz SC, Cornelius J, Schulz PM: The amphetamine challenge test in patients with borderline disorder. Am J Psychiatry 145:809–814, 1988

Siever LJ, Rotter M, Losonczy M, et al: Lateral ventricular enlargement in schizotypal personality disorder. Psychiatry Res 57:109–118, 1995

Widiger TA: Generalized social phobia versus avoidant personality disorder: a commentary on three studies. J Abnorm Psychol 101:340–343, 1992

CHAPTER 52

Treatment of Depression

Select the single best response for each question.

52.1   Hypotension is a common side effect of all of the following antidepressants *except*

    A. Trazodone.
    B. Mirtazapine.
    C. Venlafaxine.
    D. Imipramine.
    E. Maprotiline.

The correct response is option **C.**

The most common cardiac side effect of antidepressants is their effect on blood pressure. Tricyclic antidepressants (amitriptyline, imipramine, nortriptyline), tetracyclic antidepressants (maprotiline, nefazodone, trazodone), and mirtazapine all can cause decreases in blood pressure, particularly orthostatic blood pressure. Venlafaxine causes sustained *increases* in blood pressure, particularly at higher dosages (>300 mg/day). Although this may diminish over time, the effect can persist (Thase 1998). **(pp. 850, 854; see also Table 52–3)**

52.2   The two best predictors of antidepressant response are

    A. Side-effect profile and comorbid psychiatric symptoms.
    B. Gender and sedating versus activating properties.
    C. Family history of response and cost.
    D. A history of prior response to an agent and a family history of preferential response.
    E. None of the above.

The correct response is option **D.**

On average, all antidepressants have approximately equal efficacy. However, individuals may preferentially respond to a particular class of agents or even a single agent. The best predictors of such a response are a history of prior response to an agent and a family history of preferential response. **(p. 851)**

52.3   The greatest threat to treatment response to a particular antidepressant agent is

    A. Common side effects.
    B. Nonadherence.
    C. Suicidal ideation.
    D. Comorbid conditions.
    E. Idiopathic side effects.

The correct response is option **B.**

The greatest threat to treatment response is nonadherence to an agent. Dropout rates ranging from 7% to 44% have been reported in various studies of tricyclic antidepressants (TCAs) and from 7% to 23% in studies of selective serotonin reuptake inhibitors (SSRIs) (Cookson 1993). Choosing an agent that will be well tolerated by an individual increases the likelihood of adherence. In some cases, the presence of preexisting medical factors may result in relative contraindications; thus, a patient with epilepsy should not be treated with bupropion, and a conduction abnormality would be a relative contraindication to the use of TCAs. More often, an in-depth evaluation of the patient will yield an understanding of which side effects are more or less likely to be tolerated. **(p. 853)**

52.4   The two most troublesome antidepressant side effects, which can lead to drug discontinuation despite efficacy, are

   A. Weight gain and sexual side effects.
   B. Weight gain and orthostasis.
   C. Weight gain and sedation.
   D. Sexual side effects and nausea.
   E. Sexual side effects and anorexia.

The correct response is option **A.**

Weight gain and sexual dysfunction are behind many patients' decision to discontinue an antidepressant despite a reasonable antidepressant response. **(p. 857)**

52.5   Which of the following statements regarding possible pro-suicide effects of antidepressants is *true?*

   A. The phenomenon is likely not unique to any one antidepressant.
   B. Tricyclic antidepressants (TCAs) are pro-suicidal only at doses three to five times the therapeutic dose.
   C. Bupropion is the safest of the second- and third-generation antidepressants when taken in overdose.
   D. Selective serotonin reuptake inhibitors (SSRIs) have a narrow margin of safety.
   E. None of the above.

The correct response is option **A.**

In the early 1990s, a great deal of concern was generated by reports of sudden, violent suicidal ideation associated with administration of the SSRI fluoxetine (Teicher et al. 1990). This was followed by a similar report involving sertraline (Balon 1993); the result was speculation among some that the SSRIs were "suicide pills." Subsequent meta-analyses (Kapur et al. 1992; Mann and Kapur 1991) and a later prospective study (Leon et al. 1999) showed that if any pro-suicide effect exists, it is extremely rare and not unique to any one antidepressant. In fact, at least one study suggested that fluoxetine may have a protective effect in some suicidal patients (Sachetti et al. 1991). Although some concerns about potentiating suicidal behavior may remain, these should be balanced over the clear risk of suicide in patients with untreated depression. Because many suicidal patients choose to overdose on their medication, antidepressants with wide safety margins should be chosen for patients considered at high risk for suicide. For this reason, TCAs are often avoided; doses of only three to five times the therapeutic dose can be lethal in adults (and the ratio is lower in children: doses of 5 mg/kg can be toxic). Most of the second- and third-generation agents are relatively safe in overdose, but bupropion can cause seizures in about one-third of overdoses. **(pp. 855–856)**

52.6   In the event of treatment nonresponse to a first antidepressive agent, the best strategy is to

A. Augment with lithium.
B. Augment with a stimulant.
C. Augment with thyroid hormone.
D. Increase the dosage past the manufacturer's recommendations.
E. Change to an alternative agent in a different chemical/mechanism class.

The correct response is option **E.**

In cases in which little or no response is seen, a new trial of an alternative agent should be considered. Although some evidence suggests that after nonresponse to one agent within a certain class, patients may respond to a second agent within the same class (Thase et al. 1997), the best evidence continues to support changing to an alternative class of agent, and approximately half of the patients failing to respond to a first trial will respond to a trial with an antidepressant from a different class (Thase et al. 2002). In switching to an incompatible agent (e.g., from a selective serotonin reuptake inhibitor to a monoamine oxidase inhibitor), adequate time should be allowed for antidepressant clearance. Augmentation with lithium, with a stimulant, or with thyroid hormone is a treatment strategy used in the event of partial response. **(p. 859)**

References

Balon R: Case report 5: suicidal ideation during treatment with sertraline. Journal of Drug Development 6:77–78, 1993

Cookson J: Side-effects of antidepressants. Br J Psychiatry 163 (suppl):20–24, 1993

Kapur S, Mieczkowski T, Mann JJ: Antidepressant medications and the relative risk of suicide attempt and suicide. JAMA 268:3441–3445, 1992

Leon AC, Keller MB, Warshaw MG, et al: Prospective study of fluoxetine treatment and suicidal behavior in affectively ill subjects. Am J Psychiatry 156:195–201, 1999

Mann J, Kapur S: The emergence of suicidal ideation and behavior during antidepressant pharmacotherapy. Arch Gen Psychiatry 48:1027–1033, 1991

Sachetti E, Vita A, Guarneri L, et al: The effectiveness of fluoxetine, clomipramine, nortriptyline and desipramine in major depressives with suicidal behavior: preliminary findings, in Serotonin-Related Psychiatric Syndromes: Clinical and Therapeutic Links. Edited by Cassano GB, Akiskal HS. London, Royal Society of Medicine Services, 1991, pp 47–53

Teicher M, Glod C, Cole J: Emergence of intense suicidal preoccupation during fluoxetine treatment. Am J Psychiatry 147:207–210, 1990

Thase ME: Effects of venlafaxine on blood pressure: a meta-analysis of original data from 3744 depressed patients. J Clin Psychiatry 59:502–508, 1998

Thase ME, Blomgren SL, Birkett MA, et al: Fluoxetine treatment in patients with major depressive disorder who failed initial treatment with sertraline. J Clin Psychiatry 58:16–21, 1997

Thase ME, Rush AJ, Howland RH, et al: Double-blind switch study of imipramine or sertraline treatment of antidepressant-resistant chronic depression. Arch Gen Psychiatry 59: 233–239, 2002

CHAPTER 53

Treatment of Bipolar Disorder

Select the single best response for each question.

53.1   What percentage of patients treated for apparent major depression in the outpatient setting subsequently receive a diagnosis of bipolar I or II disorder?

   A. 5%–10%.
   B. 15%–30%.
   C. >40%.
   D. <5%.
   E. Unknown.

The correct response is option **B.**

Studies suggest that 15%–30% of the patients treated for apparent major depressive disorder in outpatient settings subsequently receive a diagnosis of bipolar I or bipolar II disorder (Manning et al. 1997, 1998; Rao and Nammalvar 1977; Winokur and Morrison 1973). **(p. 866)**

53.2   All of the following drugs have shown efficacy in the treatment of acute mania in randomized, placebo-controlled trials *except*

   A. Olanzapine.
   B. Chlorpromazine.
   C. Carbamazepine.
   D. Lamotrigine.
   E. Divalproex.

The correct response is option **D.**

All except lamotrigine have been shown to be efficacious in treating acute mania (Keck et al. 2002; McElroy and Keck 2000). Lamotrigine may help in depression associated with bipolar disorder (American Psychiatric Association 2002). **(p. 867)**

53.3   All of the following are associated with better response rates to lithium in the treatment of acute mania *except*

   A. Few lifetime manic episodes.
   B. Classic manic or elated symptoms.
   C. Rapid-cycling symptoms.
   D. Presentation with psychotic symptoms.
   E. Presentation with no psychotic symptoms.

The correct response is option **C**.

Lithium exerts improvement in psychotic and manic symptoms. Patients with elated or classic manic symptoms (Bowden 1995) and relatively few lifetime mood episodes (Swann et al. 1999) appear to have a better response rate to lithium than do patients with mixed episodes and rapid cycling (Dunner and Fieve 1974; McElroy et al. 1992). **(p. 867)**

53.4   In comparing lithium to divalproex in the treatment of acute mania, which of the following statements is *false*?

A. Divalproex works better in patients with depressive symptoms.
B. Divalproex works better in patients with previous multiple mood episodes.
C. Both lithium and divalproex can help with psychotic symptoms in acute mania.
D. Both are efficacious for acute mania in comparison with placebo, but lithium is generally superior to divalproex in head-to-head trials.
E. Both agents have better long-term efficacy in the treatment of acute mania in combination with other medications.

The correct response is option **D**.

Divalproex and related formulations of valproic acid had superior efficacy compared with placebo (Bowden et al. 1994; Brennan et al. 1984; Emrich et al. 1981; Pope et al. 1991) and comparable efficacy compared with lithium (Bowden et al. 1994; Freeman et al. 1992). **(p. 868)**

53.5   All of the following medications have been shown to have little to no efficacy in the treatment of acute mania *except*

A. Gabapentin.
B. Topiramate.
C. Clonazepam.
D. Carbamazepine.
E. Lamotrigine.

The correct response is option **D**.

Carbamazepine was superior to placebo in one crossover trial (Ballenger and Post 1978) and one parallel-group trial (Ketter et al. 2003), comparable to lithium in two comparison studies (Lerer et al. 1987; Small et al. 1991), and comparable to chlorpromazine in two other comparison trials (Grossi et al. 1984; Okuma et al. 1979). The other drugs listed have not yet shown efficacy in acute mania. **(p. 869)**

53.6   Recent studies suggest that the antidepressant-associated switch rate—the proportion of bipolar disorder patients who switch to manic symptoms in response to antidepressant treatment—is lower than previously believed (earlier estimated rates were as high as 70%). Which of the following best represents the current estimate of this rate?

A. 20%.
B. 30%.
C. 5%–15%.
D. <2%.
E. 50%.

The correct response is option **C**.

Until recently, some treatment guidelines suggested avoiding or minimizing use of antidepressants for bipolar depression, based on reported antidepressant-associated switch rates, which ranged widely, from 10% to 70% (see Thase and Sachs 2000 for details). However, many of these earlier estimates of the incidence of antidepressant-associated switching were based on naturalistic studies that did not control for the switch rate associated with the illness itself (Moller and Grunze 2000). The switch rates reported in recent randomized, controlled trials of lamotrigine monotherapy (Calabrese et al. 1999) and combinations of paroxetine and lithium (Nemeroff et al. 2001) or of lithium and valproate (Young et al. 2000) have ranged from 3% to 8%. In addition, Post et al. (2001) reported a switch rate of 14% (8% hypomania, 6% mania) in a 10-week acute treatment trial comparing bupropion, venlafaxine, and sertraline in combination with mood stabilizers. (pp. 871, 872)

53.7 Which of the following statements regarding the use of antidepressants in bipolar disorder is *true*?

A. Antidepressants should never be used in bipolar disorder.
B. Newer antidepressants should be considered over tricyclic antidepressants (TCAs) because of lower switch rates.
C. Lamotrigine may have effectiveness as an antidepressant and antimanic agent.
D. Olanzapine does not have antidepressant activity in acute bipolar depression.
E. None of the above.

The correct response is option **B.**

Among antidepressant options, paroxetine, venlafaxine, bupropion, and fluoxetine are the most studied in randomized controlled trials and appear to have a lower switch risk in comparison with TCAs. Combination therapy with an antidepressant can be done in patients who do not respond to mood stabilizers alone or for patients with moderate to severe bipolar depression (American Psychiatric Association 2002). Lamotrigine does not appear to have antimanic activity, and both olanzapine (Tohen et al. 2003) and quetiapine (Calabrese et al. 2005) do have some efficacy as monotherapy in cases of acute bipolar depression. (pp. 872, 873)

References

American Psychiatric Association: Practice guideline for the treatment of patients with bipolar disorder (revision). Am J Psychiatry 159 (suppl):1–50, 2002

Ballenger JC, Post RM: Therapeutic effects of carbamazepine in affective illness: a preliminary report. Commun Psychopharmacol 2:159–175, 1978

Bowden CL: Predictors of response to divalproex and lithium. J Clin Psychiatry 56 (suppl):25–30, 1995

Bowden CL, Brugger AM, Swann AC, et al: Efficacy of divalproex vs lithium and placebo in the treatment of mania. JAMA 271:918–924, 1994

Brennan MJW, Sandyk R, Borsook D: Use of sodium valproate in the management of affective disorders: basic and clinical aspects, in Anticonvulsants in Affective Disorders. Edited by Emrich HM, Okuma T, Muller AA. Amsterdam, Excerpta Medica, 1984, pp 56–65

Calabrese JR, Bowden CL, Sachs GS, et al: A double-blind placebo-controlled study of lamotrigine monotherapy in outpatients with bipolar I depression. J Clin Psychiatry 60:79–88, 1999

Calabrese JR, Keck PE Jr, MacFadden W, et al: A randomized, double-blind, placebo-controlled trial of quetiapine in the treatment of bipolar I or II depression. Am J Psychiatry 162:1351–1360, 2005

Dunner DL, Fieve RR: Clinical factors in lithium carbonate prophylaxis failure. Arch Gen Psychiatry 30:229–233, 1974

Emrich HM, von Zerssen D, Kissling W: On a possible role of GABA in mania: therapeutic efficacy of sodium valproate, in GABA and Benzodiazepine Receptors. Edited by Costa E, Dicharia G, Gessa GL. New York, Raven, 1981, pp 287–296

Freeman TW, Clothier JL, Pazzaglia P, et al: A double-blind comparison of valproate and lithium in the treatment of acute mania. Am J Psychiatry 149:108–111, 1992

Grossi E, Sacchetti E, Vita A: Carbamazepine versus chlorpromazine in mania: a double-blind trial, in Anticonvulsants in Affective Disorders. Edited by Emrich HM, Okuma T, Muller AA. Amsterdam, Excerpta Medica, 1984, pp 177–187

Keck PE Jr, Saha AR, Iwamoto T, et al: Aripiprazole versus placebo in acute mania (NR314), in 2002 New Research Program and Abstracts, American Psychiatric Association 155th Annual Meeting, Philadelphia, PA, May 18–23, 2002. Washington, DC, American Psychiatric Association, 2002

Ketter TA, Weisler RH, Kalali AH: Extended-release carbamazepine in bipolar disorders (abstract). Bipolar Disord 5 (suppl 1):60, 2003

Lerer B, Moore N, Meyendorff E, et al: Carbamazepine versus lithium in mania: a double-blind study. J Clin Psychiatry 48:89–93, 1987

Manning JS, Haykal RF, Connor PD: On the nature of depressive and anxious states in a family practice residency setting: the high prevalence of bipolar II and related disorders in a cohort followed longitudinally. Compr Psychiatry 38:102–108, 1997

Manning JS, Connor PD, Sahai A: The bipolar spectrum: review of current concepts and implications for the management of depression in primary care. Arch Fam Med 6:63–71, 1998

McElroy SL, Keck PE Jr: Pharmacological agents for the treatment of acute bipolar mania. Biol Psychiatry 48:539–557, 2000

McElroy SL, Keck PE Jr, Pope HG Jr: Clinical and research implications of the diagnosis of dysphoric or mixed mania or hypomania. Am J Psychiatry 149:1633–1644, 1992

Moller H-J, Grunze H: Have some guidelines for the treatment of acute bipolar depression gone too far in the restriction of antidepressants? Eur Arch Psychiatry Clin Neurosci 25:57–68, 2000

Nemeroff CB, Evans DL, Gyulai L, et al: Double-blind, placebo-controlled comparison of imipramine and paroxetine in the treatment of bipolar depression. Am J Psychiatry 62:906–912, 2001

Okuma T, Inanaga K, Otsuki S, et al: Comparison of the antimanic efficacy of carbamazepine and chlorpromazine: a double-blind controlled study. Psychopharmacology (Berl) 66:211–217, 1979

Pope HG Jr, McElroy SL, Keck PE Jr, et al: Valproate in the treatment of acute mania: a placebo-controlled study. Arch Gen Psychiatry 48:62–68, 1991

Post RM, Altshuler LL, Frye MA, et al: Rate of switch in bipolar patients prospectively treated with second-generation antidepressants as augmentation to mood stabilizers. Bipolar Disord 3:259–265, 2001

Rao AV, Nammalvar N: The course and outcome in depressive illness. A follow-up study of 122 cases in Madurai, India. Br J Psychiatry 130:392–396, 1977

Small JG, Klapper MH, Milstein V, et al: Carbamazepine compared with lithium in the treatment of mania. Arch Gen Psychiatry 48:915–921, 1991

Swann AC, Bowden CL, Calabrese JR, et al: Differential effect of number of previous episodes of affective disorder on response to lithium or divalproex in mania. Am J Psychiatry 156:1264–1266, 1999

Thase ME, Sachs GS: Bipolar depression: pharmacotherapy and related therapeutic strategies. Biol Psychiatry 48:558–572, 2000

Tohen M, Vieta E, Calabrese J, et al: Efficacy of olanzapine and olanzapine-fluoxetine combination in the treatment of bipolar I depression. Arch Gen Psychiatry 60:1079–1088, 2003 (erratum in Arch Gen Psychiatry 61:176, 2004)

Winokur G, Morrison J: The Iowa 500: follow-up of 225 depressives. Br J Psychiatry 123:543–548, 1973

Young LT, Joffe RT, Robb JC, et al: Double-blind comparison of addition of a second mood stabilizer versus an antidepressant to an initial mood stabilizer for treatment of patients with bipolar depression. Am J Psychiatry 157:124–127, 2000

CHAPTER 54

Treatment of Schizophrenia

Select the single best response for each question.

54.1   All of the following statements regarding positive symptoms of schizophrenia are correct *except*

A. Studies show that a high degree of positive symptoms correlates with a worse long-term prognosis.
B. Positive symptoms include hallucinations.
C. Positive symptoms respond to antipsychotic medications.
D. Positive symptoms are not the first set of symptoms that typically present in schizophrenia.
E. Positive symptoms are traditionally the focus of medication treatment.

The correct response is option **A.**

There is a growing consensus, following the seminal work of several investigators (e.g., Andreasen 1985; Crow 1985), that schizophrenia can be conceptualized as a disorder with at least two somewhat orthogonal dimensions of symptomatology: positive and negative symptoms. Positive, or psychotic, symptoms usually are the symptoms that first trigger psychiatric attention, and traditionally, the onset of schizophrenia is clinically synonymous with the emergence of overt psychosis. This concept, however, is gradually changing, because accumulating evidence indicates that the schizophrenia disease process probably begins long before the onset of psychosis. Interestingly, subtle neurological abnormalities, as well as intellectual and cognitive difficulties, have been observed in children who later show symptoms of schizophrenia (Walker et al. 1999). Positive symptoms include hallucinations, delusions, and disorganized thinking, although disorganization also can be conceptualized as an independent symptom dimension (Liddle et al. 1989). As a general rule, positive symptoms tend to respond to treatment with antipsychotic medications; traditionally, they have been the focus of treatment with these medications. Positive symptoms are dramatic, and while patients are in the midst of them, their ability to function is usually severely disrupted; however, studies have quite consistently shown that such symptoms do not appear to bear any significant association with or predict the long-term functional outcome of the illness (Green et al. 2000). **(p. 886)**

54.2   Which of the following statements about gender differences in schizophrenia is *true*?

A. The onset of illness tends to be more acute in males than in females.
B. Men tend to have a higher level of premorbid functioning than women.
C. Women generally have a more favorable outcome than men.
D. The age at onset is, on average, 5 years younger in women than in men.
E. There are no differences between men and women in onset, tempo of onset, and level of premorbid functioning.

The correct response is option **C.**

Schizophrenia is a chronic illness, with onset of psychotic symptoms usually occurring around late adolescence and early adulthood (Lewis and Lieberman 2000). The age at onset is approximately 5 years later in women than in men (Angermeyer et al. 1990; Faraone et al. 1994; Hambrecht et al. 1992; Szymanski et al. 1995). The onset of illness also tends to be more acute in women, as compared with the typically more insidious onset in men, and women tend to have had a higher level of premorbid functioning. Although there may be no clear sex differences in cross-sectional symptomatology of the illness (Hafner et al. 1993; Szymanski et al. 1995), the differences in the age at onset, tempo of onset, and level of premorbid functioning, all of which are prognostic factors, are consistent with the fact that women in general tend to have a more favorable outcome. **(pp. 888–889)**

54.3 Regarding choice of an antipsychotic for a patient with acute psychosis in schizophrenia, all of the following statements are true *except*

A. Generally, second-generation (atypical) agents are preferred.
B. All of the second-generation (atypical) agents are more effective than the first-generation (typical) agents in the treatment of positive and negative symptoms.
C. It is acceptable to use a first-generation agent if a particular patient has responded to that agent in the past.
D. The main advantage of second-generation agents is their overall lower risk of causing extrapyramidal symptoms and tardive dyskinesia.
E. Clozapine may be therapeutically superior to any other antipsychotic medications.

The correct response is option **B.**

The second-generation agents, with the exception of clozapine in treatment-resistant patients, may not be substantially better in the treatment of positive symptoms of schizophrenia compared with first-generation agents (Geddes et al. 2000). There has been evidence, albeit somewhat controversial, suggesting that some of the newer agents may improve negative symptoms and/or cognitive deficits (Chouinard et al. 1993; Claus et al. 1992; Tollefson et al. 1997). Because of the presumed clinical advantages of these agents (including their side-effect profile), they are often preferred for patients who have never been exposed to antipsychotic medication, such as those in their first episode of psychosis. However, in the following situations, first-generation drugs still may be considered "first-line": 1) when the patient has been stable on a first-generation drug, including a depot preparation, without noticeable neurological side effects; and 2) when the patient has shown a better response to these drugs than to the second-generation drugs (Marder et al. 2002). **(p. 891)**

54.4 According to findings from a meta-analysis of 15 studies, patients who are taking second-generation antipsychotics appear to demonstrate

A. Improved memory.
B. Less weight gain than with first-generation antipsychotics.
C. Better verbal fluency.
D. Better overall clinical outcome.
E. All of the above.

The correct response is option **C.**

Conventional antipsychotics do not appear to alleviate neurocognitive symptoms of schizophrenia (Cassens et al. 1990; Spohn and Strauss 1999). However, a meta-analysis of 15 studies indicated that second-generation antipsychotics have notable effects on verbal fluency and executive function, with limited improvement in memory (Bilder et al. 2002). Second-generation antipsychotics appear to be associated with more weight gain compared with first-generation antipsychotics (Allison et al. 1999; Wirshing and Wirshing 1999), and it is not clear that second-generation antipsychotics, except for clozapine, are superior overall. **(pp. 893, 897)**

54.5   The leading cause of medical morbidity in patients with schizophrenia is

   A. Obesity.
   B. Diabetes.
   C. Human immunodeficiency virus–associated hepatitis.
   D. Cigarette smoking.
   E. Lack of exercise.

The correct response is option **D.**

Cigarette smoking, which is consistently reported to be associated with cardiovascular and pulmonary diseases, is the leading cause of morbidity in schizophrenia patients (Allebeck and Wistedt 1986; Buda et al. 1988; Mortensen and Juel 1990), 90% of whom smoke. **(p. 895)**

54.6   The leading cause of premature death in patients with schizophrenia is

   A. Comorbidities associated with obesity.
   B. Alcohol and drug use.
   C. Comorbidities associated with cigarette smoking.
   D. Risky sexual behaviors.
   E. Suicide.

The correct response is option **E.**

Suicide is the leading cause of premature death in patients with schizophrenia, who have a 10% lifetime risk of suicide. **(p. 900)**

54.7   Which of the following statements best describes the usual course of illness in schizophrenia?

   A. After the acute onset, the first 2–5 years are marked by little change in severity.
   B. Negative symptoms usually respond to medication treatment better than positive symptoms.
   C. Positive symptoms usually respond to medication treatment better than negative symptoms.
   D. Positive symptoms usually become increasingly prominent during the course of illness.
   E. All of the above statements are accurate.

The correct response is option **C.**

Schizophrenia is a chronic illness, with onset of psychotic symptoms usually occurring around late adolescence and early adulthood. After the first episode of psychosis, the course of the illness is often characterized by a gradual and at times continuous deterioration, especially during the first 2–5 years (McGlashan 1998). After an initial period of functional deterioration, symptoms tend to become more or less stabilized. Some degree of amelioration of positive symptoms (and to a lesser extent of disorganized symptoms) may not be uncommon in older patients (see Davidson et al. 1995; Schultz et al. 1997). However, findings of amelioration of psychotic symptoms should be interpreted in light of the fact that these are also symptoms most responsive to neuroleptic treatment, making it difficult to distinguish between the natural course of the disorder and the accumulated response to treatment. Positive symptoms usually respond to treatment, whereas negative symptoms are believed to be relatively treatment-resistant and may tend to become increasingly prominent during the course of the illness (Breier et al. 1991). **(pp. 888, 889)**

54.8 Which of the following second-generation antipsychotics is most effective for treatment-resistant schizophrenia?

A. Clozapine.
B. Risperidone.
C. Olanzapine.
D. Quetiapine.
E. Ziprasidone.

The correct response is option **A**.

Most available data suggest that clozapine is the most effective drug for treatment-resistant schizophrenia (Kane et al. 2001). **(p. 892)**

54.9 For severe tardive dyskinesia, which of the following medications may be useful?

A. Pimozide.
B. Clozapine.
C. Haloperidol.
D. L-Serine.
E. L-Carnitine.

The correct response is option **B**.

Evidence suggests that clozapine, among the second-generation drugs, may be helpful in reducing tardive dyskinesia symptoms (Glazer 2000; Lieberman et al. 1991). **(p. 896)**

References

Allebeck P, Wistedt B: Mortality in schizophrenia: a ten-year follow-up based on the Stockholm County inpatient register. Arch Gen Psychiatry 43:650–653, 1986

Allison DB, Mentore JM, Heo M, et al: Antipsychotic-induced weight gain: a comprehensive research synthesis. Am J Psychiatry 156:1686–1696, 1999

Andreasen NC: Positive vs. negative schizophrenia: a critical evaluation. Schizophr Bull 11:380–389, 1985

Angermeyer MC, Kuhn L, Goldstein JM: Gender and the course of schizophrenia: differences in treatment outcome. Schizophr Bull 16:293–307, 1990

Bilder RM, Goldman RS, Volavka J, et al: Neurocognitive effects of clozapine, olanzapine, risperidone, and haloperidol in patients with chronic schizophrenia or schizoaffective disorder. Am J Psychiatry 159:1018–1028, 2002

Breier AF, Schreiber JL, Dyer J, et al: National Institute of Mental Health longitudinal study of chronic schizophrenia: prognosis and predictors of outcome. Arch Gen Psychiatry 48: 239–246, 1991

Buda M, Tsuang MT, Fleming JA: Causes of death in DSM-III schizophrenics and other psychotics (atypical group). Arch Gen Psychiatry 45:283–285, 1988

Cassens G, Inglis AK, Appelbaum PS, et al: Neuroleptics: effects on neuropsychological function in chronic schizophrenic patients. Schizophr Bull 16:477–499, 1990

Chouinard G, Jones B, Remington GA: Canadian multicenter placebo-controlled study of fixed doses of risperidone and haloperidol in the treatment of chronic schizophrenic patients. J Clin Psychopharmacol 13:25–40, 1993

Claus A, Bollen J, De Cuyper H, et al: Risperidone versus haloperidol in the treatment of chronic schizophrenic inpatients: a multicentre double-blind comparative study. Acta Psychiatr Scand 85:295–305, 1992

Crow TJ: The two-syndrome concept: origins and current status. Schizophr Bull 11:471–486, 1985

Davidson M, Harvey PD, Powchik P, et al: Severity of symptoms in chronically institutionalized geriatric schizophrenic patients. Am J Psychiatry 152:197–207, 1995

Faraone SV, Chen WJ, Goldstein JM, et al: Gender differences in the age at onset of schizophrenia. Br J Psychiatry 164:625–629, 1994

Geddes J, Freemantle N, Harrison P, et al: Atypical antipsychotics in the treatment of schizophrenia: systematic overview and meta-regression analysis. BMJ 321:1371–1376, 2000

Glazer WM: Expected incidence of tardive dyskinesia associated with atypical antipsychotics. J Clin Psychiatry 61 (suppl 4):21–26, 2000

Green MF, Kern RS, Braff DL, et al: Neurocognitive deficits and functional outcome in schizophrenia: are we measuring the "right stuff"? Schizophr Bull 26:119–136, 2000

Hafner H, Maurer K, Loffler W, et al: The influence of age and sex on the onset and early course of schizophrenia. Br J Psychiatry 162:80–86, 1993

Hambrecht M, Maurer K, Hafner H, et al: Transnational stability of gender differences in schizophrenia? Eur Arch Psychiatry Clin Neurosci 242:6–12, 1992

Kane JM, Handan G, Malhotra AK: Clozapine, in Current Issues in the Psychopharmacology of Schizophrenia. Edited by Breier A, Tran PV, Herrea JM, et al. Philadelphia, PA, Lippincott Williams & Wilkins, 2001, pp 209–223

Lewis DA, Lieberman JA: Catching up on schizophrenia: natural history and neurobiology. Neuron 28:325–334, 2000

Liddle PF, Barnes TR, Morris D, et al: Three syndromes in chronic schizophrenia. Br J Psychiatry 7 (suppl):119–122, 1989

Lieberman JA, Saltz BL, Johns CA, et al: The effects of clozapine on tardive dyskinesia. Br J Psychiatry 158:503–510, 1991

Marder SR, Essock SM, Miller AL, et al: The Mount Sinai conference on the pharmacotherapy of schizophrenia. Schizophr Bull 28:5–16, 2002

McGlashan TH: The profiles of clinical deterioration in schizophrenia. J Psychiatr Res 32:133–141, 1998

Mortensen PB, Juel K: Mortality and cause of death in schizophrenic patients in Denmark. Acta Psychiatr Scand 81:372–377, 1990

Schultz SK, Miller DD, Oliver SE, et al: The life course of schizophrenia: age and symptom dimensions. Schizophr Res 23:15–23, 1997

Spohn HE, Strauss ME: Relation of neuroleptic and anticholinergic medication to cognitive function in schizophrenia. J Abnorm Psychol 98:367–390, 1999

Szymanski S, Lieberman JA, Alvir JM, et al: Gender differences in onset of illness, treatment response, course, and biologic indexes in first-episode schizophrenic patients. Am J Psychiatry 152:698–703, 1995

Tollefson GD, Beasley CM, Tran PV, et al: Olanzapine versus haloperidol in the treatment of schizophrenia and schizoaffective and schizophreniform disorders: results of an international collaborative trial. Am J Psychiatry 154:457–465, 1997

Walker E, Lewis N, Loewy R, et al: Motor dysfunction and risk for schizophrenia. Dev Psychopathol 11:509–523, 1999

Wirshing DA, Wirshing WC: Novel antipsychotics: comparison of weight gain liabilities. J Clin Psychiatry 60:358–363, 1999

CHAPTER 55

Treatment of Anxiety Disorders

Select the single best response for each question.

55.1 Which of the following augmentation strategies has been found to be effective in treatment-resistant obsessive-compulsive disorder (OCD)?

A. Addition of venlafaxine to buspirone.
B. Addition of lithium to risperidone.
C. Addition of risperidone to a selective serotonin reuptake inhibitor (SSRI).
D. Addition of valproate to clomipramine.
E. Addition of gabapentin to an SSRI.

The correct response is option **C.**

The following augmentation and/or combination strategies have been reported as offering benefit. Combining fluvoxamine with clomipramine (Szegedi et al. 1995) is an approach to consider in individuals who have shown a partial response to clomipramine. Patients with OCD and comorbid tic disorders respond better to haloperidol than to placebo when added to fluvoxamine (McDougle et al. 1994). Olanzapine and risperidone have been added successfully in cases of partial SSRI response (Koran et al. 2000; Saxena et al. 1996). **(p. 914)**

55.2 A patient with panic disorder develops agitation, insomnia, and nausea while taking fluoxetine. Which of the following agents might be useful in reducing these symptoms?

A. Mirtazapine.
B. Buspirone.
C. Lithium.
D. Venlafaxine.
E. Valproate.

The correct response is option **A.**

Use of serotonin$_2$ (5-hydroxytryptamine [5-HT]$_2$) or 5-HT$_3$ antagonists, such as mirtazapine, nefazodone, and ondansetron, might be considered, to limit some of the symptoms that are mediated through these pathways (e.g., insomnia, agitation, gastrointestinal distress). **(p. 915)**

55.3 A 19-year-old woman experiences panic attack symptoms when she eats, writes, or speaks in public. Which of the following agents has been found to be effective in treating these symptoms?

    A. Atenolol.
    B. Ondansetron.
    C. Clonazepam.
    D. Buspirone.
    E. Olanzapine.

The correct response is option **C**.

Davidson et al. (1993) conducted a moderately large trial in 75 patients taking clonazepam or placebo and found a 70% response rate to clonazepam compared with a 20% response rate to placebo. **(p. 918)**

55.4 A 27-year-old man reports lifelong intermittent symptoms of worry, muscle tension, irritability, and difficulty falling asleep. Which of the following statements about possible pharmacological interventions is *true*?

    A. If a benzodiazepine is prescribed, psychic symptoms will be more effectively treated than somatic ones.
    B. If a benzodiazepine is prescribed, long-term use may be associated with development of tolerance, physiological dependence, and withdrawal.
    C. If buspirone is prescribed, alleviation of anxiety symptoms will likely occur within the first week.
    D. If venlafaxine is prescribed, alleviation of anxiety symptoms will likely occur only after the fifth week.
    E. If a tricyclic antidepressant (TCA) is prescribed, only depressive symptoms will remit.

The correct response is option **B**.

Some evidence suggests that benzodiazepines may be more effective in treating the autonomic arousal and somatic symptoms of generalized anxiety disorder (GAD) but less effective for the psychic symptoms of worry and irritability (Rickels et al. 1982; Rosenbaum et al. 1984). However, the use of benzodiazepines over longer periods is controversial, and long-term use can be associated with the development of tolerance, physiological dependence, and withdrawal (if the drug is abruptly discontinued), as well as troublesome side effects, including ataxia, sedation, motor dysfunction, and cognitive impairment. An adequate trial of buspirone in GAD would be 3–4 weeks of treatment at a dosage of up to 60 mg/day, in divided doses. In one placebo-controlled trial of venlafaxine (Allgulander et al. 2001), significant improvement was noted in symptoms of psychic anxiety by week 2 of treatment. Potential advantages of the TCAs over the benzodiazepines include their ability to treat symptoms of both anxiety and depression, their absence of potential for abuse and physiological dependence, and their effectiveness in the management of discontinuation of long-term benzodiazepine therapy (Rickels et al. 2000). **(pp. 921, 922, 923)**

References

Allgulander C, Hackett D, Salinas E: Venlafaxine extended release (ER) in the treatment of generalized anxiety disorder: twenty-four week placebo-controlled dose-ranging study. Br J Psychiatry 179:15–22, 2001

Davidson JRT, Potts NLS, Richichi EA, et al: Treatment of social phobia with clonazepam and placebo. J Clin Psychopharmacol 13:423–428, 1993

Koran LM, Ringold AL, Elliott MA: Olanzapine augmentation for treatment-resistant obsessive-compulsive disorder. J Clin Psychiatry 61:514–517, 2000

McDougle CJ, Goodman WK, Price LH, et al: Haloperidol addition in fluvoxamine-refractory obsessive-compulsive disorder: a double-blind, placebo-controlled study in patients with and without tics. Arch Gen Psychiatry 51:302–308, 1994

Rickels K, Weisman K, Norstad N, et al: Buspirone and diazepam in anxiety: a controlled study. J Clin Psychiatry 43 (12, pt 2):81–86, 1982

Rickels K, DeMartinis N, Garcia-Espana F, et al: Imipramine and buspirone in treatment of patients with generalized anxiety disorder who are discontinuing long-term benzodiazepine therapy. Am J Psychiatry 157:1973–1979, 2000

Rosenbaum JF, Woods SW, Groves JE, et al: Emergence of hostility during alprazolam treatment. Am J Psychiatry 141:792–793, 1984

Saxena S, Wang D, Bystritsky A, et al: Risperidone augmentation of SRI treatment for refractory obsessive-compulsive disorder. J Clin Psychiatry 57:303–306, 1996

Szegedi A, Wetzel H, Leal M, et al: Combination treatment with clomipramine and fluvoxamine: drug monitoring, safety and tolerability. J Clin Psychiatry 57:257–264, 1995

CHAPTER 56

Management of Noncognitive Symptoms of Dementia: Behavioral and Psychological Symptoms of Dementia

Select the single best response for each question.

56.1 An 87-year-old man with Alzheimer's disease develops chronic symptoms of depression. Which of the following treatment strategies would be the best choice for this patient?

A. Treat the patient with imipramine.
B. Treat the patient with haloperidol.
C. Treat the patient with maprotiline.
D. Treat the patient with citalopram.
E. Discontinue antidementia drugs.

The correct response is option **D.**

Nyth and Gottfries (1990) conducted a randomized, double-blind, placebo-controlled trial of the selective serotonin reuptake inhibitor (SSRI) citalopram versus placebo. The study involved a 4-week placebo trial followed by a 12-week open-label extension. After 4 weeks, the citalopram-treated patients showed significant differences from baseline on measures of emotional bluntness, confusion, irritability, anxiety, fear-panic, depressed mood, and restlessness. Between-group differences favoring citalopram were found for ratings of irritability and depressed mood. This study was followed by a larger study involving 6 weeks of treatment with citalopram compared with placebo. Patients were elderly depressed individuals with and without dementia. Citalopram-treated patients with dementia complicated by depression scored significantly better than placebo-treated patients on measures of orientation to time, recent memory, ability to increase tempo, and fear-panic. **(p. 937)**

56.2 A 93-year-old woman with Alzheimer's disease becomes acutely combative and agitated. Which of the following potential circumstances might explain these symptoms?

A. The patient may have an underlying medical illness such as a urinary tract infection.
B. The patient may be responding to a change in caregivers.
C. The patient may be responding to a recent change in medication.
D. The patient may be responding to a recent change in roommate.
E. All of the above.

The correct response is option **E.**

In addition to psychosis, predictors such as pain, acute medical illness, and poorly trained caregivers may be important clinical correlates of aggression. Acute medical illness, most commonly a urinary tract infection, was often present at the time of an aggressive attack in patients who had the most severe behavioral disturbances (Malone et al. 1993). **(pp. 941, 942)**

56.3   Which of the following drugs has been shown to be effective in the treatment of agitation and aggression in patients with dementia?

   A. Lamotrigine.
   B. Levetiracetam.
   C. Gabapentin.
   D. Valproate.
   E. Phenytoin.

The correct response is option **D.**

Anticonvulsant compounds, most notably carbamazepine and valproic acid, have been used successfully in placebo-controlled trials focusing on agitation and aggression in dementia (Porsteinsson et al. 2001; Tariot et al. 1998, 2000). **(p. 942; see also Table 56–3)**

56.4   Regarding benzodiazepine treatment of behavioral disturbances in dementia, which of the following statements is *true*?

   A. Benzodiazepines are the treatment of choice for all dementia patients with behavioral disturbances.
   B. Many clinical studies clearly show the efficacy of benzodiazepines for the treatment of behavioral disturbances in patients with dementia.
   C. Benzodiazepines can be used for short-term treatment of behavioral disturbances associated with disruptions to routines or adjustments to changes.
   D. Benzodiazepines should never be used as short-term treatment.
   E. Benzodiazepines should be given only with antipsychotics.

The correct response is option **C.**

Surprisingly little evidence supports the choice of a benzodiazepine as the first-line treatment for any behavioral symptom of Alzheimer's disease, including anxiety and sleep disturbance (Patel and Tariot 1995; Stern et al. 1991). A possible exception may be short-term use of short-acting agents with few active metabolites, such as lorazepam, to manage patients experiencing a difficult adjustment to a change in residence or other disruptions in their normal routine. **(p. 942)**

References

Malone ML, Thompson L, Goodwin JS: Aggressive behaviors among the institutionalized elderly. J Am Geriatr Soc 41:853–856, 1993

Nyth AL, Gottfries CG: The clinical efficacy of citalopram in treatment of emotional disturbances in dementia disorders: a Nordic multicentre study. Br J Psychiatry 157:894–901, 1990

Patel S, Tariot PN: Use of benzodiazepines in behaviorally disturbed patients: risk-benefit ratio, in Behavioral Complications of Alzheimer's Disease. Edited by Lawlor BA. Washington, DC, American Psychiatric Press, 1995, pp 153–170

Porsteinsson AP, Tariot PN, Erb R, et al: Placebo-controlled study of divalproex sodium for agitation in dementia. Am J Geriatr Psychiatry 9:58–66, 2001

Stern RG, Duffelmeyer ME, Zemishlani Z, et al: The use of benzodiazepines in the management of behavioral symptoms in dementia patients. Psychiatr Clin North Am 14:375–384, 1991

Tariot PN, Erb R, Podgorski CA, et al: Efficacy and tolerability of carbamazepine for agitation and aggression in dementia. Am J Psychiatry 155:54–61, 1998

Tariot PN, Dolomon PR, Morris JC, et al: A 5 month, randomized, placebo-controlled trial of galantamine in AD. The Galantamine USA-10 Study Group. Neurology 54:2269–2276, 2000

CHAPTER 57

Treatment of Childhood and Adolescent Disorders

Select the single best response for each question.

57.1 Which of the following agents or drug classes, in comparison with placebo, has demonstrated efficacy in the treatment of major depressive disorder in children and adolescents?

A. Tricyclic antidepressants (TCAs).
B. Fluoxetine.
C. Venlafaxine.
D. Mirtazapine.
E. None of the above.

The correct response is option **B**.

Fluoxetine was the first selective serotonin reuptake inhibitor (SSRI) shown to have efficacy in the treatment of children and adolescents with major depression (Emslie et al. 1997). By contrast, eight double-blind, placebo-controlled studies of TCAs in children and adolescents failed to find significant differences between TCAs and placebo (Birmaher et al. 1998; Geller et al. 1990, 1992; Keller et al. 2001; Kutcher et al. 1994; Kye et al. 1996; Tancer et al. 1992). Venlafaxine likewise has failed to demonstrate superiority to placebo in the treatment of children and adolescents with major depression (Mandoki et al. 1997). There are no published reports of the use of mirtazapine for the treatment of depression in children and adolescents. **(pp. 951, 952, 953)**

57.2 Which of the following is the only medication to have been demonstrated, in a double-blind, placebo-controlled study, to be effective in the treatment of bipolar disorder in adolescents?

A. Lithium.
B. Divalproex.
C. Carbamazepine.
D. Olanzapine.
E. Lamotrigine.

The correct response is option **A**.

Most of the available information on pharmacological treatments for bipolar disorder in youths relies on open studies, case series, and case reports. To date, only one double-blind, placebo-controlled, randomized study has examined a mood stabilizer in the treatment of adolescents with bipolar disorder (Geller et al. 1998). In this study, 25 adolescent outpatients with bipolar disorder and secondary substance dependency were randomized to receive either lithium or placebo for a 6-week trial. Lithium produced significantly greater improvement in global functioning for bipolar disorder and substance dependence than did placebo. It was found that onset of bipolar disorder preceded substance dependence by approximately 6 years. Side effects in the group treated with lithium included polyuria, thirst, nausea, vomiting, and dizziness. **(pp. 954, 955, 956)**

57.3 Published open-label treatment studies in children and adolescents with posttraumatic stress disorder (PTSD) have supported the efficacy of all of the following agents *except*

A. Citalopram.
B. Clonidine.
C. Carbamazepine.
D. Propranolol.
E. Alprazolam.

The correct response is option **E.**

Citalopram (Seedat et al. 2001, 2002), clonidine (Harmon and Riggs 1996), carbamazepine (Looff et al. 1995), and propranolol (Famularo et al. 1988) have all been shown to improve core symptoms and to be well tolerated in children and adolescents with PTSD. Alprazolam has been investigated in the treatment of generalized anxiety disorder (Simeon and Ferguson 1987; Simeon et al. 1992) and school refusal (Bernstein et al. 1990) but not that of PTSD. **(pp. 960, 961, 962)**

57.4 The evidence base is *least* supportive of which of the following agents for treatment of child and adolescent attention-deficit/hyperactivity disorder (ADHD)?

A. Psychostimulants.
B. Tricyclic antidepressants (TCAs).
C. Selective serotonin reuptake inhibitors (SSRIs).
D. Atomoxetine.
E. Bupropion.

The correct response is option **C.**

Results have been mixed regarding the efficacy of SSRIs in the treatment of childhood ADHD, with some studies showing moderate improvement (Barrickman et al. 1991; Gammon and Brown 1993) and others showing no improvement (Findling 1996). Psychostimulants in ADHD have been studied in more than 100 randomized, controlled trials (see Pliszka et al. 2000 for review); approximately 70% of school-aged subjects demonstrated significant improvement in ADHD symptoms (i.e., inattention, hyperactivity, and impulsiveness) (Spencer et al. 1996). Of the nonstimulant treatments for ADHD, TCAs have been the most widely studied in children and adolescents, with 15 double-blind, placebo-controlled studies demonstrating their efficacy (see Popper 2000 for review). Bupropion's efficacy in improving hyperactivity, impulsivity, conduct problems, and attention in ADHD has been reported in several studies (Barrickman et al. 1995; Conners et al. 1996). Atomoxetine, a selective noradrenergic enhancer being investigated for the treatment of ADHD in children, has been shown to produce statistically significant improvement in hyperactivity and inattention (Allen et al. 2001; Heiligenstein et al. 2001a, 2001b). In open-label trials of atomoxetine, response rates in children with ADHD ranged from 70% to 75% (Kratochvil et al. 2001; Spencer et al. 2001). **(pp. 964–967)**

57.5 Aside from pimozide, the only other agent that has received U.S. Food and Drug Administration (FDA) approval as a treatment for Tourette's syndrome is

A. Risperidone.
B. Fluphenazine.
C. Clonidine.
D. Haloperidol.
E. Fluoxetine.

The correct response is option **D.**

Although haloperidol and pimozide are FDA-approved medications for the treatment of Tourette's syndrome, the side-effect profile of haloperidol limits its usefulness with children. There is increasing evidence to support the efficacy of atypical antipsychotics for the treatment of children with Tourette's syndrome. **(p. 975)**

57.6 The incidence of serious rashes, including Stevens-Johnson syndrome, in pediatric patients taking lamotrigine is reported to be approximately

A. 10%.

B. 5%.

C. 1%.

D. 0.1%.

E. 0.01%.

The correct response is option **C.**

Common side effects of lamotrigine in children are ataxia, nausea, vomiting, and constipation. Of particular concern is the incidence of serious rash (reported to be 1% in pediatric patients), including Stevens-Johnson syndrome. This high incidence of serious rash may be attributable to the prior use of high doses of lamotrigine with concomitant divalproex (Messenheimer 1998). The current dosing guidelines (initiation at 25 mg/day, with slow upward titration of 25 mg every 2 weeks) may reduce the incidence of rash in pediatric patients. **(p. 1004)**

References

Allen A, Spencer T, Heiligenstein J, et al: Safety and efficacy of atomoxetine for ADHD in two double-blind, placebo-controlled trials. Poster presented at the annual meeting of the Society of Biological Psychiatry, New Orleans, LA, May 2001

Barrickman LL, Noyes R, Kuperman S, et al: Treatment of ADHD with fluoxetine: a preliminary trial. J Am Acad Child Adolesc Psychiatry 30:762–767, 1991

Barrickman LL, Perry PJ, Allen AJ, et al: Bupropion versus methylphenidate in the treatment of attention-deficit/hyperactivity disorder. J Am Acad Child Adolesc Psychiatry 34:649–657, 1995

Bernstein GA, Garfinkel BD, Borchardt CM: Comparative studies of pharmacotherapy for school refusal. J Am Acad Child Adolesc Psychiatry 29:773–781, 1990

Birmaher B, Waterman GS, Ryan ND, et al: Randomized, controlled trial of amitriptyline versus placebo for adolescents with "treatment resistant" major depression. J Am Acad Child Adolesc Psychiatry 37:527–535, 1998

Conners CK, Casat CD, Gualtieri CT, et al: Bupropion hydrochloride in attention deficit disorder with hyperactivity. J Am Acad Child Adolesc Psychiatry 35:1314–1321, 1996

Emslie GJ, Rush AJ, Weinberg WA, et al: A double-blind, randomized, placebo-controlled trial of fluoxetine in children and adolescents with depression. Arch Gen Psychiatry 54:1031–1037, 1997

Famularo R, Kinscherff R, Fenton T: Propranolol treatment for childhood posttraumatic stress disorder, acute type. A pilot study. Am J Dis Child 142:1244–1247, 1988

Findling RL: Open-label treatment of comorbid depression and attentional disorders with co-administration of serotonin reuptake inhibitors and psychostimulants in children, adolescents, and adults: a case series. J Child Adolesc Psychopharmacol 6:165–175, 1996

Gammon G, Brown T: Fluoxetine and methylphenidate in combination for treatment of attention deficit disorder and comorbid depressive disorder. J Child Adolesc Psychopharmacol 3:1–10, 1993

Geller B, Cooper TB, Graham DL, et al: Double-blind placebo-controlled study of nortriptyline in depressed adolescents using a "fixed plasma level" design. Psychopharmacol Bull 26:85–90, 1990

Geller B, Cooper TB, Graham DL, et al: Pharmacokinetically designed double-blind placebo-controlled study of nortriptyline in 6- to 12-year-olds with major depressive disorder. J Am Acad Child Adolesc Psychiatry 31:34–44, 1992

Geller B, Cooper TB, Sun K, et al: Double blind and placebo controlled study of lithium for adolescent bipolar disorders with secondary substance dependency. J Am Acad Child Adolesc Psychiatry 37:171–178, 1998

Harmon RJ, Riggs PD: Clonidine for posttraumatic stress disorder in preschool children. J Am Acad Child Adolesc Psychiatry 35:1247–1249, 1996

Heiligenstein J, Faries D, Dunn D, et al: Efficacy of tomoxetine versus placebo in school age children with ADHD who failed psychostimulant treatment. Poster presented at the 154th annual meeting of the American Psychiatric Association, New Orleans, LA, May 5–10, 2001a

Heiligenstein J, Wagner KD, Casat CD, et al: Efficacy of atomoxetine versus placebo in school-age children with attention-deficit/hyperactivity disorder, inattentive subtype. Poster presented at the 154th annual meeting of the American Psychiatric Association, New Orleans, LA, May 5–10, 2001b

Keller MB, Ryan ND, Strober M, et al: Efficacy of paroxetine in the treatment of adolescent major depression: a randomized, controlled trial. J Am Acad Child Adolesc Psychiatry 40:762–772, 2001

Kratochvil CJ, Bohac D, Harrington M, et al: An open-label trial of tomoxetine in pediatric attention deficit hyperactivity disorder. J Child Adolesc Psychopharmacol 11:167–170, 2001

Kutcher SP, Boulos C, Ward B, et al: Response to desipramine treatment in adolescent depression: a fixed-dose, placebo-controlled trial. J Am Acad Child Adolesc Psychiatry 33:686–694, 1994

Kye CH, Waterman GS, Ryan ND, et al: A randomized, controlled trial of amitriptyline in the acute treatment of adolescent major depression. J Am Acad Child Adolesc Psychiatry 35:1139–1144, 1996

Looff D, Grimley P, Kuller F, et al: Carbamazepine for PTSD. J Am Acad Child Adolesc Psychiatry 34:703–704, 1995

Mandoki MW: Olanzapine in the treatment of early onset schizophrenia in children and adolescents. Biol Psychiatry 41:S22, 1997

Messenheimer J: Rash in adult and pediatric patients treated with lamotrigine. Can J Neurol Sci 25 (4, suppl):S14–S18, 1998

Pliszka SR, Greenhill LL, Crismon ML, et al: The Texas Children's Medication Algorithm Project: report of the Texas Consensus Conference Panel on medication treatment of childhood attention-deficit/hyperactivity disorder, I: attention deficit/hyperactivity disorder. J Am Acad Child Adolesc Psychiatry 39:908–919, 2000

Popper CW: Pharmacologic alternatives to psychostimulants for the treatment of attention-deficit/hyperactivity disorder. Child Adolesc Psychiatr Clin N Am 9:605–646, 2000

Seedat S, Lockhat R, Kaminer D, et al: An open trial of citalopram in adolescents with post-traumatic stress disorder. Int Clin Psychopharmacol 16:21–25, 2001

Seedat S, Stein DJ, Ziervogel C, et al: Comparison of response to a selective serotonin reuptake inhibitor in children, adolescents, and adults with posttraumatic stress disorder. J Child Adolesc Psychopharmacol 12:37–46, 2002

Simeon JG, Ferguson HB: Alprazolam effects in children with anxiety disorders. Can J Psychiatry 32:570–574, 1987

Simeon JG, Ferguson HB, Knott V, et al: Clinical, cognitive, and neurophysiological effects of alprazolam in children and adolescents with overanxious and avoidant disorders. J Am Acad Child Adolesc Psychiatry 31:29–33, 1992

Spencer T, Biederman J, Wilens T, et al: Pharmacotherapy of attention-deficit/hyperactivity disorder across the life cycle. J Am Acad Child Adolesc Psychiatry 35:409–432, 1996

Spencer T, Biederman J, Heiligenstein J, et al: An open-label, dose-ranging study of atomoxetine in children with attention deficit hyperactivity disorder. J Child Adolesc Psychopharmacol 11:251–265, 2001

Tancer NK, Klein RG, Koplewicz HS, et al: Rate of atypical depression and tricyclic drug response in adolescents. J Am Acad Child Adolesc Psychiatry 31:576, 1992

CHAPTER 58

Treatment of Substance-Related Disorders

Select the single best response for each question.

58.1 In patients with hepatic impairment that has diminished their ability to metabolize medications, which of the following agents would be the best choice for prophylaxis of delirium tremens?

A. Diazepam.
B. Clonazepam.
C. Alprazolam.
D. Triazolam.
E. Oxazepam.

The correct response is option **E.**

The diagnosis of delirium tremens is given to patients who have marked confusion and severe agitation in addition to the usual alcohol withdrawal symptoms. Pharmacotherapy with a benzodiazepine is the treatment of choice for the prevention and treatment of the signs and symptoms of alcohol withdrawal. In outpatient settings, oxazepam may be particularly useful because it is associated with less abuse and does not require hepatic biotransformation. **(p. 1010)**

58.2 When a person taking disulfiram drinks alcohol, the subsequent toxic reaction is due to accumulation of which of the following?

A. Acetone.
B. Alcohol.
C. Acetaldehyde.
D. Glutamate.
E. Dopamine.

The correct response is option **C.**

Disulfiram inhibits a key enzyme, aldehyde dehydrogenase, involved in breakdown of ethyl alcohol. After drinking, the alcohol–disulfiram reaction produces excess blood levels of acetaldehyde, which is toxic in that it produces facial flushing, tachycardia, hypotension, nausea and vomiting, and physical discomfort. **(p. 1010)**

58.3   Although no medication has been clearly identified as effective in preventing relapse to cocaine abuse, double-blind studies have supported moderate benefit for which of the following?

A. Desipramine.
B. Bupropion.
C. Fluoxetine.
D. Amantadine.
E. Pergolide.

The correct response is option **A**.

Although no medication has been clearly identified as beneficial in the treatment of cocaine abuse, the tricyclic antidepressant desipramine, which has been studied in several double-blind studies (Arndt et al. 1992; Gawin et al. 1989; Kosten et al. 1992), appears to be moderately effective in inducing abstinence. Medications found to be ineffective include fluoxetine (Grabowski et al. 1995), bupropion (Margolin et al. 1995), amantadine (Kampman et al. 1996), risperidone (Grabowski et al. 2000), pergolide (Malcolm et al. 2001), and ecopipam (Haney et al. 2001). **(pp. 1013, 1014)**

58.4   Which of the following agents used in the treatment of opioid dependence is itself a partial agonist of the μ opioid receptor?

A. Naltrexone.
B. Buprenorphine.
C. Methadone.
D. Clonidine.
E. Hydromorphone.

The correct response is option **B**.

Buprenorphine is a partial agonist of the μ opioid receptor and is a clinically effective analgesic agent, with an estimated potency 25–40 times that of morphine (Cowan et al. 1977). Buprenorphine in sublingual formulation has been approved by the U.S. Food and Drug Administration for the treatment of opioid dependence. **(p. 1018)**

58.5   The hallucinogen methylenedioxymethamphetamine (MDMA; Ecstasy) is related to what class of drugs?

A. Amphetamines.
B. Opioids.
C. Dissociative anesthetics.
D. Cannabinoids.
E. Benzodiazepine reverse agonists.

The correct response is option **A**.

The hallucinogen MDMA is an amphetamine congener. **(p. 1020)**

58.6   Efficacy in smoking cessation has been demonstrated by all of the following *except*

    A. Transdermal nicotine.
    B. Bupropion.
    C. Nortriptyline.
    D. Propranolol.
    E. Clonidine.

The correct response is option **D.**

A placebo-controlled, double-blind trial of propranolol found it to be no better than placebo for smoking cessation (Farebrother et al. 1980). By contrast, the effectiveness of transdermal nicotine (Daughton et al. 1991; Tonnesen et al. 1991) and of the monocyclic antidepressant bupropion (Ferry et al. 1992; Hurt et al. 1997) in smoking cessation has been well documented. Clonidine, an α_2-adrenergic agonist used to treat opiate and alcohol withdrawal symptoms, has also been found to decrease nicotine withdrawal symptoms and tobacco craving (Glassman et al. 1984, 1990). Nortriptyline has been reported to produce significantly higher rates of smoking cessation, independent of depression, compared with placebo (Hall et al. 2001); this antidepressant is recommended as a second-line medication for smoking cessation by the Tobacco Use and Dependence Clinical Practice Guideline Panel, Staff, and Consortium Representatives (2000). **(pp. 1021, 1022)**

References

Arndt IO, Dorozynsky L, Woody GE, et al: Desipramine treatment of cocaine dependence in methadone-maintained patients. Arch Gen Psychiatry 49:888–893, 1992

Cowan A, Lewis JW, Macfarlane IR: Agonist and antagonist properties of buprenorphine, a new antinociceptive agent. Br J Pharmacol 60:537–545, 1977

Daughton DM, Heatley SA, Pendergast JJ, et al: Effect of transdermal nicotine delivery as an adjunct to low-intervention smoking cessation therapy. Arch Intern Med 151:749–752, 1991

Farebrother MJB, Pearce SJ, Turner P, et al: Propranolol and giving up smoking. Br J Dis Chest 74:95–96, 1980

Ferry LH, Robbins AS, Scariati PD, et al: Enhancement of smoking cessation using the antidepressant bupropion hydrochloride: abstract from the 65th Scientific Sessions of the American Heart Association, New Orleans, LA. Circulation 86 (suppl 1):671, 1992

Gawin FH, Kleber HD, Byck R, et al: Desipramine facilitation of initial cocaine abstinence. Arch Gen Psychiatry 46:117–121, 1989

Glassman AH, Jackson WK, Walsh BT, et al: Cigarette craving, smoking withdrawal, and clonidine. Science 226:864–866, 1984

Glassman AH, Helzer JE, Covey LS, et al: Smoking, smoking cessation, and major depression. JAMA 264:1546–1549, 1990

Grabowski J, Rhoades H, Elk R, et al: Fluoxetine is ineffective for treatment of cocaine dependence or concurrent opiate and cocaine dependence: two placebo controlled double-blind trials. J Clin Psychopharmacol 15:163–173, 1995

Grabowski J, Rhoades H, Siverman P, et al: Risperidone for the treatment of cocaine dependence: randomized double-blind trial. J Clin Psychopharmacol 20:305–310, 2000

Hall S, Reus VI, Munoz RF, et al: Nortriptyline and cognitive-behavioral therapy in the treatment of cigarette smoking. Arch Gen Psychiatry 55:683–690, 2001

Haney M, Ward AS, Foltin RW, et al: Effects of ecopipam, a selective dopamine D1 antagonist, on smoked cocaine self-administration by humans. Psychopharmacology (Berl) 155:330–337, 2001

Hurt RD, Sachs DP, Glover ED, et al: A comparison of sustained-release bupropion and placebo for smoking cessation (comments). N Engl J Med 337:1195–1202, 1997

Kampman K, Volpicelli JR, Alterman A, et al: Amantadine in the early treatment of cocaine dependence: a double-blind, placebo-controlled trial. Drug Alcohol Depend 41:25–33, 1996

Kosten TR, Morgan CM, Falcione J, et al: Pharmacotherapy for cocaine-abusing methadone-maintained patients using amantadine or desipramine. Arch Gen Psychiatry 49:894–898, 1992

Malcolm R, Herron J, Sutherland SE, et al: Adverse outcomes in a controlled trial of pergolide for cocaine dependence. J Addict Dis 20:81–92, 2001

Margolin A, Kosten TR, Avants SK, et al: A multicenter trial of bupropion for cocaine dependence in methadone-maintained patients. Drug Alcohol Depend 40:125–131, 1995

Tobacco Use and Dependence Clinical Practice Guideline Panel, Staff, and Consortium Representatives: A clinical practice guideline for treating tobacco use and dependence: a US Public Health Service report. JAMA 283:3244–3254, 2000

Tonnesen P, Norrezaard J, Simonsen K, et al: A double-blind trial of a 16-hour transdermal nicotine patch in smoking cessation. N Engl J Med 325:311–315, 1991

CHAPTER 59

Treatment of Eating Disorders

Select the single best response for each question.

59.1   Which of the following antidepressants is relatively contraindicated in the treatment of bulimia nervosa?

A. Bupropion.
B. Fluoxetine.
C. Imipramine.
D. Desipramine.
E. Trazodone.

The correct response is option **A.**

A study of bupropion found that a higher-than-expected proportion of patients developed grand mal seizures (Horne et al. 1988). The authors concluded that bupropion should not be used for the treatment of bulimia nervosa. **(p. 1033)**

59.2   Studies support the effectiveness in binge-eating disorder of all of the following interventions *except*

A. Fluvoxamine.
B. Phentermine + fluoxetine + cognitive-behavioral therapy (CBT).
C. Imipramine.
D. Topiramate.
E. Sibutramine.

The correct response is option **C.**

Imipramine was found not to differ from placebo in reducing binge eating (Alger et al. 1991). Fluvoxamine, in a large study (Hudson et al. 1998), was found to significantly reduce binge eating. In an open-label study examining the combination of phentermine and fluoxetine with 20 weeks of CBT (Devlin et al. 2000), 12 of 16 (75%) patients had stopped binge eating at the end of treatment. The medication combination appeared to lead to significant weight losses of, on average, 19 lbs at the end of treatment. Both sibutramine (a novel serotonin and norepinephrine reuptake inhibitor) and topiramate appeared to be useful in the treatment of binge-eating disorder in open-label studies (Appolinario et al. 2002; Shapira et al. 2000). Weight losses were relatively large with both of these medications. **(p. 1037)**

59.3 Which of the following medications has demonstrated possible benefit in reducing relapse in weight-restored patients with anorexia nervosa?

A. Pimozide.
B. Escitalopram.
C. Naltrexone.
D. Olanzapine.
E. Fluoxetine.

The correct response is option **E.**

Fluoxetine may have a role in reducing relapse in weight-restored patients with anorexia nervosa. In a randomized, controlled trial of 35 patients with anorexia nervosa who were followed up for 1 year, fluoxetine (10–60 mg/day) or placebo was started in the hospital and continued until the patient stopped taking medication or terminated the study, usually because of relapse (Kaye et al. 2001). Nonetheless, for those taking medication, there was a significant difference in the relapse rates between groups. Ten (63%) of the participants taking fluoxetine and 3 (16%) of those taking placebo remained in the trial for 1 year. Hence, it appears that fluoxetine may prevent relapse in outpatients with anorexia, because only the group continuing fluoxetine showed improvement from baseline to the end of follow-up in depression, anxiety, obsessions, compulsions, and core eating disorder symptoms. **(p. 1038)**

59.4 Complications of bulimia nervosa include all of the following *except*

A. Dental caries.
B. Pulmonary hypertension.
C. Potassium depletion.
D. Salivary gland enlargement.
E. Exercise injuries.

The correct response is option **B.**

Medical complications of bulimia nervosa are relatively rare; the most serious are potassium depletion and dental caries. Other complications include salivary gland enlargement and exercise injuries. **(p. 1032)**

59.5 Which of the following statements about anorexia nervosa is *true*?

A. Diagnostic criteria require that a patient's weight be at least 75% below ideal body weight.
B. Amenorrhea is uncommon in anorexia nervosa.
C. Anorexia nervosa is the most lethal psychiatric disorder.
D. Fluoxetine has proven effective in treating hospitalized patients with anorexia.
E. Patients with anorexia tend to be especially cooperative with treatment.

The correct response is option **C.**

Anorexia nervosa is a relatively rare disorder characterized by marked weight loss (at least 15% below ideal body weight), an intense fear of gaining weight, a disturbance in the experience of body shape (i.e., feeling fat in the face of marked weight loss), and (in females) amenorrhea. Anorexia nervosa is the most lethal psychiatric disorder. Follow-up studies document an aggregate mortality rate of about 5.6% per decade; about half of these deaths are a result of suicide, and the remainder are largely due to cardiac arrest (Sullivan 1995). Fluoxetine was not found to be effective in hospitalized patients with anorexia nervosa (Attia et al. 1998). Treatment of anorexia nervosa can be quite difficult because of the patient's reluctance to gain weight. Weight should be monitored at every outpatient visit, and it is important that the patient be weighed in a hospital gown to prevent the use of lead weights, to which some patients with anorexia resort. Other methods of inflating weight are less easy to detect, such as drinking large quantities of water before being weighed. **(pp. 1037, 1038)**

References

Alger A, Schwalberg D, Bigaouette JM, et al: Effect of a tricyclic antidepressant and opiate antagonist on binge-eating behavior in normoweight bulimic and obese, binge-eating subjects. Am J Clin Nutr 53:865–871, 1991

Appolinario JC, Godoy-Matos A, Fontenelle LF, et al: An open-label trial of sibutramine in obese patients with binge eating disorder. J Clin Psychiatry 63:28–30, 2002

Attia E, Haiman C, Walsh BT, et al: Does fluoxetine augment the inpatient treatment of anorexia nervosa? Am J Psychiatry 155:548–551, 1998

Devlin MJ, Golfein JA, Carino JS, et al: Open treatment of overweight binge eaters with phentermine and fluoxetine as an adjunct to cognitive-behavioral therapy. Int J Eat Disord 28:325–332, 2000

Horne RL, Ferguson JM, Pope HG Jr, et al: Treatment of bulimia with bupropion: a multicenter controlled trial. J Clin Psychiatry 49:262–266, 1988

Hudson JI, McElroy SL, Raymond NC, et al: Fluvoxamine in the treatment of binge-eating disorder: a multicenter placebo-controlled, double-blind trial. Am J Psychiatry 155:1756–1762, 1998

Kaye WH, Nagata T, Weltzin TE, et al: Double-blind placebo-controlled administration of fluoxetine in restricting- and restricting-purging-type anorexia nervosa. Biol Psychiatry 49:644–652, 2001

Shapira NA, Goldsmith TD, McElroy SL: Treatment of binge-eating disorder with topiramate: a clinical case series. J Clin Psychiatry 61:368–372, 2000

Sullivan PF: Mortality in anorexia nervosa. Am J Psychiatry 152:1073–1074, 1995

CHAPTER 60

Treatment of Agitation and Aggression in the Elderly

Select the single best response for each question.

60.1   Which of the following statements regarding tardive dyskinesia in elderly patients is *true*?

A. It may develop more rapidly and at lower doses than with younger patients.
B. It is more common in patients with cortical atrophy.
C. It is less likely to disappear when neuroleptics are discontinued.
D. All of the above.
E. None of the above.

The correct response is option **D.**

In elderly patients who have not previously taken conventional antipsychotics, tardive dyskinesia may develop more rapidly and at lower doses than in younger patients (Caligiuri et al. 1997; Jeste et al. 1999; Karson et al. 1990; Lieberman et al. 1984; Saltz et al. 1989; Yassa et al. 1988). Tardive dyskinesia is also more common in patients with evidence of cortical atrophy (Sweet et al. 1992). When neuroleptics are discontinued, tardive dyskinesia symptoms are less likely to disappear in older patients than in younger adults (De Veaugh-Geiss 1988; Smith and Baldessarini 1980; Yassa et al. 1984). **(p. 1042)**

60.2   Which group of elderly patients is at increased risk for neuroleptic malignant syndrome from conventional antipsychotics?

A. Patients with cardiac disease.
B. Patients with Parkinson's disease.
C. Patients with cerebrovascular disease.
D. Patients with hypertension.
E. Patients with diabetes.

The correct response is option **B.**

Neuroleptic malignant syndrome may occur in older patients taking conventional antipsychotics. This syndrome was found to be more common among elderly patients with dementia or Parkinson's disease (Addonizio 1992). **(p. 1042)**

60.3 Side effects associated with clozapine use include which of the following?

A. Agranulocytosis.
C. Orthostasis.
D. Anticholinergic symptoms.
E. All of the above.
E. None of the above.

The correct response is option **D.**

Clozapine produces a high frequency of side effects, which means that it should not be a first-choice atypical antipsychotic for elderly patients (Salzman et al. 1995). Common side effects of clozapine include an increased incidence of agranulocytosis, as well as sedation, orthostatic hypotension, and anticholinergic and pulmonary side effects. **(p. 1042)**

60.4 Which of the following atypical antipsychotics has been found to effectively and safely treat agitation in the elderly?

A. Ziprasidone.
B. Quetiapine.
C. Olanzapine.
D. Aripiprazole.
E. Risperidone.

The correct response is option **C.**

Olanzapine has been widely used to treat agitation in the elderly. In elderly nursing home residents who had psychotic and/or behavioral symptoms, dosages of 5, 10, and 15 mg/day were found to be significantly superior to placebo and well tolerated (Street et al. 2000). The lower dosages (5 and 10 mg/day, compared with 15 mg/day) were associated with fewer side effects. In a second study, olanzapine was compared with risperidone or haloperidol for the treatment of behavioral symptoms of dementia in 2,747 individuals. Olanzapine produced an overall greater improvement than did the other two medications and also was associated with greater improvement in aggression (Edell and Tunis 2001). In smaller studies, olanzapine was effective in treating mild to moderate psychosis and behavioral symptoms of Alzheimer's disease (Kennedy et al. 1999) and schizophrenia (Sajatovic et al. 1998) in elderly patients without producing a decrement in cognitive functioning. **(p. 1043)**

60.5 Which of the following agents has been found to rapidly and safely treat sexual acting-out behavior in elderly men with dementia?

A. Lithium.
B. Buspirone.
C. Trazodone.
D. Medroxyprogesterone.
E. Lorazepam.

The correct response is option **D.**

Medroxyprogesterone has been reported to rapidly and safely treat sexual acting-out behavior in elderly men with dementia (Cooper 1987). **(p. 1044)**

References

Addonizio G: Neuroleptic malignant syndrome in the elderly, in Psychopharmacological Treatment Complications in the Elderly. Edited by Shamoian CA. Washington, DC, American Psychiatric Press, 1992, pp 63–70

Caligiuri MP, Lacro JP, Rockwell E, et al: Incidence and risk factors for severe tardive dyskinesia in older patients. Br J Psychiatry 171:148–153, 1997

Cooper AJ: Medroxyprogesterone acetate (MPA) treatment of sexual acting out in men suffering from dementia. J Clin Psychiatry 48:368–370, 1987

De Veaugh-Geiss J: Clinical changes in tardive dyskinesia during long-term follow-up, in Tardive Dyskinesia: Biological Mechanisms and Clinical Aspects. Edited by Wolf ME, Mosnaim AD. Washington, DC, American Psychiatric Press, 1988, pp 89–105

Edell WS, Tunis SL: Antipsychotic treatment of behavioral and psychological symptoms of dementia in geropsychiatric inpatients. Am J Geriatr Psychiatry 9:289–297, 2001

Jeste DV, Lacro JP, Palmer B, et al: Incidence of tardive dyskinesia in early stages of low-dose treatment with typical neuroleptics in older patients. Am J Psychiatry 156:309–311, 1999

Karson CG, Bracha HS, Powell A, et al: Dyskinetic movements, cognitive impairment, and negative symptoms in elderly neuropsychiatric patients. Am J Psychiatry 147:1646–1649, 1990

Kennedy JS, Basson BR, Zagar AJ, et al: The effects of olanzapine on Alzheimer's Disease Assessment Scale scores in patients with mild to moderate Alzheimer's disease with psychosis and behavioral disturbances. Poster presented at the 38th American College of Neuropsychopharmacology Annual Meeting, Acapulco, Mexico, December 12–16, 1999

Lieberman J, Kane JM, Woerner M, et al: Prevalence of tardive dyskinesia in elderly samples. Psychopharmacol Bull 20:22–26, 1984

Sajatovic M, Perez D, Brescan D, et al: Olanzapine therapy in elderly patients with schizophrenia. Psychopharmacol Bull 34:819–823, 1998

Saltz BL, Kane JM, Woerner MG, et al: Prospective study of tardive dyskinesia in the elderly. Psychopharmacol Bull 25:52–56, 1989

Salzman C, Vaccaro B, Lieff J, et al: Clozapine in older patients with psychosis and behavioral disruption. Am J Geriatr Psychiatry 3:26–33, 1995

Smith JM, Baldessarini RJ: Changes in prevalence, severity and recovery in tardive dyskinesia with age. Arch Gen Psychiatry 37:1368–1373, 1980

Street JS, Clark WS, Gannon KS, et al: Olanzapine treatment of psychotic and behavioral symptoms in patients with Alzheimer's disease in nursing care facilities. Arch Gen Psychiatry 57:968–976, 2000

Sweet RA, Benoit H, Mulsant MD, et al: Dyskinesia and neuroleptic exposure in elderly psychiatric inpatients. J Geriatr Psychiatry Neurol 5:156–161, 1992

Yassa R, Nair V, Schwartz G: Tardive dyskinesia: a two-year follow-up study. Psychosomatics 25:852–855, 1984

Yassa R, Nastase C, Camille Y, et al: Tardive dyskinesia in a psychogeriatric population, in Tardive Dyskinesia: Biological Mechanisms and Clinical Aspects. Edited by Wolf ME, Mosnaim AD. Washington, DC, American Psychiatric Press, 1988, pp 125–133

CHAPTER 61

Treatment of Personality Disorders

Select the single best response for each question.

61.1   Regarding use of antidepressants in treating borderline personality disorder patients, which of the following statements is *true*?

   A. Tricyclic antidepressants (TCAs) and monoamine oxidase inhibitors (MAOIs) pose serious risks of overdose and dangerous adverse effects that are of particular concern in an unstable and an impulsive population.
   B. Selective serotonin reuptake inhibitors (SSRIs) lose efficacy for aggression and irritability after 2 months of treatment.
   C. SSRIs have not been found to decrease suicidality and self-injury in borderline personality disorder patients.
   D. Phenelzine is far more effective than placebo in the treatment of borderline personality disorder patients in all behavioral and mood-sphere domains studied.
   E. All of the above.

The correct response is option **A**.

Regardless of efficacy, both TCAs and MAOIs pose serious overdose and dangerous adverse effect risks that are of particular concern in this unstable, impulsive population. Compared with placebo, fluoxetine at dosages of 20–60 mg/day led to a consistent and significant decrease in aggression and irritability and to global improvement apparent by the second month of treatment, and this effect was independent of changes in depression or anxiety (Coccaro and Kavoussi 1997). Twenty-three borderline personality disorder patients were treated openly for an initial 12-week period with sertraline 200 mg/day, and about half the patients showed improvement in self-injurious behavior, anxiety, depression, and suicidality (Markovitz 1995). Cornelius et al. (1993) found that phenelzine had only modest efficacy in borderline personality disorder and was superior to placebo only against anger and hostility and not on measures of depression, atypical depression, psychoticism, impulsivity, or global borderline severity. By contrast, a crossover placebo-controlled study of four classes of medications in borderline personality disorder (Cowdry and Gardner 1988) found that the MAOI tranylcypromine was significantly superior to placebo, according to both clinicians and patients, in global ratings and in most domains that were measured, including depression, anxiety, anger, rejection sensitivity, impulsivity, and suicidality. **(pp. 1053, 1055; see also Table 61–1)**

61.2   The three most useful classes of medications in the treatment of borderline personality disorder are

   A. Benzodiazepines, azapirones, and serotonergic and noradrenergic reuptake inhibitors (SNRIs).
   B. Selective serotonin reuptake inhibitors (SSRIs), mood stabilizers, and atypical antipsychotics.
   C. Mood stabilizers, SSRIs, and stimulants.
   D. Benzodiazepines, stimulants, and azapirones.
   E. Benzodiazepines, nonbenzodiazepine hypnotics, and conventional antipsychotics.

The correct response is option **B.**

Three classes of medications have emerged as the most useful in treating borderline personality disorder: SSRIs, mood stabilizers, and atypical antipsychotics. Of these, the fewest controlled data to date are available for the atypical antipsychotics. Thus far, the SSRI fluoxetine and the mood stabilizer valproate have the most data documenting their efficacy. Comparison trials of these three classes of medications, including combination strategies, have not been reported and would be of great interest in the future. **(p. 1059)**

61.3   Which of the following statements regarding comorbid personality disorders and Axis I disorders is *true?*

A.   In one community survey, most patients (approximately 80%) with personality disorders who were deemed in need of treatment of Axis I disorders were not receiving such treatment.
B.   Personality disorder comorbidity is strongly associated with poor medication compliance in bipolar patients.
C.   In a large study, anxiety disorder patients with comorbid borderline personality disorder were more likely than those without a personality disorder diagnosis to be receiving multiple medications.
D.   All of the above.
E.   None of the above.

The correct response is option **D.**

A community survey, conducted as part of a 1981 epidemiological study that used DSM-III (American Psychiatric Association 1980) diagnostic criteria, examined the association between Axis I and Axis II disorders and the need for and likelihood of treatment (Samuels et al. 1994). In essence, although individuals with comorbid personality disorders were proportionately more likely to be receiving some type of psychiatric treatment if in need of it, about 80% of the total individuals with personality disorders who were identified as needing treatment were not receiving it. A study examining various factors affecting medication compliance among 200 bipolar I and II disorder patients found that personality disorder comorbidity was the factor most strongly associated with poor compliance (Colom et al. 2000). A large study examined the amount of psychiatric treatment received by anxiety disorder patients as a function of comorbid personality disorder (Phillips et al. 2001). The investigators examined several hundred anxious patients with a variety of Axis I diagnoses: panic disorder, generalized anxiety disorder, social phobia, obsessive-compulsive disorder, posttraumatic stress disorder, and agoraphobia. Despite minor discrepancies between the two time-point assessments (1991 and 1996), the findings were fairly consistent: similar percentages of anxious subjects with and without personality disorders received medication treatment. If medicated, the patients with personality disorders, and especially those with borderline personality disorder, were likely to be receiving a greater number of medications, specifically heterocyclic antidepressants. **(pp. 1062, 1063)**

61.4   Conventional antipsychotics may be helpful in borderline personality disorder for which of the following problems?

A.   Suicidality.
B.   Ideas of reference.
C.   Social functioning.
D.   All of the above.
E.   None of the above.

The correct response is option **D.**

In one large trial (Serban and Siegel 1984) in personality disorder patients, treatment with thiothixene (9.4 mg/day) or haloperidol (3 mg/day) resulted in improvement on multiple domains, including cognitive disturbance, derealization, ideas of reference, anxiety, depression, and self-esteem and social functioning, suggesting that medicating target symptoms may have a wide-reaching effect. In a placebo-controlled study (Montgomery and Montgomery 1982) in patients with personality disorders, mostly borderline, presenting acutely with a suicide attempt and with a history of at least two prior attempts, treatment with a low-dose depot antipsychotic (flupenthixol 20 mg every 4 weeks) was highly effective in reducing suicide attempts at 4–6 months of treatment. **(p. 1052)**

61.5   Which of the following is the main indication for use of medications in the treatment of personality disorders?

   A. During periods of acute decompensation.
   B. For longer-term management of symptom clusters that are maladaptive and that may be responsive to medication.
   C. To treat reappearance or worsening of comorbid Axis I conditions.
   D. All of the above.
   E. None of the above.

The correct response is option **D**.

The main indications for using medications in treating personality disorders are periods of decompensation, crises, and hospitalizations; the longer-term management of symptom clusters that are maladaptive and may be responsive to medication; and the reappearance or worsening of comorbid Axis I conditions. **(p. 1049)**

References

American Psychiatric Association: Diagnostic and Statistical Manual of Mental Disorders, 3rd Edition. Washington, DC, American Psychiatric Association, 1980

Coccaro EF, Kavoussi RJ: Fluoxetine and impulsive aggressive behavior in personality-disordered subjects. Arch Gen Psychiatry 54:1081–1088, 1997

Colom F, Vieta E, Martinez-Aran A, et al: Clinical factors associated with treatment noncompliance in euthymic bipolar patients. J Clin Psychiatry 61:549–555, 2000

Cornelius JR, Soloff PH, Perel JM, et al: Continuation pharmacotherapy of borderline personality disorder with haloperidol and phenelzine. Am J Psychiatry 150:1843–1848, 1993

Cowdry RW, Gardner DL: Pharmacotherapy of borderline personality disorder: alprazolam, carbamazepine, trifluoperazine, and tranylcypromine. Arch Gen Psychiatry 45:111–119, 1988

Markovitz PJ: Pharmacotherapy of impulsivity, aggression, and related disorders, in Impulsivity and Aggression. Edited by Hollander E, Stein DJ. New York, Wiley, 1995, pp 263–288

Montgomery SA, Montgomery D: Pharmacological prevention of suicidal behaviour. J Affect Disord 4:291–298, 1982

Phillips KA, Shea MT, Warshaw M, et al: The relationship between comorbid personality disorders and treatment received in patients with anxiety disorders. J Personal Disord 15:157–167, 2001

Samuels JF, Nestadt G, Romanoski AJ, et al: DSM-III personality disorders in the community. Am J Psychiatry 151:1055–1062, 1994

Serban G, Siegel S: Response of borderline and schizotypal patients to small doses of thiothixene and haloperidol. Am J Psychiatry 141:1455–1458, 1984

C H A P T E R 6 2

Psychiatric Emergencies

Select the single best response for each question.

62.1 Psychiatric emergencies can be divided into 1) those that do not require pharmacological intervention, 2) those in which pharmacological interventions are adjunctive, and 3) those in which medications are required. An example of the second class of psychiatric emergency would be

A. Assaultive or aggressive behavior.
B. Acute grief or trauma.
C. Neuroleptic-induced dystonia.
D. Ethanol withdrawal.
E. Anticholinergic delirium from tricyclic antidepressants.

The correct response is option **B.**

Psychiatric emergencies requiring minimal or adjunctive pharmacological intervention occur in many different situations, although many share a common thread of developing in response to some discrete, identifiable stressor. Included in this class are psychiatric emergencies associated with adjustment disorder or acute grief; rape, assault, or trauma; borderline personality disorder; and panic disorders. By contrast, management of severe behavioral emergencies nearly always requires psychopharmacological intervention. Episodes of disorganized, disinhibited, agitated, aggressive, or violent behaviors can occur in patients who are psychotic, manic, or intoxicated and also in those who have organic syndromes such as dementia or delirium. Patients who are experiencing severe medication side effects and adverse events also require pharmacological interventions, as do patients with substance use disorders in withdrawal states. **(pp. 1068, 1073; see Table 62–2)**

62.2 Which of the following groupings represent psychotropic medications available for intravenous administration?

A. Buspirone, nefazodone, diazepam.
B. Trazodone, buspirone, lithium.
C. Lorazepam, diazepam, haloperidol.
D. Pimozide, lorazepam, sertraline.
E. Midazolam, venlafaxine, haloperidol.

The correct response is option **C.**

Three medications suitable for use in behavioral emergencies are available for intravenous administration: lorazepam, diazepam, and haloperidol. **(p. 1076)**

62.3 Which of the following groupings represent psychotropic medications available for intramuscular administration?

    A. Lorazepam, haloperidol, olanzapine.
    B. Ziprasidone, diazepam, nefazodone.
    C. Haloperidol, bupropion, lorazepam.
    D. Clonazepam, lithium, amitriptyline.
    E. Pimozide, paroxetine, ziprasidone.

The correct response is option **A**.

As of 2003, five medications suitable for use in behavioral emergencies are available for intramuscular administration: lorazepam, diazepam, the typical antipsychotic haloperidol, and the atypical antipsychotics olanzapine and ziprasidone. **(p. 1077)**

62.4 Acute *severe* dystonic reactions (e.g., oculogyric crisis or laryngospasm) should be treated with

    A. Intramuscular thiamine.
    B. Intravenous diphenhydramine.
    C. Oral benztropine.
    D. Intravenous β-blockers.
    E. Oral buspirone.

The correct response is option **B**.

Dystonic reactions are characterized by extreme muscle contraction and rigidity in a patient with stable vital signs and a clear sensorium; they occur most frequently as an adverse effect of high-potency, first-generation antipsychotics. Most dystonic reactions are extremely uncomfortable and frightening to the patient. Treatment of these reactions is typically 1–2 mg of benztropine via the oral or intramuscular route. An alternative is diphenhydramine in doses of 25–50 mg via the oral or intramuscular route. Dystonias that include the eyes, the so-called oculogyric crises, are particularly frightening, as are dystonias that cause laryngeal spasms, which can compromise the airway. These reactions should be treated with 50 mg of intravenous diphenhydramine, which provides rapid relief. Maintenance treatment of 1–2 mg of benztropine twice a day or 25–50 mg of diphenhydramine twice a day should be initiated after the acute reaction has resolved (Keepers et al. 1983). **(p. 1079)**

62.5 Which of the following symptoms is present in neuroleptic malignant syndrome (NMS)?

    A. Autonomic instability.
    B. Altered consciousness.
    C. Lead-pipe rigidity.
    D. Elevated creatine phosphokinase (CPK).
    E. All of the above.

The correct response is option **E**.

NMS is a potentially fatal delirium that develops in some patients in response to antipsychotic agents (Sussman 2001). The diagnosis is made on the triad of symptoms of altered level of consciousness, muscular rigidity (often described as lead-pipe rigidity), and autonomic instability. The autonomic instability includes hyperthermia, tachycardia, labile blood pressure, diaphoresis, incontinence, and occasional dysphagia and bowel obstruction. Associated findings include elevated CPK, elevated white blood cell count, and metabolic acidosis. **(p. 1080)**

62.6   The serotonin syndrome is a delirium characterized by which of the following?

   A. Neuromuscular abnormalities and autonomic instability.
   B. Sedation and hyporeflexia.
   C. Altered consciousness and flaccidity.
   D. Agitation and hyporeflexia.
   E. None of the above.

The correct response is option **A.**

The serotonin syndrome is a delirium characterized by altered level of consciousness, autonomic instability, and neuromuscular abnormalities, including myoclonus, hyperreflexia, nystagmus, akathisia, and muscle rigidity (Martin 1996; Mason et al. 2000). Several different drugs, usually administered in combination, can cause this adverse event. Drugs reported to provoke the serotonin syndrome include selective serotonin reuptake inhibitors, venlafaxine, trazodone, nefazodone, monoamine oxidase inhibitors, lithium, tryptophan, meperidine, sumatriptan, buspirone, and amphetamines. Discontinuation of the offending agent and general supportive measures are the principal interventions. In contrast to its usefulness in treating neuroleptic malignant syndrome, bromocriptine can worsen the serotonin syndrome. Drugs useful in treating this condition are benzodiazepines, cyproheptadine, chlorpromazine, methysergide, and propranolol. **(p. 1080)**

References

Keepers GA, Clappison VJ, Casey DE: Initial anticholinergic prophylaxis for neuroleptic-induced extrapyramidal syndromes. Arch Gen Psychiatry 40:1113–1117, 1983

Martin T: Serotonin syndrome. Ann Emerg Med 28:520–526, 1996

Mason PJ, Morris VA, Balcezak TJ: Serotonin syndrome: presentation of 2 cases and review of the literature. Medicine (Baltimore) 79:201–209, 2000

Sussman VL: Clinical management of neuroleptic malignant syndrome. Psychiatr Q 72:325–336, 2001

CHAPTER 63

Treatment During Late Life

Select the single best response for each question.

63.1 Which of the following pharmacokinetic functions do not change with age?

 A. Absorption.
 B. Distribution.
 C. Metabolism.
 D. Excretion.
 E. None of the above.

The correct response is option **A.**

The rate and extent of passive drug absorption do not appear to be affected by normal aging. Antacids, high-fiber supplements, and cholestyramine may significantly diminish the absorption of medications. For most psychotropics that are lipid soluble, the loss of lean body mass with aging will lead to increases in drug volumes of distribution, resulting in longer half-lives and drug accumulation. This is because a drug's half-life is directly proportional to its apparent volume of distribution. Conversely, for water-soluble drugs such as lithium and digoxin, volumes of distribution will be diminished in older patients, reducing the margin of safety after acute increases in plasma drug concentration. Reductions in hepatic mass and blood flow with aging place greater emphasis on interindividual differences in drug metabolic capacity. Drugs metabolized by cytochrome P450 3A4, such as alprazolam, triazolam, sertraline, mirtazapine, and nefazodone, appear to be cleared less well in elderly patients (Barbhaiya et al. 1996; Greenblatt et al. 1991; Ronfeld et al. 1997; Timmer et al. 1996). The well-established age-associated decline in renal clearance may affect excretion of psychotropic drug metabolites and lithium in older patients. **(pp. 1083–1085)**

63.2 Which of the following brain imaging findings is associated with late-onset (after age 60 years) depression?

 A. Enlarged ventricles.
 B. Significant cerebrovascular disease.
 C. Cortical atrophy.
 D. Frontal lobe lesions.
 E. Central pontine myelinolysis.

The correct response is option **B.**

Depression in late life probably represents a heterogeneous group of disorders with distinct etiologies; for example, late-onset depression, defined as having a first episode after age 60 years, is associated with brain imaging findings consistent with significant vascular disease (Figiel et al. 1991), and late-life dysthymia in men is associated with low testosterone levels (Seidman and Roose 2000). **(p. 1086)**

63.3 Regarding use of tricyclic antidepressants (TCAs) versus selective serotonin reuptake inhibitors (SSRIs) in the treatment of late-life depression, which of the following statements is *true*?

A. TCAs are the most prescribed class of antidepressants in the elderly population.
B. SSRIs can be safely used in post–myocardial infarction patients.
C. In elderly subjects, dropout rates with paroxetine have been found to be higher than rates with nortriptyline.
D. SSRIs pose a significant risk of urinary retention and confusion.
E. None of the above.

The correct response is option **B.**

The SSRIs are the most prescribed class of antidepressants for both earlier-onset *and* late-life depression. In contrast to the TCAs, the SSRIs have a relatively benign cardiovascular profile; specifically, they have no effect on blood pressure, heart rate, cardiac conduction, or cardiac arrhythmias, and there is no indication that they carry significant cardiac risk. In a randomized, controlled trial of post–myocardial infarction depressed patients who received sertraline or placebo, the patients treated with sertraline had significantly fewer major cardiovascular events than did those receiving placebo (Glassman et al. 2002). In a 12-week trial comparing nortriptyline with paroxetine in 116 inpatients and outpatients (mean age: 72 years) (Mulsant et al. 2001), the rate of dropout due to side effects in the nortriptyline group was significantly higher than that in the paroxetine group (33% vs. 16%; $P = 0.04$). The anticholinergic effects of TCAs result in dry mouth, constipation, and blurred vision; more important, the geriatric population is particularly susceptible to anticholinergic-induced urinary retention and confusional states. **(pp. 1087–1089)**

63.4 Regarding use of atypical antipsychotic drugs in the elderly, which of the following statements is *true*?

A. Diabetic ketoacidosis is less common with clozapine and olanzapine compared with other atypicals.
B. Fasting lipid levels have been reported to rise more with olanzapine than with risperidone.
C. Higher doses of atypical antipsychotics are necessary to treat elderly patients.
D. Extrapyramidal symptoms and tardive dyskinesia are less common in the elderly.
E. All of the above.

The correct response is option **B.**

New-onset type 2 diabetes mellitus or diabetic ketoacidosis may be *more* common with clozapine and olanzapine compared with other antipsychotics, and blood glucose levels need to be monitored in elderly patients (Jin et al. 2002). Fasting lipid levels have been reported to rise more with olanzapine than with risperidone (Meyer 2002). Although neurological side effects are less of a concern with most atypical antipsychotics, lower doses are still needed because of the older patient's susceptibility to the other side effects of antipsychotics, including anticholinergic and cardiovascular side effects. Up to 50% of all patients between 60 and 80 years old receiving conventional antipsychotic medications develop either extrapyramidal symptoms or tardive dyskinesia (Jeste et al. 1999). **(p. 1092)**

63.5 Which antipsychotic drug is best tolerated by Parkinson's disease patients with psychosis?

A. Haloperidol.
B. Olanzapine.
C. Clozapine.
D. Thioridazine.
E. Quetiapine.

The correct response is option **E.**

In a series of five patients with Parkinson's disease who developed psychosis, olanzapine treatment was not effective in treating psychosis and was associated with worsening motor function and sedation (Marsh et al. 2001), and two double-blind, placebo-controlled trials did not find an advantage for olanzapine over placebo in these patients (Breier et al. 2002). Clozapine may be of some value in patients with Parkinson's disease (Friedman and Fernandez 2002), but quetiapine may be the preferred antipsychotic in this disorder. Long-term quetiapine use is generally well tolerated in patients with Parkinson's disease or diffuse Lewy body disease (Fernandez et al. 2002). **(p. 1100)**

References

Barbhaiya RH, Buch AB, Greene DS: A study of the effect of age and gender on the pharmacokinetics of nefazodone after single and multiple doses. J Clin Psychopharmacol 16:19–25, 1996

Breier A, Sutton V, Feldman P, et al: Olanzapine in the treatment of dopamimetic-induced psychosis in patients with Parkinson's disease. Biol Psychiatry 52:438–447, 2002

Fernandez HH, Trieschmann ME, Burke MA, et al: Quetiapine for psychosis in Parkinson's disease versus dementia with Lewy bodies. J Clin Psychiatry 63:513–515, 2002

Figiel GS, Krishnan KRR, Doraiswamy PM, et al: Subcortical hyperintensities on brain magnetic resonance imaging: a comparison between late age onset and early onset elderly depressed subjects. Neurobiol Aging 26:245–247, 1991

Friedman JH, Fernandez HH: Atypical antipsychotics in Parkinson-sensitive populations. J Geriatr Psychiatry Neurol 15:156–170, 2002

Glassman AH, O'Connor CM, Califf RM, et al: Sertraline treatment of major depression in patients with acute MI or unstable angina. JAMA 288:701–709, 2002

Greenblatt DJ, Harmatz JS, Shader RI: Clinical pharmacokinetics of anxiolytics and hypnotics in the elderly: therapeutic considerations. Clin Pharmacokinet 21:165–177, 1991

Jeste DV, Lacro JP, Palmer B, et al: Incidence of tardive dyskinesia in early stages of low-dose treatment with typical antipsychotics in older patients. Am J Psychiatry 156:309–311, 1999

Jin H, Meyer JM, Jeste DV: Phenomenology of and risk factors for new-onset diabetes mellitus and diabetic ketoacidosis associated with atypical antipsychotics: an analysis of 45 published cases. Ann Clin Psychiatry 14:59–64, 2002

Marsh L, Lyketsos C, Reich SG: Olanzapine for the treatment of psychosis in patients with Parkinson's disease and dementia. Psychosomatics 42:477–481, 2001

Meyer JM: A retrospective comparison of weight, lipid, and glucose changes between risperidone- and olanzapine-treated inpatients: metabolic outcomes after 1 year. J Clin Psychiatry 63:425–433, 2002

Mulsant BH, Pollock BG, Nebes R, et al: A twelve-week, double-blind randomized comparison of nortriptyline and paroxetine in older depressed patients and outpatients. Am J Geriatr Psychiatry 9:406–414, 2001

Ronfeld RA, Tremaine LM, Wilner KD: Pharmacokinetics of sertraline and its N-demethyl metabolite in elderly and young male and female volunteers. Clin Pharmacokinet 32 (suppl 1):22–30, 1997

Seidman SN, Roose SP: The relationship between depression and erectile dysfunction. Curr Psychiatry Rep 2:201–205, 2000

Timmer CJ, Paanakker JE, Van Hal HJM: Pharmacokinetics of mirtazapine from orally administered tablets: influence of gender, age and treatment regimen. Hum Psychopharmacol 11:497–509, 1996

C H A P T E R   6 4

Psychopharmacology During Pregnancy and Lactation

Select the single best response for each question.

64.1   Which of the following antidepressants has received a Category B use-in-pregnancy rating?

   A. Sertraline.
   B. Fluoxetine.
   C. Nortriptyline.
   D. Desipramine.
   E. Bupropion.

The correct response is option **E.**

Despite a paucity of data, U.S. physicians are increasingly prescribing bupropion to treat depression during pregnancy, apparently as a consequence of its B risk category for pregnancy by the U.S. Food and Drug Administration. **(p. 1120)**

64.2   Which selective serotonin reuptake inhibitor (SSRI) has the largest evidence base demonstrating safety during breastfeeding?

   A. Fluoxetine.
   B. Sertraline.
   C. Paroxetine.
   D. Fluvoxamine.
   E. Citalopram.

The correct response is option **B.**

As of 2004, published reports pertaining to SSRIs and lactation consisted of 173 maternal–infant nursing pairs constituting 121 sertraline exposures, 86 fluoxetine exposures, 52 paroxetine exposures, 7 fluvoxamine exposures, and 5 citalopram exposures. Although infant follow-up data are limited, only a few isolated cases of adverse effects have been reported. The package insert for citalopram, however, does report a case of an infant who experienced a transient apneic episode. Long-term neurobehavioral studies of infants exposed to SSRI antidepressants during lactation have not been conducted, although a study of 12 infants who were exposed to sertraline during nursing detected no adverse effects on growth or on achievement of developmental milestones at age 24 months (see Llewellyn et al. 1997 for details). **(pp. 1119, 1120)**

64.3   Which tricyclic antidepressant (TCA) has been found to be present at considerably higher levels in breastfeeding infants than other TCAs and is thus relatively contraindicated during breastfeeding?

A. Clomipramine.
B. Imipramine.
C. Amitriptyline.
D. Doxepin.
E. Desipramine.

The correct response is option **D.**

TCAs have been widely used during lactation. The only adverse event reported to date is respiratory depression in a nursing infant exposed to doxepin, leading the authors to conclude that doxepin should be avoided but that most TCAs are safe for use during breastfeeding (Matheson et al. 1985). **(p. 1121)**

64.4   If valproate must be used during pregnancy, which of the following nutritional supplements is strongly recommended?

A. Vitamin B$_6$ (pyridoxine).
B. Vitamin B$_1$ (thiamine).
C. Folate.
D. Vitamin E (tocopherol).
E. Vitamin C (ascorbic acid).

The correct response is option **C.**

If valproate must be used during pregnancy, its risk may be reduced by being careful not to exceed 1,000 mg/day or a serum concentration of 70 µg/mL. Folate supplementation (4–5 mg/day) is also recommended, although no evidence shows that this reduces the risk of valproate-associated anomalies. Because nearly half of the pregnancies in the United States are unplanned, and women with unplanned pregnancies typically recognize that they are pregnant during the sixth week of gestation or even later (2 full weeks after neural tube closure), all women of childbearing potential who are taking valproate should receive concomitant folate supplementation, regardless of whether they plan to conceive. The preliminary evidence that aspects of fetal valproate syndrome other than neural tube defects may be associated with valproate's antagonism of folate metabolism suggests that folate supplementation should be administered not only in the first trimester but also throughout gestation. **(p. 1125)**

64.5   Clonazepam has received which of the following use-in-pregnancy category ratings?

A. Category A.
B. Category B.
C. Category C.
D. Category D.
E. Category X.

The correct response is option **C.**

Clonazepam, with a U.S. Food and Drug Administration Category C rating, appears to have minimal teratogenic risks (Sullivan and McElhatton 1977). **(p. 1133)**

64.6   Which of the following statements about fluctuations of medication levels during pregnancy is *true*?

    A. Nortriptyline doses are likely to require increases in order to maintain stable maternal blood levels as pregnancy progresses.

    B. Maternal–fetal lithium concentration ratios at delivery are roughly 10 to 1.

    C. Maternal valproate concentrations increase as pregnancy progresses.

    D. Lamotrigine clearance decreases as pregnancy progresses.

    E. None of the above.

The correct response is option **A.**

In a pharmacokinetic investigation addressing nortriptyline dosage management during gestation, Wisner et al. (1993) reported that dosages approximately 1.6 times higher than the preconception dose might be required in late pregnancy to maintain therapeutic serum concentrations and thereby sustain clinical benefit. Pharmacokinetic studies in women with epilepsy indicate that maternal valproate concentrations steadily *decline* across pregnancy, reaching levels as much as 50% lower than preconception concentrations (Yerby et al. 1990, 1992). Several reports collectively indicate that lamotrigine clearance steadily *increases* across gestation (Pennell et al. 2000; Rambeck et al. 1997; Sathanandar et al. 2000; Tran et al. 2002). Although no cases of agranulocytosis have been reported in the infants of women taking clozapine during pregnancy or lactation, this theoretical risk and the consequent requirement for monitoring of leukocyte counts in newborns and nursing infants limit the utility of clozapine during the peripartum period. **(pp. 1121, 1124, 1127, 1129, 1130)**

References

Llewellyn AM, Stowe ZN, Nemeroff CB: Infant outcome after sertraline exposure (abstract). Paper presented at the 150th annual meeting of the American Psychiatric Association, San Diego, CA, May 17–22, 1997

Matheson I, Pande H, Alertsen AR: Respiratory depression caused by N-desmethyldoxepin in breast milk (letter). Lancet 2(8464):1124, 1985

Pennell P, Gleba J, Clements S: Antiepileptic drug monitoring during pregnancy in women with epilepsy. Epilepsia 41:200, 2000

Rambeck B, Kurlemann G, Stodieck SR, et al: Concentrations of lamotrigine in a mother on lamotrigine treatment and her newborn child. Eur J Clin Pharmacol 51:481–484, 1997

Sathanandar S, Blesi K, Tran T, et al: Lamotrigine clearance increases markedly during pregnancy. Epilepsia 41:246, 2000

Sullivan FM, McElhatton PR: A comparison of the teratogenic activity of the antiepileptic drugs carbamazepine, clonazepam, ethosuximide, phenobarbital, phenytoin, and primidone in mice. Toxicol Appl Pharmacol 40:365–378, 1977

Tran TA, Leppik IE, Blesi K, et al: Lamotrigine clearance during pregnancy. Neurology 59:251–255, 2002

Wisner KL, Perel JM, Wheeler SB: Tricyclic dose requirements across pregnancy. Am J Psychiatry 150:1541–1542, 1993

Yerby MS, Friel PN, McCormick K, et al: Pharmacokinetics of anticonvulsants in pregnancy: alterations in plasma protein binding. Epilepsy Res 5:223–228, 1990

Yerby MS, Friel PN, McCormick K: Antiepileptic drug disposition during pregnancy. Neurology 42:12–16, 1992

CHAPTER 65

Treatment of Insomnia

Select the single best response for each question.

65.1   Which of the following treatments may relieve high-altitude insomnia?

   A. Continuous positive airway pressure.
   B. Acetazolamide.
   C. Tricyclic antidepressants.
   D. Benzodiazepines.
   E. Shifting of the sleep-cycle schedule.

The correct response is option **B.**

Travel from sea level to higher altitudes, even those of several North American ski areas, can be associated with disruptions in sleep. Altitude-induced changes include frequent awakenings, periodic breathing with associated arousals (Reite et al. 1975), and, in more severe cases, related symptoms of acute mountain sickness. The periodic breathing per se can fragment sleep and produce an insomnia complaint; acute mountain sickness also includes insomnia as a component. The pathophysiology of acute mountain sickness is not well understood, but it may include disturbances of fluid balance associated with tissue hypoxia. Acetazolamide (250 mg twice daily) can prevent or reduce symptoms of acute mountain sickness and improve sleep at high altitudes (Roberts 1994). Short-half-life nonbenzodiazepine hypnotics (e.g., zolpidem 5–10 mg) can also temporarily relieve high-altitude insomnia. **(p. 1150)**

65.2   Which of the following antidepressive agents increases rapid eye movement (REM) sleep?

   A. Bupropion.
   B. Clomipramine.
   C. Phenelzine.
   D. Venlafaxine.
   E. Sertraline.

The correct response is option **A.**

Antidepressants that increase REM sleep include bupropion and nefazodone. Clomipramine, phenelzine, venlafaxine, and sertraline all decrease REM sleep (Winokur and Reynolds 1994). **(pp. 1155, 1156; see Table 65–2)**

65.3   Which of the following agents is considered the first-line treatment for periodic limb movements in sleep (PLMS) and restless legs syndrome (RLS)?

A. Lorazepam.
B. Clomipramine.
C. Zolpidem.
D. Ropinirole.
E. Selective serotonin reuptake inhibitors.

The correct response is option **D.**

Dopaminergic agents are currently used as first-line treatment of PLMS and RLS (Hening et al. 1999). Dopamine agonists such as carbidopa/levodopa and pergolide have been shown to be effective treatments in a large percentage of patients with RLS or PLMS. Newer-generation dopaminergic agents such as pramipexole and ropinirole also have been used successfully. Alternative treatments have included benzodiazepines and anticonvulsant agents. **(p. 1158)**

65.4   Which of the following sleep-related disorders increases in frequency with increasing age?

A. Sleep-related breathing disturbances.
B. Depression.
C. Periodic limb movements in sleep (PLMS).
D. Insomnia due to a medical condition.
E. All of the above.

The correct response is option **E.**

Sleep complaints are more prevalent in elderly persons than in other age groups (Ganguli et al. 1996). More than 50% of persons older than 65 years report poor sleep (Ancoli-Israel 1997). Whereas it was once thought that elderly persons require less sleep, it now appears that they in fact get less sleep, primarily because the conditions known to disrupt sleep and produce insomnia complaints increase with age. The incidence of sleep-related breathing disturbances (Ancoli-Israel et al. 1991), depression, PLMS (Ancoli-Israel and Kripke 1991), and medical conditions increases with age, as does that of associated insomnia complaints. **(p. 1163)**

65.5   Which of the following antidepressive agents reduces rapid eye movement (REM) sleep yet causes little or no sedation?

A. Amitriptyline.
B. Bupropion.
C. Phenelzine.
D. Nefazodone.
E. Trazodone.

The correct response is option **C.**

Of the antidepressants listed, only phenelzine greatly decreases REM sleep and has no sedative effect. Both bupropion and nefazodone increase REM sleep; amitriptyline and trazodone reduce REM sleep but have significant sedative effects (Winokur and Reynolds 1994). **(p. 1156)**

References

Ancoli-Israel S: Sleep problems in older adults: putting myths to bed. Geriatrics 52:20–30, 1997

Ancoli-Israel S, Kripke DF: Prevalent sleep problems in the aged. Biofeedback Self Regul 16:349–359, 1991

Ancoli-Israel S, Kripke D, Klauber M: Sleep-disordered breathing in community-dwelling elderly. Sleep 14:486–495, 1991

Ganguli M, Reynolds CF, Gilby JE: Prevalence and persistence of sleep complaints in a rural older community sample: the MoVIES project. J Am Geriatr Soc 44:778–784, 1996

Hening W, Allen R, Earley C, et al: The treatment of restless legs syndrome and periodic limb movement disorder: an American Academy of Sleep Medicine review. Sleep 22:970–999, 1999

Reite M, Jackson D, Cahoon RL, et al: Sleep physiology at high altitude. Electroencephalogr Clin Neurophysiol 38:463–471, 1975

Roberts MJ: Acute mountain sickness—experience on the Roof of Africa expedition and military implications. J R Army Med Corps 140:49–51, 1994

Winokur A, Reynolds C: Overview of effects of antidepressant therapies on sleep. Prim Psychiatry 1:22–27, 1994